WORK STRESS

Health Care Systems in the Workplace

Edited by
James C. Quick, Rabi S. Bhagat,
James E. Dalton,
and Jonathan D. Quick

PRAEGER

New York
Westport, Connecticut
London

Library of Congress Cataloging-in-Publication Data

Work Stress.

    Includes index.
    1. Job stress.   2. Work–Psychological aspects.
3. Psychotherapy.   4. Employee assistance programs.
5. Job stress–Prevention.   I. Quick, James C.
HF5548.85.W67   1987   616.85'2   86–30636
ISBN 0–275–92329–0 (alk. paper)

Library of Congress Catalog Card Number: 86–30636
ISBN: 0–275– 92329–0

First published in 1987

Praeger Publishers, One Madison Avenue, New York, NY 10010
A division of Greenwood Press, Inc.

Printed in the United States of America

The paper used in this book complies with the Permanent Paper Standard issued by the National Information Standards Organization (Z39.48–1984).

10 9 8 7 6 5 4 3 2 1

Contents

Tables and Figures

TABLES

FIGURES

Contributors

Gilbert T. Adams, Jr.	Attorney-at-Law; Adams, Adams Jr., and Clarkson, Beaumont, Texas
William B. Baun	Manager of Tenneco Health & Fitness Center, Tenneco Corporation, Houston, Texas
E. J. Bernacki	Corporate Medical Director, Tenneco Corporation, Houston, Texas
Rabi S. Bhagat	Professor of Organizational Behavior and International Management, University of Texas at Dallas, Dallas, Texas
Ronald J. Burke	Professor of Organization Behavior, Faculty of Administrative Studies, York University, Downsview, Ontario, Canada
Margaret A. Chesney	Director, Department of Behavioral Medicine, Center for Health Studies, SRI International, Menlo Park, California
James E. Dalton, Jr.	Divisional Vice President of Hospital Corporation of America, Arlington, Texas
Richard S. DeFrank	Assistant Professor, Department of Preventive Medicine and Community Health, University of Texas Medical Branch, Galveston, Texas
T. E. Dielman	Department of Post-Graduate Medicine, University of Michigan, Ann Arbor, Michigan
James L. Francek	Manager, Employee Health Advisory Program, Medicine and Environmental Health Department, Exxon Corporation, New York, New York
Bertil Gardell	Professor of Social Psychology of Work, Department of Psychology, University of Stockholm, Sweden
William R. Harlan	Department of Post-Graduate Medicine, University of Michigan, Ann Arbor, Michigan
R. Van Harrison	Director, Continuing Medical Education, Department of Post-Graduate Medicine, University of Michigan, Ann Arbor, Michigan
Suzanne G. Haynes	Department of Epidemiology, University of North Carolina, Chapel Hill, North Carolina
J. Alan Herd	Medical Director, Institute for Preventive Medicine, Methodist Hospital, Houston, Texas

William J. Horvath   Mental Health Research Institute, University of Michigan, Ann Arbor, Michigan

James S. House   Professor of Sociology, Survey Research Center, and Associate Research Scientist, Department of Epidemiology, Univeristy of Michigan, Ann Arbor, Michigan

John M. Ivancevich   Cullen Distinguished Professor of Organizational Behavior, Department of Organizational Behavior and Management, University of Houston, Houston, Texas

Robert L. Kahn   Professor, Institute for Social Research, University of Michigan, Ann Arbor, Michigan

Stanislav V. Kasl   Professor of Epidemiology, Yale School of Medicine, New Haven, Connecticut

Andrea Z. LaCroix   Department of Epidemiology, University of North Carolina, Chapel Hill, North Carolina

Tobi Lippin   Coordinator, North Carolina Occupational Safety and Heath Project, Durham, North Carolina

Michael T. Matteson   Professor of Management, College of Business Administration, University of Houston, Houston, Texas

Alan A. McLean   Clinical Associate Professor, Cornell University Medical College, New York, New York

Gordon E. Moss   Department of Sociology, Eastern Michigan University, Ypsilanti, Michigan

Rita E. Numerof   Assistant Professor, George Warren Brown School of Social Work, Washington University, St. Louis, Missouri

Judith E. Pliner   Vice President and Counseling Psychologist, Drake, Beam, Morin, Inc., Dallas, Texas

James C. Quick   Professor of Organizational Behavior, University of Texas at Arlington, Arlington, Texas

Jonathan D. Quick   Staff Associate, Management Sciences for Health, Boston, Massachusetts

Thomas Robischon   Philosophy Faculty and Medical Writer, Antioch University, Los Angeles, California

Robert M. Rose   Professor and Chairman, Department of Psychiatry and Behavioral Sciences, University of Texas Medical Branch, Galveston, Texas

Bonnie C. Seamonds   Occupational Medicine Consultant, B. Seamonds and Associates, Westport, Connecticut, and Paddington, NSW, Australia

Raymond R. Suskind   Director Emeritus, Institute of Environmental Health, University of Cincinnati Medical Center, Cincinnati, Ohio

William W. Winpisinger   President, International Machinist Union, Washington, D.C.

John C. Wolfe   President and Chief Executive Officer, AMI Psychiatric Services, Inc., Culver City, California

Steering Committee

Michael J. Colligan, Ph.D.   Research Psychologist, Department of Health and Human Services, Public Health Service, Robert A. Taft Laboratories, Cincinnati, Ohio

J. Alan Herd, M.D.   Medical Director, Institute for Preventive Medicine, Methodist Hospital, Houston, Texas

Joseph C. Hutts, M.H.A.   Senior Vice President, Hospital Corporation of America, Nashville, Tennessee

Stanislav V. Kasl, Ph.D.   Professor of Epidemiology, School of Medicine, Yale University, New Haven, Connecticut

Alan A. McLean, M.D.   Clinical Associate Professor, Cornell University Medical College, New York, New York

Charles B. Mullins, M.D.   Executive Vice Chancellor for Health Affairs, The University of Texas System, Austin, Texas

Foreword

For years I have been involved in medical care delivery, the education of young physicians, and the management of health science centers in Texas. Health care management has become an increasingly complex, expensive, and difficult activity. This has been especially true with the changes in the health care environment of the last few years. We all need to learn how to be healthier and we need to develop more effectiveness and efficiency in health care management.

"Stress" is a magnetic word that has moved into our language with rich imagery but not with great scientific precision. Nevertheless, there are a host of stressors, symptomatic stress reactions, and individual stress responses that are important to attend to in the maintenance of health and well-being. The identification of these various stress factors in the workplace has become a major concern of management, labor, legal authorities, health care providers, researchers, and practitioners. The conference, Work Stress and the Role for Health Care Delivery Systems, which our Steering Committee organized, and the resulting book reflect a unique spectrum of leaders in a variety of disciplines who have come together to contribute their individual expertise to addressing work stress and health care management.

It is critical for all of us to bridge the boundaries of our own disciplines in learning what others have to offer in the complex and confusing area of stress. This book takes a first step in establishing a strong interdisciplinary dialogue and it provides a basic framework for our thinking. First, we need to continue our research activities so that we learn more about the causes and consequences of work stress. Our efforts to extend our knowledge must never cease. Second, we must take action to prevent work stress from becoming distress. The action must be taken by medical professionals, managers, and other experts in specific change activities. Third, we must help heal those who suffer distress. Despite our best-laid plans, some people get in trouble with distress and our health care systems must help these people out of trouble.

This book is an excellent contribution to our knowledge in many different fields. Therefore, it is most fitting that the U.T.A. College of Business Administration has honored both the conference and this book with the 1987 Distinguished Service Award.

Charles B. Mullins, M.D.

Acknowledgments

We would like to thank many people, especially the Steering Committee, for helping make possible the conference, Work Stress and the Role for Health Care Delivery Systems. The Steering Committee consisted of Michael J. Colligan, J. Alan Herd, Joseph C. Hutts, Stanislav V. Kasl, Alan A. McLean, and Charles B. Mullins. Joseph C. Hutts, Senior Vice President of Hospital Corporation of America, was instrumental in the fall of 1983 by hosting the planning session for the conference and providing essential support and resources to carry out the plan of the Steering Committee. Bob F. Perkins, Dean of the Graduate School at the University of Texas at Arlington (UTA), was most helpful in committing Organized Research Funds to the conference. Eirik G. Furubotn, Professor of Economics and Eunice and James L. West Chair of Private Enterprise and Entrepreneurship, was equally supportive with resources from his endowed chair. Michael Hitt, Chairman of the Department of Management, and Walter E. Mullendore, Dean of the College of Business Administration, were most supportive throughout the execution of the plan. Mike was particularly supportive in working out some of the knotty, final details. Dr. Wendell Nedderman was a wonderful host as President of UTA.

Martha Gamblin deserves a special round of thanks for her long hours of careful and detailed work in putting everything together to make the conference a wonderful success. The participants were especially complimentary, and so are we. She did a marvelous job. Linda Lee Richardson was full of good ideas during the time of the conference and in editorial work on the book.

Rebecca S. Horn was industrious, thoughtful and helpful in the editorial work on the manuscripts for the book. Her careful and detailed work helped immensely in assembling the total package for publication. Kathryn Dunton was helpful in adding the finishing touches of copy and page proof corrections. Sheri Schember Quick helped with proof reading.

Michele Bock was most helpful in working with all of us in preparing several chapters for publication. John Trapani, Tiff Hawks, Jane Giacobbe, Steve Premack, Edwin Gerloff, Wayne Bodensteiner, and Joseph Rosenstein hosted the invited speakers. Jack Feldman was encouraging and supportive in the final stage of conducting the conference and David A. Gray was most supportive in the final preparation of the book.

xvii

I Work stress: research and practice

1   *Introduction*

James C. Quick, Jonathan D. Quick,
Rabi S. Bhagat, and James E. Dalton, Jr.

The management of health care costs in the United States and around the world has been an important concern over the last several years. One of the hidden culprits identified as a source of health problems in recent years is "stress." Actually, it is the bad side of stress—distress—that is the real culprit. Because it is often difficult to trace the origins and adverse effects of stress, it has been very difficult to identify the real health care costs associated with the mismanagement of stress at work. Therefore, academicians and practitioners joined forces to develop a conference and set of papers that would address the causes, consequences, prevention, and therapy of stress at work. The conference, Work Stress and the Role of Health Care Delivery Systems, was held at the University of Texas at Arlington in October 1985.

The purpose of this book is to present an interdisciplinary panel of authorities on work stress and health care so as to provide a basic framework for cross-disciplinary dialogue, learning, questioning, and practice. Certainly this should in no way be an end, in one sense, but a beginning. Our intention is to stimulate a blending of knowledge and ideas from different professions so as to achieve greater synergy, as opposed to fragmentation, in the area of work stress. The blending ultimately will require a series of individual and collective efforts such as this one if real progress is even hoped to be achieved in the pooling of knowledge, resources, and practices concerning work stress and health care.

In this Introduction we will discuss the relationship between work stress and health care; the conceptual framework for both the conference and the book; the practitioner-researcher dialogue of the conference that is needed in the field; and the interdisciplinary synergy that will lead to good stress theory, research, and practice.

WORK STRESS AND HEALTH CARE

Why do some people die prematurely? Why do some people suffer disease and disability when others do not? Why do some organizations become ineffective and inefficient while others thrive?

Fielding (1984) has argued that our national health care system is not cost-effective in improving the health of the population. But why? Part of the issue is related to how we define health and who is responsible for it. Culturally, we have assigned much of that responsibility to the medical profession and the health care system. This has been based on a definition of health that is largely medical and physiological as opposed to one that is holistic (physical-psychological-spiritual). Stress has become a rubric through which we look at how individuals adjust to the demands of work and personal life. It gives us a new perspective on defining health and the responsibility for health.

Lawyers and theologians have been among the most critical of the current state of affairs in health care. The phrase "the end of medicine" was used by a lawyer, Rick Carlson (1975), as a title of a book in which he argued that advances in medicine and clinical models of diagnosis have failed to reduce mortality, and that a new comprehensive approach to a healthy life should be an important focus for the rest of the decade.

Ivan Illich, a theologian, had set forth the intellectual and philosophical underpinnings for this argument in a book originally entitled *Medical Nemesis* when published in London in 1975, but retitled *The Limits of Medicine* when reprinted in New York in 1976. Illich's message in this book is clear and straightforward: the medical establishment itself has become a major threat to health.

The writings of Carlson and Illich have attracted considerable attention. Reactions to their thesis of the somewhat disabling and disturbing impact of professional control over medicine were loud and swift, ranging from the medically naive to the progressive sociomedical scientists and health care researchers. One of the strongest critiques of this view was in the art of marshalling statistics for the inefficacy of a medical model of health care. Carlson and Illich have fallen prey to the *insensitivity* of the measures that were and still are normally used for assessing the impact of medical care (Elinson, 1977). However, the impact of Illich's book in the development of the roots of a biobehavioral science of health care has been considerable.

In organizing the conference, the members of the Steering Committee focused not only on the etiology of work stress and health outcomes, but also on some of the currently unmet needs of health care in contemporary organizations. The Illich announcement of the "end of medicine" has since proved premature, if not unfounded (Elinson, 1977; Horrobin, 1980). But the sense of inquiry into biobehavioral and context-based factors of health care delivery systems and management that it encouraged is remarkable and, in our opinion, healthy. In the decade following its publication, health care-related research has continued to expand dramatically. Currently, medical care expenditures account for the highest proportion of gross national product (GNP)—over 10 percent in the United States. From 1981 to 1983 health care costs equaled almost 25 percent of after-tax profits for the Fortune 500 industrial companies and the 250 largest nonindustrial companies. It is individuals and organizations who pay this price. The rate of expansion of the health care facilities along with innovations in medical technology and more recently into biotechnology and robotics account for the fastest growing sector of the U.S. economy (*Newsweek*, October 13, 1983).

Unprecedented profits are being made by the delivery of medical care as reflected in the growth of what we would term corporate medicine, managed care, and wellness programs. Specialty medical establishments such as office prognostication and surgery, urgent health care systems, preventive health care management systems and practices (for example, Kenneth Cooper's Aerobic Center in Dallas, chiropractic care, transcendental meditation techniques of some of the Eastern countries, neighborhood stop smoking clinics, and so on, and health maintenance organizations (HMOs) are flourishing at an astonishing rate. Federal financial support of preventive issues in the delivery of health care as well as its effective management shows no signs of abatement. Consider the following:

- New York Telephone Company saves at least $2.7 million annually from a well-designed wellness program (*Business Insurance*, September 21, 1981).
- HCA has invested over $50,000 annually in cash awards to employees who participate in an aerobic exercise program (personal communication with Debbie Meredith, Public Relations Office, HCA Corporate Headquarters, November 17, 1986).
- The Los Angeles Fire Department has a program of teaching meditation to its trainees (*Newsweek*, November 5, 1984, p. 97).
- General Motors figures that in 1985, health care costs accounted for $400 of the cost of every car they produced (*Medical World News*, January 13, 1986, p. 52).
- Johnson and Johnson and IBM have instituted comprehensive programs of health checkups and exercise and "life-style" classes for smoking cessation and stress management (*Newsweek*, November 5, 1984, p. 96).
- Aerobics Center in Dallas is a focal point for corporate physical fitness programs. Some 60 corporations are members and there is a waiting list of over 20 more (*Dallas Life Magazine*, September 30, 1984, p. 9).
- Employer contributions for employee health insurance have gone from $1.8 billion in 1955 to $101.0 billion in 1985, nearly a hundredfold increase in 30 years (*Medical World News*, January 13, 1986, p. 52).

The above-mentioned examples, signal the beginning of an important era in the study of human stress and strain in work organizations, its etiological significance, and the role of preventive management in its governance. Health promotion and effective management of work stress in terms of encouraging both preventive and therapeutic interventions are slowly becoming important parts of today's corporation's strategic mission.

The picture of a lean chief executive officer (CEO) who is a nonsmoker and a marathon runner and who pays his employees to jog is very comforting for us as symposium coordinators to imagine, but we have not yet reached that point in our evolutionary history in understanding the scientific principles governing causes, consequences, and prevention of work stress and the role of health care delivery systems.

THE CONCEPTUAL FRAMEWORK

This book is based upon the notions of research, prevention, and therapy, which are depicted in Figure 1.1. Taken together, the chapters in the book are organized in a framework that makes a great deal of theoretical sense. One of the current difficulties in the whole stress area is the proliferation of "quick fixes" without a sufficiently solid theoretical framework for thinking through the problems as a solid empirical research basis for prevention and therapy. The conceptual framework here provides us with a better rationale for understanding how work stresses affect health, how they could be prevented, and how, if they are not prevented, therapeutic interventions become absolutely crucial to implement.

Part II focuses on the issues of theory and research, primarily dealing with causes of stress and overviews of work done in Canada and Sweden. There are substantial cross-cultural differences in research, theory, and practice as may be seen through Chapters 5 and 6 by Ronald Burke and Bertil Gardell, respectively. Thus, while the experience of stress is universal, there are important cultural and individual factors that determine what causes stress for different people and how the experience of stress turns out for different people. As Margaret Chesney points out in Chapter 9, an individual's personality-behavior pattern is a personal characteristic that affects the degree of stress a person experiences as well as their symptoms of distress. On the other hand, Harrison et al. point out in Chapter 7 that one must consider environmental factors and the person's fit in their environment to determine one's experience of stress and distress.

Good theory and research can give us frameworks for understanding the phenomena of stress and the course of various disease processes associated with distress. However, part of our purpose in studying the stress process is so that intervention and action may be taken to channel stress-induced energy and stressful situations in constructive avenues. This purpose motivates the chapters in Part III, which are directed at prevention.

Preventive action is aimed at heading off both symptomatic and asymptomatic disease. The occurrence of symptoms in either the individual or the organization are only a cue that the system (either individual or organization) is not in balance, either within itself or with its environment.

Figure 1.1.   The conceptual framework

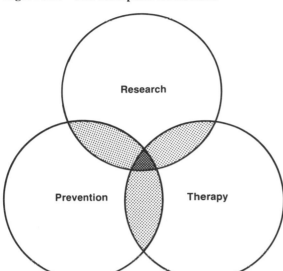

Source: Compiled by the authors.

The proper functioning of the system results in effective and constructive responses by the system to its environmental and internalized stressors. In this way, little if any residual energy is left for destructive purposes. The exception would occur in the case of a catastrophically stressful event that overwhelmed the system before a constructive response could be developed.

Ongoing theoretical and empirical work is needed to evaluate, refine, improve, and alter our preventive activities. It is essential that preventive action is taken based upon the best available information, as opposed to waiting for foolproof evidence about efficacy. That in part is the difference between the practitioner and the researcher. Those who are engaged in the design and implementation of preventive stress management methods fall more into the arena of practice than theory-research, although there is an overlap in prevention and theory-research that may be seen in Figure 1.1.

There is also some overlap between prevention and therapy, although the arenas are rather separable. The focus of therapy is on the process of healing already existent distress. Regardless of the best laid plans for prevention, there are vulnerabilities and risk factors that result in distress. When this occurs, it is essential to have strategies, methods, and techniques that may be employed to heal the organizational, medical, or psychological distress that exists. It is for that reason that Part IV of the book contains a set of chapters aimed at therapeutic activities. These chapters are more clinically oriented in nature, but do overlap also with the arena of theory-research.

Taken together, these three arenas—theory-research, prevention, and therapy—are an excellent way of organizing our knowledge in the area of work stress. They give us not only a good organizing scheme but also a solid basis for extending our knowledge in each arena. That was a key function of the conference. Another key feature of the conference was the practitioner-researcher dialogue that was generated—and that dialogue is important.

THE PRACTITIONER–RESEARCHER DIALOGUE

The practitioner and the researcher in any discipline need each other, though for different reasons. Because they need each other, it is essential that a dialogue develop and be maintained between the two. That sort of dialogue did occur in the framework of the conference and our hope is that it will be extended and expanded.

The practitioner needs the researcher to: establish causal relationship through good research designs; test interventions to affirm the utility of those that work and discard those that do not prove out; guide practitioners to invest energy in those methods and activities that are more likely to succeed; and suggest new techniques and methods for which there is preliminary theoretical or empirical evidence of efficacy. The researcher generates new ideas and knowledge for the practitioner. It is the researcher who extends and affirms our understanding of the techniques and methods of prevention and therapy. The researcher is not accountable for the same results a practitioner is, and therefore is free to be more creative and hypothetical in the search for and extension of knowledge.

The researcher, in turn, needs the practitioner to: apply those methods that are effective in solving problems and in healing; identify key individual and organizational problems that need solutions to be developed and tested; insure that techniques are methodologically sound and practical in application; and provide feedback on technique feasibility and implementation. It is through the practitioner that the researcher makes the rubber meet the road. It is through the practitioner that the best ideas and techniques are put into action, achieving utilitarian value. It is the practitioner who makes theory and research useful to those in need.

The difference between researchers and practitioners is an underlying theme in this book. When these differences are blended together through a dialogue between the two, the result is greater than the sum of the two alone. This is also true of the differences in professional disciplines, which was a more overt theme in the conference. It is an important one.

INTERDISCIPLINARY SYNERGY

One of the complications in developing a cohesive body of theory, research, and practice in the area of work stress is that there is a wide diversity of disciplines and professions which are involved in various aspects of work stress. Their disciplines are generally concerned primarily with either work organizations or health care delivery.

Work organizations have a vested interest in work stress owing to the increasing awareness that its improper management can be extremely costly, either in direct or indirect ways, for an organization. In this regard, the concerns of management, labor, and law are both direct and pragmatic. General managers, personnel specialists, and management consultants are interested in the identification of interventions that will be of benefit in managing work-related stress. This includes, for example, four chapters within this preventive stress management vein. These are Rita Numerof's chapter (13), which talks about team-building interventions for preventing work-related distress and encouraging healthy working relations; the Baun, Bernacki, and Herd chapter (16), which addresses the preventive role of physical fitness programs in the workplace; Bonnie Seamond's chapter (20) which focuses on risk factor screening as a preventive activity; and James Francek's chapter (19), which looks at the role of employee assistance programs in the workplace.

The managers in work organizations are not the only organizational constituencies or concerned parties who address work stress and health care. As we see from Chapter 15 by William Winpisinger, labor has a vested interest in stress because of the health and well-being of its unionized constituency. In addition, Chapter 17 by Gilbert Adams shows how the legal professionals are increasingly involved in cases dealing with work stress and health care issues.

Bottom-line results, action, and performance are major concerns for the management, labor, and legal professional. They have their own value schemes, languages, and rules of behavior. They are not necessarily compatible in all cases with those of the academic or clinical disciplines. Yet they are players in the arena and their legitimate concerns must be responded to effectively.

Health care delivery systems are also quite concerned with stress in general and work stress in particular. Because of the cultural emphasis upon the medical community as the guardians of health and well-being in the society, their legitimate role with regard to work stress focuses on how stress presents a risk factor that may lead to either asymptomatic or symptomatic disease. That is at a global level. Within medicine, there are a number of subspecialties that have specific emphases or concerns. These include occupational medicine, psychiatry, public health and epidemiology, primary care disciplines such as family practice and internal medicine, and specialties such as cardiology and neurology. Even though they fall within the umbrella of medicine, there is a substantial diversity of conceptual frameworks, professional jargon, and research methodologies employed by each. This spectrum is reflected in the diversity of medically authored papers in this volume, to include Robert Rose's chapter (10), which examines neuroendocrinological issues and their implications for health and well-being; Chapter 16, which addresses the fitness issue from the standpoint of a physician in industry; Raymond Suskind's chapter (21), which focuses on the occupational physician's role.

Healing and health have been the province of these medical specialists. They are concerned not only with procedures, therapies, and techniques for healing the sick, but they are also concerned with the prevention of illness through the identification of risk factors that precede the development of frank disease. The physician's values, standards, and technical language are not always comprehensible to those outside of the profession. Clearly there is cultural benefit to bounded definition of the profession and those who practice within it, but there are also some drawbacks when attempting to achieve integration with other disciplines with other values.

Psychologists have worked with the stress phenomena for over three decades now in work stress for both research and clinical reasons. Within psychology, as in medicine, there are a number of subspecialities that have specific concerns with regard to work stress. These include organizational and industrial, health care, occupational, and clinical psychology. Again as in the case of medicine, even though there is a rather well-defined profession of psychology, there is diversity within the subspecialties. This spectrum is reflected in the diversity of psychologically oriented papers in this volume, to include Gardell's chapter (6) about Swedish thrusts in the workplace to deal with stress; Chesney's chapter (9) that considers behavioral aspects of the stress process at work; Michael Matteson's chapter (12) examining individual-organizational fit issues in preventive work stress management; and the concluding chapter (24) by Robert Kahn, which integrates this book and also includes some distinctively original material.

The establishment of an interdisciplinary dialogue in the area of work stress and health care delivery is essential. The difficulties in achieving an interdisciplinary dialogue are numerous, not only because of language and nomenclature issues, but also because of value, orientation, belief, and rules of evidence issues. We fall prey to the common organization disorder of suboptimization unless each profession, discipline, and subspecialty is able to transcend its own provincial interests and accept a commitment to the much more significant objectives of (1) better defining and measuring the assortment of constructs embedded within the ecological model posited at the outset; (2) evaluating preventive intervention strategies aimed at ameliorating the risk factors associated with the various aspects of work stress; and (3) evaluating the diversity of therapeutic intervention strategies aimed at either asymptomatic or symptomatic disease, either in the individual or the organization.

REFERENCES

Carlson, R. 1975. *The End of Medicine*. New York: Wiley Interscience.
Elinson, J. 1977. Intensive health statistics and the dilemma of the health system agencies. *American Journal of Public Health*, 67: 417–418.
Fielding, J. E. 1984. Health promotion and disease prevention at the worksite. *Annual Review of Public Health*, 5: 237–265.
Horrobin, D. F. 1980. *Medical Hubris: A Reply to Ivan Illich*. Westmount, Quebec: Eden Press.
Illich, I. 1976. *The Limits to Medicine*. New York: Pantheon Press.

2 *The practitioner's perspective*

Alan A. McLean

Work stress issues are pervasive in our society. From the perspective of the individual at risk of exposure to stressors at work, I want to give focus to clinical and administrative issues that will be elaborated in many of this book's chapters. My focus does not minimize the importance of organizational issues. Rather, in the division of labor that was created during the development of the conference, it was clear that Stanislav Kasl could far better introduce research and organizational issues. We therefore divided Part I to fit the perspectives of the organizational researcher and the practitioner concerned with occupational health issues.

THE INDIVIDUAL AND THE ORGANIZATION

I would point out that clinicians, concerned with patients reacting to stressors on the job, recognize the importance of organizational variables in the lives of their patients. They are vitally aware that the work organization creates both the stressors and the context in which the work stress–stress response reaction takes place. I am also interested, as are my colleagues, in those aspects of the world of work that can buffer those same stressors; that can be succoring, caring, and therapeutic.

The potentially powerful interaction between individual and the organization is illustrated by the case of Mr. MacKenzie, who began work for General Motors at the age of 15. After 41 years, in 1965, he took early retirement when he was 56.

For five years prior to his retirement he worked on the day shift in a General Motors Fisher Body salvage department. His job was to count, keep track of, and ship back to vendors red-tagged defective parts. During his last two or three years he became anxious and irritable because the afternoon shift would take defective parts from his department and install them on cars being manufactured on the assembly line. He was particularly concerned about the safety of the cars put together with parts he knew to be potentially dangerous. He also had to recount the remaining parts and to account to his supervisor for the missing parts. Further, he felt the poor work habits of his co-workers required Mr. MacKenzie to work harder, which, in turn, added to his anxiety.

The stress of this job was a major determinant in his decision to retire. For several years he stewed about his strong feelings of unfair treatment. Eventually, some years later, he sued General Motors under the Michigan Workers Compensation statutes.

After a referee-awarded compensation (finding that, although the stresses of the job were not great enough to cause ill effects in an average person, the stress did cause Mr. MacKenzie to become disabled), General Motors appealed. Thus began a long series of hearings and decisions before the Worker Compensation Appeal Board, the Court of Appeals, and, eventually, the Supreme Court of the State of Michigan.

Let me quote from excerpts of the lengthy Opinion of the Court:

At the hearing before the referee, MacKenzie's psychiatrist, Dr. Dreyer, testified that MacKenzie suffered from a long-standing personality defect of compulsive perfectionism that centered on his job, and that eventually the job pressures disabled him. This was subjective analysis based on MacKenzie's view of his job.

General Motors' psychiatrist, Dr. Fink, testified that it was MacKenzie's perfectionistic need in conflict with the impairments of aging that produced his anxiety and that although MacKenzie perceived the stresses of the job as causing his anxiety, these stresses were usual occurrences and did not cause his emotional problems. This was an objective analysis based on the normal worker's view of MacKenzie's job (394 Mich 473–474).

To continue to quote from the closely reasoned Opinion of the Court:

The referee-awarded compensation finding that, although the stresses of the job were not great enough to cause ill effects in an average person, the stress did cause MacKenzie to become disabled.

The Appeal Board in its five to two majority opinion reversed the referee and rejected the subjective analysis in favor of an objective analysis and ruled that an actual mental injury caused by the claimant's perception of his work environment is not compensable when that environment is not injurious to the average worker.

The Michigan Supreme Court, however, reversed this opinion, agreeing with the referee, and held that, since Mr. MacKenzie *honestly believed* that the stress of work had caused his disability, worker compensation benefits must be awarded—and they were.

This provocative case clearly interrelates work stress and disabling psychiatric illness and clearly presents a complex challenge to the health care delivery system (that is, how to treat a patient the courts *pay* to reinforce a false and delusional belief).

WORK STRESS AND HEALTH CARE MANAGEMENT

While there is not time to develop fully the practitioner frame of reference here, I would like to suggest three variables that must be considered in any individual case or administrative situation involving work stress. The first variable is the nature of the individual stressor and its meaning for the individual or work organization. Why do some events and conditions provoke a symptomatic reaction in some people and not in others? Second, what is the context in which the stressor-stress response takes place? Is it protective or destructive of the individual or organization? We need to know. Finally, and most important, how vulnerable is either the individual or the organization at the time the stressor hits? Keeping in mind that vulnerability is ever-changing, the assessment of this variable in any work-up becomes key. We need to know and understand.

Now, then, how do all these issues relate to health care delivery systems? If one thinks narrowly of hospitals, acute care facilities, and the doctor in his office—all treating sick and injured patients—one can make some associations between them and the individual with an occupational injury or illness. One can also identify a relationship between work stress and health care in the patient being treated for physical symptoms encountered in response to stressful demands at work. So even at this level, some degree of relationship can be found.

Yet as I see it, every author of a chapter in this book is involved in the health care delivery system in this country. Perhaps John Ivancevich (Chapter 11) would not so identify himself, since his doctorate is in business administration and he is a professor. But his article in the March/April 1985 issue of *Harvard Business Review* stimulated, I am sure, greater interest in intervention strategies by employers in stress-related matters. I suggest this is an important element in stimulating more efforts by those providing service.

Robert Rose, and his work with air traffic controllers, and more recently with neuroendocrine effects of work stress (Chapter 10) may not see himself as part of the health care delivery system, but that work has taught us much about organizational stressors and feeds important information to those of us on the front line in occupational health. His data suggest where to look, how to interpret the information, and what credence to give to the stressors our patients face.

Gilbert Adams, a distinguished attorney, speaks to compensation payments made by employers for stress-disabled workers (Chapter 17). A part of "health care delivery"? You had better believe it! Employers are paying out many millions of dollars each year for disability growing out of the course of employment. The costs are rising rapidly and an increasing percent are for claims related to job stress.

William Winpisinger has a labor perspective on stress management (Chapter 15). The emphasis may be on bargaining for less stressful working conditions, but the effect should be on reducing costs for the health care delivery systems of this country.

And so it goes: The health care system is not only an essential partner in treating the consequences of work stress, but a potentially important beneficiary of reduced costs through reduced stress-related illness. Similarly, the workplace is not simply a source of stress, but also an important component in a growing network of institutions and organizations concerned with the preventive management of stress.

REFERENCE

Ivancevich, J. M., Matteson, M. T., and Richards, E. P. III. 1985. Who's liable for stress on the job? *Harvard Business Review*, 64(2): 60–72.

3   *The researcher's perspective*

Stanislav V. Kasl

In thinking through the possible content of my introductory remarks for this volume on *Work Stress*, I felt that I had a couple of options open to me. The first seemed to be to provide an overview of the subject from a very broad perspective, which would encompass and integrate divergent views and approaches and would be, in some sense, accomodating to whatever is going on in the field of work stress. The second option seemed to be to give an overview from a single narrower perspective that could give my commentary greater sharpness and coherence, if not a bit of abrasiveness as well. Given my own background and interests, I have chosen the latter alternative: My perspective will be that of an investigator or researcher in occupational epidemiology.

OCCUPATIONAL EPIDEMIOLOGY

If one surveys the field of work stress, one finds that investigators are working with five types of variables:

1. Those that describe the *objective* environmental conditions in the work setting
2. Those that deal with *subjective* descriptions—perceptions and evaluations—of the work setting
3. Those that represent *intermediate outcome* variables, such as biological indicators
4. Those that might be described as the more *distal outcome variables* in which the investigator is interested, such as coronary heart disease, or major depression, or burnout, or being fired
5. Those variables that help us understand *modifying* influences and *mediating* processes in the overall work stress dynamics.

The majority of studies do not, in fact, encompass all five types of variables in a single design. Many studies are less ambitious, necessarily so. Hence, we confront the issue of priorities. From the perspective of occupational epidemiology I would like to argue that our primary goal should be to identify linkages between exposure to some aspect of the *objective* work environment and adverse (or, possibly, positive) health outcomes. We should design our studies, and conduct our analyses, so as to optimize our chances of demonstrating that such linkages represent, in fact, cause-effect relationships. Additional effort that goes into designing the study (such as additional data collection or data analysis) should be in the service of the primary goal; for example, we can work on design changes that would serve to reduce biases due to self-selection into specific work conditions.

However, there are two second goals that are eminently worthwhile: (1) to identify variables that explain additional variance in the adverse health outcomes and that, thereby, indicate differential reactivity to the environmental exposure; and (2) to provide information on the underlying mechanisms involved in the overall association. Obviously, the two additional goals are well intertwined: advancing one is likely to advance the other.

This perspective of occupational epidemiology is pertinent both to basic etiological studies dealing with adverse health effects of stress at work and to intervention studies at the worksite, which attempt to modify some link in the overall causal process.

I think we should use the above perspective as a rock-bottom basis for thinking about various conceptual and methodological issues and for evaluating diverse studies. I recognize that there are other perspectives that could be articulated and defended. I put forward this one only for the "stress and disease in the workplace" domain; it is likely to be much less suitable for the general stress and disease area, and is certainly unsuitable for a "psychology of stress" orientation in which one seeks to reconstruct the phenomenology of the stress process.

RESEARCH PRIORITIES AND RECOMMENDATIONS

Applying the perspective of occupational epidemiology on research priorities to a survey of what actually goes on reveals a different picture, a different implicit set of priorities.

Above all, we have numerous studies—they constitute the majority—in which the only independent variable is the subjective measure of exposure to the work setting, the subjective perceptions and evaluations. Now this creates two major difficulties: (1) we don't know to what objective environmental conditions these subjective perceptions link up; and (2) we don't know any more how cleanly we have been able to separate—conceptually and methodologically—the measurement of the dependent variable from the measurement of the subjective independent variable.

In fact, the subjective measures of exposure are richly embedded in a matrix of state and trait influences, thereby complicating our interpretive task enormously.

I believe that the primary reason for this state of affairs is that the currently dominant theoretical formulation on stress is an excessively phenomenological one. It tells us, essentially, that it is perfectly fine to drop the objective indicators of environmental exposure—if they are too difficult to obtain— and to keep only the subjective ones, since all causal processes are mediated by the subjective exposure.

My own position is that a theory that deals primarily with the phenomenological experience of stress is an unsuitable model for research that aims to describe the health consequences of different exposures in the work setting. There is only so much one can do in one piece of research and priorities need to be set. The priorities that come to us from the model of stress that emphasizes the subjective phenomenology of the process are inappropriate and we end up with research designs that are unable to provide the etiological links between the work environment and the distal disease outcomes.

It might be mentioned in passing that there is a small side benefit to the occupational epidemiology perspective I espouse: There is no need to wait for the stress field to straighten out the severe terminological and conceptual confusion regarding the term "stress", since the term can drop out of our conversation altogether.

The emphasis on the study of health consequences of exposures to objectively defined conditions in the workplace is a recommendation not without its difficulties of implementation. The development of assessment techniques for the measurement of specific (discrete) aspects of the objective work environment has lagged far behind the development (nay, proliferation) of the subjective measures. It has been exceedingly difficult to dimensionalize the work setting adequately, to identify reasonably convenient measurement strategies, and to develop a commensurate pairing of the objective and the subjective measures so that one could examine the theory that the eventual consequences of exposure operate through the subjective perceptions.

The recommended emphasis on objective work environment as the basic starting point for our etiological research is vulnerable to misunderstanding and distortion. For example, there is nothing in this emphasis that should discourage the inclusion of person variables, such as in a Person-Environment Fit model approach: objective environmental demands paired with the person's capabilities (skills, resources). The inclusion of individual difference variables is independent of whether we measure the environment objectively or subjectively. Similarly, there is nothing in the emphasis that forces us to translate this into an exclusively physicalistic measurement of only the physical reality. It may be fully appropriate to wish to study, for example, the effects of perceived exposure to carcinogens (independent of actual physical reality). However, we should strive to measure this "objectively" (for example, announcements by the union, distribution of pamphlets, screening program started by company), rather than rely on purely subjective assessments; the latter might be too seriously contaminated by stable trait characteristics, such as neuroticism.

It should also be acknowledged that subjective measures of environmental exposure do have their usefulness when they are embedded in a strong research design—for example, a prospective study of an initially healthy cohort in which known biological risk factors are included as covariates. Hence we may have a reasonable confidence that our subjective exposure variable has etiological significance in the disease outcome. However, even a strong design like that leaves us in the dark regarding the appropriate objective conditions (if any) that link up with the subjective measure.

I would like to use the epidemiological perspective to make some comments about intervention studies at the work site and their relevance to the study of work stress.

Since just about all of our work stress research is based on passive observation—that is, quasi-experimental field research—one naturally looks toward intervention studies as the only practical opportunity for full experimental control. When the experimentally induced modification of a risk factor is followed by reduced risk for disease, then we have powerful supplementary evidence in the best tradition of public health.

When I look at the current intervention research—health promotion and risk reduction at the workplace—I do not feel that it links up in any way with the stress research. That is, I feel that such studies do not provide the supplementary experimental evidence on risk factors identified in the quasi-experimental stress studies.

I think there are two related reasons why the intervention studies do not illuminate stress-disease processes that have been tentatively identified in the observational stress research. One reason is that the overwhelming majority of intervention studies *avoid* attempting to modify some aspect of the actual work environment and concentrate instead on the response side of the assumed causal dynamics. For example, the few studies that do address the issue of environmental modification—such as those that deal with flextime—do not study the dimensions that are prominent in the observational stress studies. Only the European investigators (particularly the Swedes) retain an abiding interest in the possibility of modifying the actual work environment.

A second reason that the intervention studies do not illuminate the stress process is that they target for modification outcomes—such as high blood pressure, or distress, or alcohol consumption problems—which are not in any unique way attributable to stress at work. People are selected, or self-selected, into these programs because they are high on these outcomes, not because these outcomes came about in a certain documented way that links them to a certain work environmental dimension.

I recognize that the goals of the health promotion and risk reduction activities are completely worthwhile in their own right: It is proper to attempt to manage hypertension control in the work setting, and it doesn't have to address the issue of etiology. However, I have made my comments for two reasons: First, there is a common misperception that these interventions—particularly those labeled "stress reduction"—somehow do explicitly address the alteration of the linkage between the exposure to some work conditions and some outcome variables. Second, I believe there is a missed opportunity here in not linking up explicitly the intervention efforts with the stress research.

When I was scanning the literature on interventions in the workplace, I expected that even if I didn't find the close link between observational stress studies and experimental interventions, I would at least learn something about the unique advantages of conducting health promotion and risk reduction in the work setting. That is, that such studies would illuminate the special dynamics of the workplace and would document the special effectiveness of the programs in that setting. I confess that I have been disappointed on this account as well. The preventive health behavior literature pays minimal attention to the setting (and its dynamics) in which the intervention is done. Comparative conceptual analyses of advantages and disadvantages of different settings for conducting intervention and health promotion are rare, and comparative evaluative research is even rarer. The worksite is seen as a good place for health promotion but aside from the issue of cost-effective access to target individuals and vague references to social support systems in the workplace, one learns little about the interplay of workplace dynamics and health promotion dynamics. On intuitive grounds one would certainly expect that different targets of intervention—dietary modification, exercise, blood pressure control—may be differentially suitable for the workplace setting. So, I believe, there is another missed research opportunity here as well.

In conclusion, I hope that the epidemiological perspective I have been urging upon you will help us keep track of certain important issues in the work stress area, will remind us of alternative ways of formulating the problems and the research design solutions, and will highlight the unfulfilled research promises in this fascinating and challenging field.

II Work stressors

4   *Research on work stress and health*

James S. House

This book, and the conference from which it derives, were designed to promote the integration of research and practice in the area of work stress and health. The goal has been to focus attention on work stress as a threat to health and effective functioning in the workplace, and to promote both better utilization of research in preventive or therapeutic health programs and increased relevance of research to the pressing practical issues of stress and health in the workplace.

THE INTERPLAY OF RESEARCH AND PRACTICE

I welcomed the opportunity to help organize a set of conference presentations and papers on research in the area of work stress and health. The researchers involved similarly welcomed the opportunity to disseminate their ideas to an audience of health care professionals in work organizations and the medical care system. We all welcomed the opportunity to get the perspectives of management, labor, and health care professionals on current and future directions for research.

The potential relevance of research to practice seems obvious but is often difficult to actualize. Development of effective programs to promote health and prevent disease in the workplace must be based on sound knowledge of the determinants of health in the workplace. Good research can also be invaluable for assessing the effectiveness of preventive interventions designed to reduce stress, promote health, or prevent disease in the workplace. Chapter 9 by Margaret Chesney provides an excellent illustration of how research can guide the design and evaluation of preventive interventions, and Chapter 6 by Bertil Gardell of Sweden indicates how research can be used as the basis for policy at the level of organizations and even entire societies. These chapters also alert us to problems in the utilization and implementation of research, to which I will return below.

The potential relevance of practice to research is perhaps less obvious, yet often very real if inadvertent. The distinctions between basic research, applied research, and practice are often artificial and overdrawn. I think one can argue, particularly in scientific fields related to health, that many advances in basic knowledge have their genesis in attempts to understand and deal with very practical problems. The plagues of infectious disease that once ravaged human populations stimulated research that led to our present knowledge of basic physiology, bacteriology, virology, and cellular biology. Similarly, one can see in the chapters by Ronald Burke (5), Suzanne Haynes, and Andrea La Croix (8), Robert Rose (10), and Bertil Gardell ways in which applied problems of health in the workplace have stimulated important lines of basic research.

Increasingly in the area of work stress and health, we need knowledge from longitudinal and quasi- or true experimental studies to better understand basic causal mechanisms of processes in the interplay between work stress and health. Research done in conjunction with preventive intervention programs can be a source of this kind of needed basic research knowledge while also providing a better basis for evaluating and improving such interventions. This is another, currently utilized, way in which applied preventive and therapeutic health programs can make a contribution to basis research.

OBJECTS OF RESEARCH AND PRACTICE

Research is also important to a volume and conference concerned with applied prevention and therapy, because research raises fundamental and important questions about the appropriate objects of both research and practice in the area of work stress and health. Research and theory on stress and health have long recognized that stress is not really a single concept or entity, but rather a rubric or process that focuses attention on the manifold ways in which psychosocial factors at the level of interpersonal relationships, groups, organizations, and even societies can affect the psychological and physiological functioning of individuals. Thus research or practice on work stress can focus on processes at the level of individual psychology or physiology, interpersonal relationships or small groups, organizations, or the larger society.

The medical care system in our society is heavily focused on dealing with health at the level of individual psychology and physiology. Health care providers typically work with individual clients or patients, and the sources and solutions to health problems are often defined as individual in nature. Preventive and therapeutic health programs generally focus on individuals rather than on the interpersonal, organizational, or societal contexts in which they are located. Yet stress research, as exemplified in all of the chapters here, teaches us that the sources of stress-related health problems are also likely to be found in the social environment as in the individual. Thus a major lesson of stress research for preventive and therapeutic medical care is that we must make greater efforts to modify interpersonal, organizational, or societal contexts rather than simply focusing on individuals.

THE POLITICS OF RESEARCH AND PRACTICE

A final major issue that these chapters raise is why we do not see more extensive or intensive efforts in our society to identify and alleviate stress-related threats to health in the workplace. Here the comparative perspective provided by Chapter 5 by Ronald Burke on Canadian stress research and especially Chapter 6 by Gardell on research in Scandinavia are particularly instructive. One can argue that there has been somewhat more interest in environmental and social policy approaches to problems of work stress and health in Canada than in the United States and, clearly, Sweden and the other Scandinavian countries have gone much further in these directions than either Canada or the United States.

It is sometimes argued that research on work stress has not had great impact on preventive or therapeutic medical care in the United States because this is a relatively new area of research and does not provide sufficient knowledge to guide practice. Yet neither Canada nor Sweden know any more about problems of stress and health than we do. Therefore, greater knowledge is clearly not a prerequisite for greater utilization of research in practice. Rather, we must recognize that the extent and manner of utilization of research on work stress in preventive or therapeutic programs is substantially a function of the sociopolitical context in which such efforts at utilization occur. If we wish to see greater utilization of research, we need not only more and better research, but also greater willingness of practitioners and policy makers to act on the basis of existing research (also generating, as noted above, important new opportunities for research).

OVERVIEW OF CHAPTERS

The six chapters in this section provide an excellent overview of research on work stress as it relates to problems of the design and implementation of preventative and therapeutic health programs. Burke's chapter (5) provides an excellent overview of stress research in general as well as the unique contributions that Canadian researchers have made to the literature. Chapter 8 by Suzanne Haynes and Andrea La Croix immediately makes clear that the health of women as well as men is increasingly threatened by stressors in the work environment, and that new technological changes have the potential to both alleviate some stressors and create still others. Robert Rose's chapter (10) clearly shows that the effects of work stress on individuals can be physiological as well as psychological or behavioral. Thus effective research and practice in this field must simultaneously consider physiological, psychological, social, and technological factors. This makes research and practice in the area of work stress and health an exceedingly complex phenomena—as R. Van Harrison et al. illustrated in Chapter 7. The interdisciplinary nature of this field is indicated by the representation of epidemiologists, physicians, psychologists, and sociologists in this segment of the book and conference.

The chapters by Margaret Chesney (9) and Bertil Gardell (6) show that even though research on work stress and health is complex, interdisciplinary, and relatively new, it can and has yielded knowledge that is important and useful in planning and evaluating preventive and therapeutic intervention. Chesney's review of her own research and that of others on workplace-based programs for controlling hypertension exemplifies the role that research has played in relation to practice in the United States, while Gardell's review of the Scandinavian experience provides a very different model of research, practice, and public policy for us to ponder.

5   Issues and implications for health care delivery systems: a Canadian perspective

Ronald J. Burke

The area of work stress has developed almost faddish aspects in Canada during the past five years. Many occupational groups (police officers, teachers, child care workers, air traffic controllers) seem eager to claim the high-stress label that they can then use to demand higher pay from their employers. In addition, a large stress industry has developed, offering the latest work stress reduction techniques (TM, TA, relaxation, yoga, exercise) to members of the general public and to organizations, to help them understand and manage work stress. *The Joy of Stress* (Hanson, 1985) topped the nonfiction best-seller list as this chapter was being written. This heightened interest in work stress shown by lay individuals is matched by increasing research attention within the academic community. It is not an exaggeration to conclude that work stress has become a central variable in the field of organizational behavior. Thus interest in work stress in Canada continues to remain high.

WHY AN INTEREST IN WORK STRESS?

There are several legitimate reasons why interest in the effects of work stress continues to remain high. Some of these reasons relate to financial costs borne by individuals, organizations, and Canadian society as a whole. An individual who develops a physical or an emotional illness, either of short or long duration, usually requires some form of health care and is likely to be absent from work for some period of time. The direct and indirect costs borne by society as a whole as a consequence of work-related illness are staggering (Lalonde, 1974). In addition, organizations endure a cost since individuals experiencing greater work stress are likely to be less productive, to have more work-related accidents, to be absent or late for work more often, and to more frequently quit their organization and have to be replaced (Quick and Quick, 1984). Thus work stress is likely to be related to lowered individual and organizational performance. There has also been an increasing trend in North America to place legal responsibility on the organization for the emotional and physical well-being of its employees (Ivancevich, Matteson, and Richards, 1985). Finally, there has developed a widespread belief among senior management in organizations that employees indeed represent assets that must be supported and developed if their organization is to be effective. Organizations that search for excellence care about the health and well-being of their staffs (Peters and Waterman, 1982).

THE CANADIAN CONTEXT

It is important to understand the larger Canadian context as it relates to health and health care delivery systems before we examine work stress. There have been four important developments that have had an impact on the general level of health and welfare of Canadians: the development of a health care system of high quality, support for health promotion through identifying and changing environmental and behavioral risks, the existence of the Canadian Mental Health Association (CMHA), and the recent creation of the Canadian Center for Occupational Health and Safety (CCOHS).

The Canadian Health Care System

The federal and the ten provincial governments have long recognized that good physical and mental health are necessary for the quality of life. They have developed a health care system that, although not perfect, is the equal of any in the world. This system involves a program of prepaid health services that makes it possible for everyone to obtain medical and hospital care, hospitals to be built, and physicians and other health professionals to be trained.

There is general agreement (Lalonde, 1974) on three indicators of the level of health service: the ratio of various health professions to the total population, the ratio of treatment facilities to the population, and the extent of prepaid medical coverage. In hospital and medical insurance coverage, Canada equaled the best of the five countries chosen for comparison; it led in physicians, was in the middle rank in terms of hospital beds, and second in terms of nurses. Thus Canada compared favorably with other countries that have high-quality health care services.

Changing Environmental and Behavioral Risks

In spite of the great strides that Canada has made over the past few years in health care delivery, major problems, including costs and access, still exist. Canada is now approaching the point where health care costs are beyond the capacity of our country to finance them. Despite the huge investments in health care delivery, health care services are still not equally available to all segments of the population.

The traditional view of the health field is that the science of medicine has led to whatever improvements in health have occurred, and most individuals equate the level of health with the quality of medicine. As a result of this view, most direct expenditures on health are physician-centered, including medical care, laboratory tests, and prescription drugs. If one adds dental care and service of other professionals, over $10 billion per year are spent on a personal health care system that is mainly oriented to treating existing illness.

But there are limitations to the traditional view (Knowles, 1980). Historical analyses have indicated that the most important past influences on health improvements have, in fact, involved behavioral and environmental changes and these factors will continue to be important for further advances (McKeown, 1971).

Thus a new strategy is needed. The government of Canada has made a decision to promote improvements in the environment and in life-style (Lalonde, 1974). This is where the concern with work stress comes into play. Work stress research has typically included both work environment and life-style variables.

Canadian Mental Health Association

CMHA is a national voluntary organization begun in 1918 and has been working to improve the care and rehabilitation of the mentally ill, to prevent mental illness, and to promote mental health (Morwood, 1984). CMHA expanded rapidly between 1950 and 1970. By 1983, it comprised about 30,000 volunteers and 250 staff working through a network of 190 community-based branches, 12 provincial/territorial divisions, and a national office. CMHA has historically been interested in the care and rehabilitation of the mentally ill, but has almost been forced to consider prevention in light of recent developments in its environment.

One priority program initiative that CMHA has undertaken, in attempting to achieve its objectives, is Mental Health and the Workplace. The purpose of this nationwide education and development project was to promote the availability of programs and strategies through the workplace, aimed at: maintaining and enhancing the mental health of employees, providing early identification and access to counselling services for employees experiencing trouble, and developing employment preparation and job opportunities for mentally disabled persons. Funded by Health and Welfare Canada, the project developed and made available practical resource information, educational materials, and program models and guidelines. Service users and service providers were engaged in an exploration of mental health needs and issues and were involved in the design of program strategies to meet identified needs. CMHA acted as a catalyst by bringing interested parties together, by providing a forum for the exchange of views and information, and by encouraging the development of specific plans and programs that responded to local needs. The participatory process used throughout the project established a climate conducive to attitudinal, structural, and policy changes in the workplace (Morwood, 1984).

CMHA has also undertaken a research project on the effects of the workplace on mental health in five communities across Canada. First CMHA volunteers in each community completed a telephone survey to gather information on the attitudes, opinions, and knowledge of mental health resources of working people. Then CMHA volunteers personally interviewed individuals representing employers, unions, self-help groups, and human service professionals. This information was then put together into reports for each of the five communities, along with an overall summary of the research project. These products have served to highlight the potential effects of the workplace on health and well-being and to assist the citizens of each of the five communities and CMHA plan follow-up actions for the betterment of mental health in the workplace. Finally CMHA has also been active in the promotion of employee assistance programs in the workplace. These initiatives, taken together, have created a widespread grass-roots interest in the causes and consequences of work stress and its prevention.

Canadian Center for Occupational Health and Safety

Another recent development was the passage by the federal government of Canada of the Canadian Center for Occupational Health and Safety Act in April 1978. The purpose of this act was to promote the basic right of Canadians to a healthy and safe working environment by creating a national institute concerned with the study, encouragement, and cooperative advancement of occupational health and safety.

The objectives of the Center are: (1) to promote health and safety in the workplace in Canada and the physical and mental health of working people in Canada; (2) to facilitate cooperation among various levels of government, and between labor and management, in establishing and maintaining high standards of occupational health and safety; (3) to assist in the development and maintenance of policies and programs aimed at the reduction or elimination of occupational hazards; and (4) to serve as a national center for statistics and other information relating to occupational health and safety.

CCOHS has emphasized the gathering and distributing of information and statistics during its short history. It has both sponsored and undertaken research projects emphasizing the physical work environment almost exclusively. CCOHS also provided technical advice to other initiatives (external committees, educational activities, training courses), created a national information clearinghouse, published a quarterly newsletter, and primarily responded to inquiries from the public.

Job Loss, Unemployment, and Health

The unemployment rate in Canada reached a peak of almost 13 percent in 1982, at the height of the recent recession, and it continues to remain high. It is presently about 10 percent. In a curious way, research on the effects of unemployment on health, coupled with social activism highlighting the plight of the unemployed, has emphasized the role of work in contributing to health in a positive way. The media have dramatized these findings, often in a simplistic and exaggerated manner, serving to strengthen the work/well-being link in the minds of many Canadians. As a result, all levels of government face continuing pressure to create jobs.

WORK STRESS RESEARCH

There are at least five important bodies of research findings, or research thrusts, that can be identified in Canadian work stress research: (1) replications and extensions of the work environment and well-being framework developed by the Institute for Social Research at the University of Michigan, (2) studies of coronary-prone or Type A behavior, (3) investigations of burnout in work settings, (4) examinations of various effects of social support on work stress and well-being, and (5) studies of work stress among working women.

Work Stress and Individual Well-Being

Several studies have been conducted to establish links between work stresses of various kinds and several different aspects of individual well-being. Most of these studies have used the person-environment fit model developed by the Institute for Social Research and discussed in this volume by Harrison and his associates in Chapter 7. Tests of the model have included samples such as male and female administrators of correctional institutions (Burke and Weir, 1980b), female managers (Greenglass, 1984), female nurses (Jamal, 1984), males and females employed in a variety of jobs in hospitals (Arsenault and Dolan, 1982), male air traffic controllers (MacBride, 1978), and male and female managers (Nicholson and Goh, 1983). They have examined a range of work stresses such as role ambiguity (Howard, Cunningham, and Rechnitzer, in press; Nicholson and Goh, 1983), role conflict (Greenglass, 1984), shiftwork (Jamal and Jamal, 1982), and responsibility for people and things (Burke and Weir, 1980b). In addition, they have included several different measures of emotional and physical well-being. These include: psychosomatic symptoms (Burke and Weir, 1980b); Greenglass, 1984), job satisfaction (Arsenault and Dolan, 1982; Greenglass, 1984), and biochemical and cardiovascular responses (Howard, Cunningham, and Rechnitzer, in press). Given the number of studies that have used the same (or similar) measures the time has come to undertake a meta-analysis of their findings. These studies have generally shown modest statistically significant associations between measures of work stress and individual well-being.

Coronary-Prone or Type A Behavior

Empirical research on Type A behavior has been ongoing in Canada for almost a decade. The first programmatic effort was undertaken by John Howard and his colleagues (Howard, Cunningham and Rechnitzer, 1976).

Their work examined work and health patterns associated with Type A behavior. They found that Type As worked more hours per week, traveled more days per year, but were not necessarily more job satisfied than their Type B counterparts. Another important conclusion they noted was that some organizations in their sample of twelve had a greater proportion of Type As than others. This raised the intriguing question of whether phenomena such as Type A organizations, Type A professions, or Type A work exist; that is, might Type As be more attracted to particular professions and organizations than are Type Bs?

Burke and his associates (Burke and Weir, 1980b; Burke, Weir, and DuWors, 1980) examined the influence of Type A behavior of job incumbents on their nonwork or family lives, and on the experiences of their spouses. They found, consistent with anecdotal reports of Friedman and Rosenman (1974), that Type As were less satisfied in their marriages and reported that their jobs had a greater negative impact on their family, home, and personal lives than did Type Bs. This pattern was also present among the Type A wives. Thus spouses of Type As also reported less marital satisfaction and a more negative impact of their spouse's job on home, family, and personal lives. In addition, these women reported less emotional and psychological support (social support) from others and fewer friendships and less social participation. Thus not only did these women experience greater stress in their lives, they had fewer resources to deal with this situation.

Greenglass (1985a) has replicated some of the previous studies of career and organizational experiences of Type A men using female professionals and managers. This focus, though relatively neglected to date, will become increasingly important as more women enter the work world and nontraditional occupations in particular. Greenglass (1985c) has also recently investigated the role of anger in Type A behavior and specifically how anger is evoked in the female manager.

The final area of Canadian research dealing with Type A behavior that will be discussed involves attempts to reduce Type A behavior. Roskies (1983) and Roskies and associates (1979, 1985) have devoted the last ten years to developing and evaluating various treatment approaches. She has shown that both behavior modification and traditional psychotherapy can produce alterations in Type A behavior among individuals who have already had coronary heart disease. She has attempted to reduce Type A behavior among healthy males with less success however.

Burnout in Work Settings

Three recent Canadian contributions to our understanding of burnout are noteworthy: (1) attempts to validate the Cherniss (1980) process model of burnout, (2) an examination of the existence of progressive phases of burnout, and (3) conducting longitudinal studies of burnout.

Cherniss (1980) proposed perhaps the only comprehensive model of burnout. He and his associates interviewed 28 beginning professionals in four fields (mental health, poverty law, public health nursing, and high school teachers). All individuals were interviewed several times over a one- to two-year period of time. The process model he proposed is shown in Figure 5.1. The variables in the model were distilled from interviews and observations of these new professionals.

This model proposes that individuals having particular career orientations and extra-work support and demands interact with particular work-setting characteristics. The coming together of these factors results in the experience of particular sources of stress. Individuals cope with these stresses in different ways. Some individuals employ techniques and strategies that might be termed active problem solving while others cope by exhibiting the negative attitude changes Cherniss identified in his concept of burnout. Burnout, for Cherniss, occurs over time (it is a process) and represents one way of adapting to, or coping with, particular sources of stress.

A second contribution examines the notion of progressive stages or phases of burnout. Golembiewski and his colleagues (Golembiewski, 1984; Golembiewski and Munzenrider, 1984) proposed the existence of eight progressive phases of burnout.

Recent research (Golembiewski, Munzenrider, and Carter, 1983; Golembiewski and Munzenrider, 1984; Burke and Greenglass, 1985) has validated the notion of progressive phases of burnout by comparing individuals in the various phases of burnout on other measures. In general, these studies provide support for the preparation that individuals at different phases of burnout also differ on antecedents and consequences of burnout.

The third contribution is a longitudinal test of the Cherniss model. Burnout is a process—that is, it develops over time. Thus the most appropriate research on burnout would be conducted over time. We were able to collect data from half of the teacher sample one year later using

Figure 5.1.   Cherniss process model of burnout

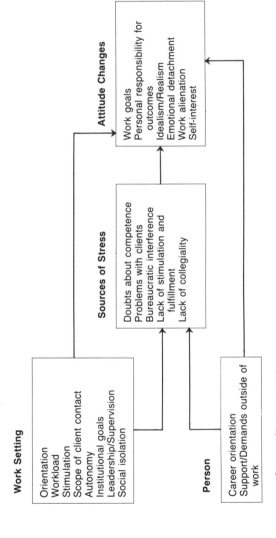

Work Setting

Orientation
Workload
Stimulation
Scope of client contact
Autonomy
Institutional goals
Leadership/Supervision
Social isolation

Person

Career orientation
Support/Demands outside of
work

Sources of Stress

Doubts about competence
Problems with clients
Bureaucratic interference
Lack of stimulation and
fulfillment
Lack of collegiality

Attitude Changes

Work goals
Personal responsibility for
outcomes
Idealism/Realism
Emotional detachment
Work alienation
Self-interest

Source: Cherniss, 1980.

34

essentially the same measures. My associate, Jacob Wolpin, is currently analyzing this data and the results of the longitudinal examination of the Cherniss process model of burnout will be available soon. This project will also determine what changes, if any, take place in the phases of burnout individuals occupy over a one-year period of time.

Social Support

The Clarke Institute of Psychiatry, a teaching and research center in Toronto, has conducted a series of studies on the role of social support in stressful life situations (Freeman and Sheldon, 1984). These studies involved an examination of work stress and psychological distress among Canadian air traffic controllers (ATCs), a two-year study of adjustment following conjugal bereavement, a comparative study of depressed versus nondepressed university students, and an investigation of work stress and psychological distress among government employees. All four studies used the same outcome measure, the General Health Questionnaire (GHQ), developed by Goldberg (1972) to assess emotional health.

Let us consider some of the specific findings. First, in the ATC study (MacBride, 1978) each measure of social support was significantly and negatively associated with emotional distress. Second, in the longitudinal conjugal bereavement study (Vachon et al., 1982) women with deficits in social support reported greater distress on the GHQ. These two studies, while indicating a direct effect of social support on distress, did not measure stress in any way.

Burke and his associates have undertaken intensive examinations of social support as it exists in work settings. Burke and Weir (1975) first examined help-seeking in managers, the people they turned to, and their motivations for help-seeking. Data from three groups of professional males indicated that help was sought from a wide range of relationships both within and without their work settings. However, spouses and co-workers were relied on as the primary sources of help. The most common reasons given for selecting a particular helper involved his or her skill in the areas of emotional support and clarification, and personal validation. A later study (Burke, Weir, and Duncan, 1976) obtained a detailed picture of supportive interventions at work of 53 managers from a variety of organizations. The findings indicated that: status appeared to dictate to whom an individual at work would go for help, an attitude of noninvolvement in the affairs of others characterized work relationships unless explicit requests for help were made, the helping activity itself was more problem-centered than person-centered, with greater attention given to external aspects of the problem and less to dealing with the feelings and emotions of the person helped.

Work Stress of Women

Studies of work stress have focused mainly on men. However, with the dramatic rise in women's employment in recent years and their increasing visibility in nontraditional areas such as management, there is a growing need for the systematic investigation of factors related to women's work stress. Moreover, evidence suggests that even in the same employment situation, men and women may experience different stressors (Greenglass, 1982).

In a study of female managers, Greenglass (1985a) observed a relationship between stressors in female managers such as perceived sex discrimination, inequity of pay, and underutilization of skills, as well as depression, anxiety, and psychosomatic symptoms. Further research by Greenglass (1985b) has demonstrated the psychological consequences of token status associated with the female managerial role. Data collected from a sample of managerial women indicated that female managers tended to perceive their jobs as primarily socially evaluative. These women's reactions to their jobs may be a reflection of their "token" status, one that leads to greater scrutiny and evaluation of their work. Thus these data point to another source of stress in female managers, a subtle source whose psychological implications have only begun to be studied.

Additional research by Greenglass (1985a) has investigated the antecedents and consequences of role conflict in female workers. Role conflict was conceptualized as simultaneous demands for action and emotional involvement from various spheres such as home and work. Rigid work schedules and work overload were significantly related to role conflict, which in turn was associated with depression, irritation, and anxiety. The research by Greenglass (1985a) has demonstrated the deleterious effects of role conflict on women's health—both physical and psychological.

In a study of female managers, Greenglass (1984) found that the Type A behavior pattern plays a moderating role in these women's stress reactions to challenges in the work environment. This research extended Type A theory to women by showing that Type A women, like their male counterparts, respond with more distress to challenges in the work environment than did Type B women. In response to stress, Type A women were significantly more likely than their Type B counterparts to want to quit their jobs—an action-oriented type of coping. Moreover, intention to turnover was significantly associated with stressful consequences to a greater extent in Type As than in Type Bs.

Research by Greenglass (1985c) with women who occupy faculty and managerial roles has reported greater role conflict for Type A women than for Type B. Type A women, as expected, had greater difficulty meeting all of their self-imposed demands both in the home and at work. These data suggest that, in women, the Type A behavior pattern is reflected in both family and work roles as Burke and Weir (1980b) report for men. These data also indicate an even greater health risk associated with Type A behavior in women—a health risk that is considerably heightened given that it is significantly and positively associated with role conflict between home and work roles.

The relationship between anger and Type A behavior among female managers was the subject of another study conducted by Greenglass (1985c). Increasingly, anger and hostility have been identified as critical components of Type A behavior in contributing to the etiology of cardiovascular heart disease. Results showed a positive relationship between state and trait anger (Spielberger et al., 1983) in Type As but not in Type Bs. This suggests that trait anger is a mediator of state anger in Type As—the higher the trait anger in Type As, the more easily provoked to anger in situations. Contrary to the assumption that anger and hostility always characterize Type As, these data suggest that Type As vary in their predisposition to anger provocation according to their level of trait anger. While all respondents reacted with anger to high role conflict and underutilization of skills, only Type As showed a positive association between perceived sex discrimination on the job and state anger.

INTERVENTIONS TO REDUCE WORK STRESS

Canadian organizations have taken four approaches in assisting their employees to deal with work stress. The first involves the area of *physical fitness*. Many Canadian organizations will pay for their employees (mostly professional and managerial) to join fitness clubs. The widely held belief is that an individual who is fit and healthy will both experience less stress (prevention) and be able to cope better with whatever stress he or she encounters. A few organizations have built first-rate facilities on their premises, complete with qualified staff. Although great claims are often made about the benefits of these programs, the basis for such evaluations are often weak (Burke and Weir, 1980a).

Cox and his colleagues have conducted an excellent evaluation of the benefit of a fitness program introduced into an organization (Cox, Shephard, and Corey, 1981; Shephard, Cox, and Corey, 1981). The head offices of two large Canadian Assurance Companies located in Toronto participated in the research. One, with 1,281 employees, served as the test company, while the other, with 579 employees, served as the control. A professionally directed employee fitness program was initiated at the test company for a six-month period, repeat measures of fitness and worker satisfaction were undertaken, quarterly departmental records of productivity were provided by both companies, absenteeism was noted on a bimonthly basis, and employee turnover at the test company was reported only retrospectively.

About 20 percent of the test company employees participated in the exercise class. The general attitudes of employees toward their work improved. Employee turnover during a ten-month period was substantially lower in exercise adherents than in the remainder of company employees. Productivity showed small gains in both test and control companies. Absenteeism of high adherents was reduced by 22 percent relative to other employees.

The researchers (Shephard et al., 1983) also examined the effects of this program on health care costs. At the test company, health care cost data were collected for one year before and one year after implementation of the employee fitness program. Health care costs were obtained from the government-controlled Ontario Health Insurance Plan (OHIP). Initially, hospital utilization was somewhat greater for employees at the test company. This trend underwent a dramatic reversal with the institution of the employee fitness program. The total cost of medical care was initially very similar for test and control companies. At the control company, costs showed a substantial jump from 1977 to 1978, while there was little change at the test company.

The second intervention to reduce work stress is an *educational* one. It involves exposing employees in organizations to material on work stress and coping. Some of these also involve the spouses of job incumbents (Burke, 1980), either together with or separate from their partners. Although the participants are almost uniformly positive about these experiences, there is little other evidence that these offerings make any difference.

A third type of organizational intervention involves *changes in policies, work design, and organizational roles and structure.* The Children's Aid Society of Metropolitan Toronto developed an interesting intervention to reduce burnout among entering frontline social workers in child welfare. This program differed radically in many ways from routine orientation practices involving (1) hiring frontline workers in batches; (2) keeping these newly hired workers in small groups (N = 5 or 6) for their first six months of employment; (3) gradually increasing their case load so that it eventually reached 60 percent of the normal case load by the six-month point; (4) an enhanced supervisor's role emphasizing education (accompanied by a reduction of other supervisory duties); (5) an improved training program (one to two days of training every two weeks); (6) an increased social support for the group; and (7) attempts to deal with stressors found to be associated with burnout in previous research (for example, promoting clear, consistent, and specific feedback; clarifying rules, policies, and roles; allowing for autonomy and innovation).

The research employed a pretest extended posttest design with a nonequivalent comparison group. The project designed to run for 2.5 years was cut short because of budget cutbacks resulting from the general economic recession. The resulting sample sizes rendered the quantitative data of little use. Qualitative data indicated general satisfaction with the program and beliefs that the goals of the program were realized. Supervisors felt that frontline workers in the program achieved a level of skill during the six months comparable to that achieved in one year under the traditional program.

The fourth organizational intervention that appears to offer much potential in reducing work stress are *employee assistance programs* (EAPs) (Santa Barbara, 1984). EAPs developed in the 1960s to assist alcoholic employees. They then broadened their focus to assist employees with a wider range of personal problems. Anything that interfered with the capacity of the employee to perform his job became a legitimate problem for discussion. Organizations made appropriate referrals to external agencies or hired qualified professionals as internal counselors. Some EAPs now include the family of job incumbents under their umbrella. In addition, some encourage employees to deal with sources of work stress, as well as sources of nonwork stress. EAPs appear to be able to offer assistance to those in need and to offer help in preventing work stress from leading to negative outcomes.

Much more research effort is needed to evaluate the strengths and weaknesses of each of these organization-sponsored efforts to deal with work stress.

SOME ISSUES RESULTING FROM WORK STRESS RESEARCH

Let us now step back from a discussion of specific findings from Canadian work stress research and consider some broader issues raised by the interpretation and implementation of these findings. These issues involve: definition (high stress versus high risk); appropriate targets for invention (job components versus job categories); the distinction between job content versus work environment; the importance of changing what can be changed; stereotypes, myths, and work stress realities; and the importance of bridging research and practice.

High Stress versus High Risk

The terms "high stress" and "high risk" are often used interchangeably. High stress is used to describe both the stressful conditions (stressors) and an individual's reaction to these stressors (strain, or stress responses). The term "high stress" implies that an increase in work stressors automatically increases the incidence of various strains (physical, physiological, and psychological) that, in turn, automatically increase the risk of showing various negative outcomes (divorce, mental illness, alcoholism). These assumptions follow from equating high stress with high risk. MacBride (1984) highlights the need to clarify the relationship among terms. She proposes that distinctions be made between *work stresses*, the experience of *strain*, and various *outcomes* of stress. An individual may experience high stress but low strain and low risk of showing negative outcomes. High stress does not necessarily equal high risk.

Job Components versus Job Categories

MacBride (1984) also emphasizes the need for a shift in attention away from the examination and discussion of high-stress jobs (what she terms job categories) toward an emphasis on the stressfulness of various job components that may exist in varying degrees in any occupation. This change in emphasis is aimed more at the interventionist and the lay audience than at the work stress researcher. Most researchers have been identifying and describing job components or job characteristics that are associated with greater job dissatisfaction and lower health and well-being. Their findings, however, have been misinterpreted to apply to jobs as a whole.

Job Content versus Work Environment

Research being conducted at the Clarke Institute of Psychiatry in Toronto is relevant to this distinction. MacBride and her colleagues (1981) have reported that air traffic controllers were quite similar to noncontrollers in the same department on a number of outcome measures. The researchers then examined the major sources of work stress reported by the ATCs. Interestingly, the stress of their job was only weakly related to the actual nature of their work—that is, the task of controlling air traffic. Only two of the five most stressful work stresses were related to the job itself (peak traffic situations, fear of causing an accident). The other three (poor equipment, poor relationships with management, and the issue of bilingualism in air traffic control) were in some senses either avoidable or external sources of stress rather than unavoidable integral parts of the actual job.

The ATCs, both in their questionnaire and in interview comments, often made a distinction between *unavoidable* work stress directly related to the actual nature of their job and avoidable work stress that was artificially imposed on them by the job environment. Although it was not possible to make direct comparisons between ATCs and non-ATCs on sources of work stress, MacBride (1978), using impressionistic and anecdotal information, noted striking similarities between the two groups. The most common complaints among non-ATCs included management relations, government inefficiency, and lack of opportunities for career growth—all of which were noted frequently by ATCs. In addition, both groups reported common sources of job satisfaction, sense of accomplishment, feelings of responsibility, service or pride derived from the satisfactory performance of their actual jobs.

This same point is present in other research findings. Vachon has been involved for several years in a qualitative phenomological study of work stress in the care of the critically ill, dying and bereaved. She reports data gathered from men and women caring for the critically ill and dying (Vachon, 1984). Respondents indicated that sources of stress came primarily from four areas: illness, patient/family, occupational role, and environment. Interestingly, the actual exposure to dying patients accounted for only a small proportion of the work stressors (14 percent). Occupational role and work environment were cited as work stresses more often than illness of patients and families (69 percent versus 31 percent).

INTERVENTIONS IN ORGANIZATIONS: CHANGE THE THINGS THAT CAN BE CHANGED

If the work stresses of air traffic control are viewed as both inevitable and inherent in the job itself, then there is little that can be done to reduce the work stress of ATCs. In these circumstances, organizations see their role as identifying applicants with the best possibility of handling the inherent work stress (a selection problem). MacBride (1978) observed these beliefs to be widely held in both management and among ATCs.

Her research findings suggest that such an approach would be both insufficient and impractical. It would be insufficient in that only about 10 percent of the ATCs displayed periodic stress symptoms. In addition, there did not appear to be any demographic or personality characteristics that reliably distinguished those ATCs that experienced their work as chronically stressful from those who did not.

Another strategy consistent with the person-environment model of work stress is to examine the ability of the job to meet the needs, motivation, and abilities of job incumbents. MacBride found that ATCs frequently complained about organizational structure and management practices that interfered with their needs for career advancement, participation in decision making, and poor communication with management. There are many things that can be done to reduce the work stress of ATCs when the sources of stress are *not* seen as inevitable and inherent in the job itself (hence unchangeable). Thus even if some (or many) of the sources of work stress are unavoidable, improvements can be made in job components that are avoidable.

In addition, many of the sources of work stress reported by ATCs were also common to non-ATC job incumbents. Thus intervention efforts need not be limited to ATCs. Too much special attention has been devoted in the past to ATCs. MacBride (1984) recommends that those involved in intervention with ATCs should downplay the emphasis on ATCs as a high-stress job and highlight stressful job components within ATC and non-ATC employees.

High-Stress Occupations—Myth versus Reality

Professionals in the work stress field often come across listings of so-called high-stress occupations. These listings compare jobs on indicators of stressfulness or include professions that are widely acknowledged to be highly stressful. These studies serve a useful purpose in supporting the belief that individuals' jobs can and do have an impact on their physical and emotional well-being, but they often serve to perpetuate myths about particular jobs.

Recent Canadian research has been conducted on two such high-stress profile jobs: air traffic controllers and police officers. The Social and Community Psychiatry Section of the Clarke Institute of Psychiatry conducted a series of studies of psychosocial stress among Canadian ATCs and other public-sector employees within the same government department (MacBride, 1981). Let us consider some of the findings. First, the group ATC data did not support the stereotype of ATCs as a universally stressed or distressed group of employees. Only 10 percent of the ATCs had Goldberg GHQ scores of 5 or more on all three questionnaire administrations. During normal working periods, only between 25 and 30 percent had GHQ scores above 5 at any one point in time. In addition, when the GHQ scores of all the ATCs were compared with those of non-ATC personnel, no significant differences were found. The same was true when a more closely matched non-ATC subsample was examined. Similarly, there were no significant differences between the ATCs and the non-ATCs in terms of self-reported number of medical visits, ATCs and other males in their age group in the general population in use of OHIP services, or rate of marital separation, divorce, or remarriage. In fact ATCs reported themselves as being in significantly better health and significantly less anxious than their non-ATC co-workers did. However, in terms of perceived job impact on their health, psychological well-being, and relationships with their spouses and children, the ATCs consistently rated their jobs as having a more negative impact on their lives.

Let us now consider some findings on men and women in police work. We conducted two studies of burnout in which identical measures were used with 828 police officers (Burke, 1985) and 833 public school teachers (Burke and Greenglass, 1985). The two studies were based on the process model of burnout proposed by Cherniss (1980). The two samples were compared on more than 30 measures. Very few differences were found between the two occupations. One possible explanation for these findings is that teaching, like policing, is a very stressful occupation. A second explanation is that the stereotype that police work is a stressful occupation is not warranted. This conclusion was reached by health research that used police samples to examine work stress.

High-Stress Jobs and the Self-Fulfilling Prophecy

The work of MacBride and her colleagues suggests that individuals working on jobs thought to be high stress/high risk may come to believe the stereotype. Thus, although there were no data indicating a higher incidence of physical, emotional, or family concerns among ATCs, they were more likely to see their job as having a negative impact on their health, psychological well-being, and family relationships. In interviews with ATCs, personnel administrators and management respondents repeatedly made reference to the belief that ATCs had a higher incidence of physical and emotional problems, divorce, and suicide. These statements were made in spite of the absence of empirical support for them.

MacBride (1984) suggests that one explanation for ATCs reporting negative impacts of their job on various areas of their lives, even though they were not experiencing difficulties in these areas, was that they had fallen victim to their own image of the stereotype. She writes:

This explanation is reinforced by frequent comments by the controllers, both in questionnaires and in interviews, about the dangers of beginning to "believe their own myth." They often commented that they had been told so often that their job was expected to have such severe negative consequences on their health and home-life and that they would "burn out" at an early age, that they began looking for these problems where they might not otherwise have existed. Furthermore, they frequently complained about the pressure and frustration of having others around them also expecting and looking for signs in them of their inevitable deterioration and breakdown. (It is interesting to note that over 40 percent of the controllers felt that the stress of their job was "over-rated" or "very over-rated" by the media and by the general public.)

Doing the Right Thing for the Wrong Reasons

There is a considerable body of research on work stress in policing (Kroes, 1976; Territo and Vetter, 1981). These data indicate that, in general, police work is not more demanding than the vast majority of jobs. Police officers believe, however, that they are in a very demanding job. This concern is evident in the great interest shown by police departments in both individual and organizational-level interventions. Some police forces in Canada have been very concerned about and active in the work stress and health area. The belief that police work is stressful has been used to develop a wide range of both preventive and therapeutic programs.

Many of these initiatives are aimed at individual police officers: assessments of physical fitness and health, support for exercise and fitness programs, courses on financial management and retirement planning. Other initiatives are aimed at the spouses of police officers: courses on work stress and stress management, orientation of spouses to the job of their partners, and a spouse association that may satisfy social and support group motives.

Police officers occasionally get involved in incidents of a potentially traumatic nature (for example, killing another individual, shooting another individual, being shot or shot at, dealing with homicide and suicide). All police forces provide some form of trauma counseling, usually mandatory, to members of the force encountering such events. Counselors may come from inside or outside the force. A few forces have created teams of trained peer counselors to deal with these circumstances. Every large police force has some form of EAP. In the smaller forces EAPs deal mainly with alcoholic employees. Some of these police forces have broadened the EAP umbrella to deal with work stress problems as well. Thus although the research evidence may indicate that police work is no more demanding than most other jobs, because police officers themselves believe their work is stressful, their organizations have been active in supporting stress management programs for their members.

Research and Practice—Two Cultures Again?

The preparation of this chapter has highlighted a potentially large gap between Canadian work stress researchers and practitioners. This gap can be seen perhaps most clearly between work stress researchers and clinicians or applied psychologists, but it also exists between work stress researchers and organizational consultants.

The following examples are representative and illustrate the point. I participated in a symposium at the 1985 annual meeting of the Canadian Psychological Association entitled "Type A Behavior and Coronary Heart Disease—Psychological Implications." The audience, comprised primarily of Ph.D.-level clinical psychologists working in clinical or hospital settings, was large. Few were themselves actively engaged in Type A research although many were working with coronary patients. The discussion that followed was animated. It was rich in description of technique in treating coronary patients but there was little awareness of a connection to the available research literature. The same phenomenon occurs when work stress research is discussed with organizational development consultants. They seem to be unaware of work stress research findings as they undertake their task of assisting organizations.

There seems to be a gap between the producers and the consumers of work stress research. Bridging this gap would appear to be an important concern for readers of this volume. The result would be better informed research *and* practice.

This gap is not unique to the area of work stress, however (Kilmann et al., 1983). The field of organizational behavior is currently engaged in an examination of ways of doing research that is useful for both theory and practice (see *Administrative Science Quarterly*, 1982, 1983; Lawler, et al., 1985). Both researchers and consumers of research findings would benefit from an examination of this literature. It is possible to combine research and intervention in the area of work stress (Gardell, 1982) to produce findings of value for policy formulation.

WHAT IS UNIQUELY CANADIAN
IN WORK STRESS RESEARCH?

An examination of Canadian work stress research identified only one factor that would not be present in research conducted in the United States. Canada is officially a bicultural and bilingual country, anglophones and francophones having equal status. Thus there have been a few studies in which language group has been a variable (Zaleznik, Kets de Vries, and Howard, 1977; Howard, 1984; Jamal, 1984; Dolan and Arsenault, 1980). Unfortunately, researchers have not developed a theoretical rationale for comparing anglophones and francophones and none of these studies have been replicated.

Canadian work stress research has, to date, not unearthed much of significance that could be termed uniquely Canadian. It appears that the similarities between the United States and Canada have had a much greater influence on the character of work stress research in Canada than the differences that exist.

CONCLUSION

The broader Canadian environment in which work stress research is conducted and discussed was characterized by both a high degree of support for health and health care delivery and a high degree of interest in work stress and health. Much of the Canadian research replicated and extended research conducted in the United States and elsewhere. There appeared to be little that was uniquely Canadian. Two thrusts seemed to have particular importance. The first involved Type A or coronary-prone behavior—Canadian researchers were in on the forefront in exploring both work and extrawork variables in adding to our knowledge of this self-imposed health risk. The second involved research on burnout in work settings. Canadian research in this area tended to be more comprehensive (model based) and captured the process aspects of the phenomenon.

Canadian organizations supported activities designed to help individuals who were casualties of work stress and often provided considerable resources to assist individuals in their efforts to manage their own work stress. The one area in which there appeared to be limited activity in Canada involves efforts to reduce work stressors. Interventions at department or organizational levels need to be undertaken.

There is also a critical need to bridge the gap between the researcher and the practitioner. The area of intervention provides an excellent opportunity to apply some of the accumulated knowledge of work stress to the alleviation of one of the most pressing psychological and social problems of our time, namely, work stress.

Acknowledgments: Preparation of this chapter was supported in part by the Faculty of Administrative Studies, York University. I would like to acknowledge the assistance of Anita Citron in the preparation of the manuscript, the helpful comments of Esther Greenglass, Jim House, John Howard, and Jim Quick on an early draft, and my Canadian colleagues for sharing their research activities with me.

REFERENCES

Administrative Science Quarterly, Special Issue, Part I: The Utilization of Organizational Research. 1982. *Administrative Science Quarterly*, 27: 588–685.

Administrative Science Quarterly, Special Issue, Part II: The Utilization of Organizational Research. 1983. *Administrative Science Quarterly*, 28: 63–144.

Arsenault, A. and Dolan, S. 1982. Organizational and individual consequence of work stress. Final Report to Quebec Institute for Research on Health and Safety.

Burke, R. J. 1980. Examining the work-family interface: An idea of whose time has come. *Canadian Training Methods*, 11: 12–14.

Burke, R. J. 1985. Burnout among men and women in policing: An examination of the Cherniss Model. Unpublished manuscript.

Burke, R. J. and Greenglass, E. R. 1985. Correlates of burnout phases among teachers. Unpublished manuscript.

Burke, R. J. and Weir, T. 1975. Giving and receiving help with work and non-work related problems. *Journal of Business Administration*, 7: 51–65.

————. 1980a. Coping with the stress of managerial occupations. In Cooper, C. L. and Payne, R. L. (Eds.). *Current Concerns in Occupational Stress*. New York: John Wiley.

————. 1980b. The Type A experience: Occupational and life demands, satisfaction, and well-being. *Journal of Human Stress*, 6: 28–38.

Burke, R. J., Weir, R., and Duncan, G. 1976. Informal helping processes in work settings. *Academy of Management Journal*, 19: 370–377.

Burke, R. J., Weir, T., and DuWors, R.E. 1980. Perceived Type A behavior of husbands' and wives' satisfaction and well-being. *Journal of Occupational Behavior*, 1: 139–150.

Cherniss, C. 1980. *Professional Burnout in Human Service Organizations*. New York: Praeger.

Cox, M., Shephard, R. J., and Corey, P. 1981. Influence of an employee fitness program upon fitness, productivity, and absenteeism. *Ergonomics*, 24: 795–806.

Dolan, S. and Arsenault, A. A. 1980. *Stress, Health, and Performance at Work*. Monograph No. 5, School of Industrial Relations, University of Montreal.

Freeman, S. J. J. and Sheldon, A. 1984. Social support as a modifier of stress. In Burke, R. J. (Ed.). *Current Issues in Occupational Stress: Research and Intervention*. Toronto: York University Press.

Friedman, M. and Rosenman, R. H. 1974. *Type A Behavior and Your Heart*. New York: Knopf.

Gardell, B. 1982. Scandanavian research on stress in working life. *International Journal of Health Services*, : 31–40.

Goldberg, D. 1972. *The Detection of Psychiatric Illness by Questionnaire*. London: Oxford University Press.

Golembiewski, R. T. and Munzenrider, R. 1984. Active and passive reactions to psychological burnout: Toward greater specificity in a phase model. *Journal of Health and Human Resources Administration*, 7: 264–289.

Golembiewski, R. T., Munzenrider, R., and Carter, D. 1983. Phases of progressive burnout and their work-site covariants. *Journal of Applied Behavioral Science*, 19: 461–482.

Greenglass, E.R. 1982. *A World of Difference: Gender Roles in Perspectives*. Toronto: John Wiley.

———. 1984. Type A behavior and job-related stress in managerial women. Paper presented at the annual meeting of the Academy of Management, Boston, August.

———. 1985a. Psychological implications of sex bias in the workplace. *Academic Psychology Bulletin*, 7: 227–240.

———. 1985b. An interactional perspective on job-related stress in managerial women. *The Southern Psychologist*, 2: 42–48.

———. 1985c. Type A behavior and anger: Implications for coronary heart disease. Paper presented at the annual meeting of the Canadian Psychological Association, Halifax.

Hanson, P. G. 1985. *The Joy of Stress*. Islington, Ontario: Hanson Stress Management Organization.

Howard, J. H. 1984. Sociocultural patterns of stress in a Canadian organization. In Burke, R. J. (Ed.). *Current Issues in Occupational Stress: Research and Intervention*. Toronto: York University Press.

Howard, J. H., Cunningham, D. A., and Reichnitzer, P.A. 1976. Health patterns associated with Type A behavior-managerial population. *Journal of Human Stress*, 2(1): 24–31.

———. 1977. Work patterns associated with Type A behavior: A managerial population. *Human Relations*, 30: 825–836.

————. In press. Role ambiguity, Type A behavior and job satisfaction: The moderating effects on cardiovascular and biochemical responses associated with coronary risk. *Journal of Applied Psychology*.

Ivancevich, J. M., Matteson, M. T., and Richards, E. P. 1985. Who's liable for stress on the job? *Harvard Business Review*, 64: 60–68.

Jamal, M. 1984. Job stress and outcome relationship: Employees' cultural background as a moderator? In Burke, R. J. (Ed.). *Current Issues in Occupational Stress: Research and Intervention*. Toronto: York University Press.

Jamal, M. and Jamal, S. M. 1982. Work and non-work experiences of employees on fixed and rotating shifts: An empirical assessment. *Journal of Vocational Behavior*, 20: 282–293.

Kilmann, R. H. (Ed.) 1983. *Producing Useful Knowledge for Organizations*. New York: Praeger.

Knowles, J. H. 1980. *Doing Better and Feeling Worse: Health in the United States*. New York: Norton.

Kroes, W. H. 1976. *Society's Victim—The Policeman*. Springfield, Ill: Charles C. Thomas.

Lalonde, M. 1974. *A New Perspective on the Health of Canadians*. Ottawa: Government of Canada, Cat. No. 1131–1374.

Lawler, E. E., Mohrman, A. M., Mohrman, S.A., Ledford, G. E., and Cummings,T. G. 1985. *Doing Research That Is Useful for Theory and Practice*. San Francisco: Jossey-Bass.

MacBride, A. 1978. *Psychosocial Stress among Ontario Air Traffic Controllers*. Report to Transport Canada and the Canadian Air Traffic Control Association.

————. 1984. High stress occupations: The importance of job components versus job categories. In Burke, R. J. (Ed.). *Current Issues in Occupational Stress: Research and Intervention*. Toronto: York University Press.

MacBride, A., Cochrane, J., Sheldon, A., Lancee, W. A., Dolgoy, D., and Freeman, S. J. J. 1981. *Occupational Stress Among Canadian Air Transportation Administration Employees*: Ontario Region. Final Report to Transport Canada.

McKeown, T. 1971. A historical appraisal of the medical task. In *Medical History and Medical Care*. Ontario: Ontario University Press.

Morwood, G. 1984. The role of a national voluntary organization: The Canadian Mental Health Association. In Lumaden, D. P. (Ed.). *Community Mental Health Action*. Ottawa: Canadian Public Health Administration.

Nicholson, P. J. and Goh, S. C. 1983. The relationship of organization structure and interpersonal attitudes to role conflict and ambiguity in different work environments. *Academy of Management Journal*, 26: 148–155.

Peters, T. J. and Waterman, R. 1982. *In Search of Excellence*. New York: Harper & Row.

Quick, J. C. and Quick, J. D. 1984. *Organizational Stress and Preventive Management*. New York: McGraw-Hill.

Roskies, E. 1983. Stress management for Type A individuals. In Meichenbaum, D. and Jaremko, M. (Eds.). *Stress Reduction and Prevention*. New York: Plenum.

Roskies, E., Kearney, H., Spevack, M., Surkis, A., Cohen, C., and Gilman, S. 1979. Generalizability and durability of treatment effects in an intervention program for coronary-prone Type A managers. *Journal of Behavioral Medicine*, 2: 195–207.

Roskies, E., Seragaian, P., Oseasohn, R., Smilga, C., Martin, N. and Hanley, J. A. 1985. Treatment of psychological stress responses in healthy Type A men. In Neufield, R. W. J. (Ed.). *Advances in the Investigation of Stress*. New York: John Wiley.

Santa-Barbara, J. 1984. Employee assistance programs: An alternative resource for mental health service delivery. *Canada's Mental Health*, 32: 35–38.

Shephard, R. J., Corey, P., Renzland, P., and Cox, M. 1983. The impact of changes in fitness and lifestyle upon health care utilization. *Canadian Journal of Public Health*, 74: 51–54.

Shephard, R. J., Cox, M., and Corey, P. 1981. Fitness program participation: Its effect on worker performances. *Journal of Occupational Medicine*, 23: 359–363.

Spielberger, C. D., Jacobs, G., Russell, S., and Crane, R. S. 1983. Assessment of anger: The State-Trait Anger Scale. In Butcher, J. N. and Spielberger, C.D. (Eds.). *Advances in Personality* (Vol. 2). Hillsdale, N.J.: Lawrence Erlbaum Associates.

Territo, L. & Vetter, H. J. 1981. *Stress and Police Personnel*. Boston: Allyn & Bacon.

Vachon, M. L. S. 1984. Occupational stress in the care of the critically ill and dying. In Burke, R. J. (Ed.). *Current Issues in Occupational Stress: Research and Intervention*. Toronto: York University Press.

Vachon, M. L. S., Rogers, J., Lyall, W.A., Lancee, W. J., Sheldon, A., and Freeman, S. J. J. 1982. Predictors and correlates of adaptation to conjugal bereavement. *American Journal of Psychiatry*, 139: 998–1002.

Zaleznik, A., Kets deVries, M., and Howard, J. H. 1977. Stress reactions in organizations: Syndromes, causes, and consequences. *Behavioral Science*, 22: 151–162.

6 Efficiency and health hazards in mechanized work

Bertil Gardell

This chapter discusses different research strategies and summarizes the knowledge that has influenced Scandinavian legislation and trade union policies regarding the psychosocial aspect of the working environment. These problems are also often discussed under the heading of stress at work. The efficiency models used hitherto have resulted in mental and physical ill-health through their reliance on the advanced division and simplification of labor, the systems control of work pace and methods, the individualization of tasks, the introduction of shift work or incentive pay, and authoritarian and detailed supervision. Research has shown (1) that there is a direct relation between these objective working conditions and physiological and psychological stress and ill-health and (2) that these working conditions can also cause fatigue and/or passivity in the individual, thus making it harder for people to play an active part in processes of change in the workplace that might result in better working conditions and thus prevent ill-health. These latter findings are especially important in relation to preventive work with a view to bringing about changes in production methods and the organization of work. Such changes require active involvement and a will for change in the people at the workplace, as well as support from management and/or in statutes and in collective agreements.

RESEARCH AND REFORM WORK

Working conditions associated with highly rationalized and technically advanced production methods were the subject of study, debate, and reform work in Scandinavia throughout the 1960s and 1970s. Besides physical and chemical hazards, attention was given to working conditions created by mechanization and administration rationalization and the possible effects of these conditions on job satisfaction, health, and general quality of life in industrial society.

In the debate and in efforts toward reform the problems have been grouped under two headings: the working environment and industrial democracy. In Sweden, as a result of the high priority accorded to both these questions by unions and later by politicians, the industrial relations system has been placed on a new statutory basis that aims to give the employee the right and the means to influence the organization of work in a very broad sense. The most important laws in this connection are the Codetermination Act, in force since January 1, 1977, and the Working Environment Act, in force since July 1, 1978.

This legislation gives employees quite new possibilities of calling for attention to be given not only to physical and chemical hazards but also to psychosocial risk factors at the workplace. The *travaux preparatoires* to the Working Environment Act discuss in considerable detail the psychosocial risk factors associated with the advanced division and mechanization of labor, such as monotony, mental strain, fatigue, social isolation, and low job satisfaction. The act builds upon research carried on in recent decades in the fields of psychology, sociology, epidemiology, and psychosomatic medicine. This chapter attempts to summarize the knowledge that has influenced developments in the Scandinavian countries. It also discusses various strategies of research in this field in relation to work reform and concludes with remarks on preventive programs in the work environment.

PSYCHOSOCIAL RESEARCH AND VALUES

In order to understand the importance of stress research and other research on psychosocial aspects of the organization of work, it is necesary to analyze the concept of stress and evaluate the findings of research in relation to various sets of values. At least four such sets of values can be meaningfully defined and distinguished (even though the boundaries between them are understandably diffuse):

1. humanistic/idealistic value related to conceptions of "the good society"
2. health and safety at work
3. democratic values related to the individual's level of activity and to his ability to control his own environment
4. economic values related to the profitability and viability of the firm and our current economic system.

The importance of psychosocial research for society and for the organization of work depends to a great extent on what political priorities are attached to these different sets of values. Quite evidently, economic values represent "hard currency" in Western societies and hence there is a temptation for the scientist to refer primarily to these values. The more anxious a scientist is to have his research put to practical use, the more important it is that his research should tend to promote efficiency. The traditional models of efficiency—based on the advanced division of labor and on central planning and control—have long been considered to yield good economic returns. The fact that psychosocial environmental research has shown that the rationalization ideals adhered to hitherto are associated with heavy psychological and social costs has been taken as indicating that the practical application of the findings of this research would result in increased costs to the firm.

There exists, too, an unfortunate tendency in much psychosocial environmental research to avoid coming in conflict with the technical efficiency on which our present-day production system is based. This sometimes results in research being formulated and its practical application being organized exclusively with a view to changes on the individual level. It is, of course, reasonable that both individuals and groups who so wish should receive expert help in coping with the increasingly apparent mental demands that modern working life makes. However, this type of activity, in my opinion, has very little to do with occupational health in the modern sense. To explain and deal with stress problems exclusively with reference to the individual is the same as transforming a social problem in the working environment into a private problem of the individual. Psychosocial research must therefore place itself clearly and explicitly within a framework in which social values such as health, well-being, and the use of people's own creative resources are vital aims in themselves. It is therefore important for psychosocial research to be formulated in such terms that it can give us knowledge of a general nature about the way working conditions affect people in general. Such research can be used to raise the awareness of firms, of unions, and of politicians as to what can be gained by good work organization and to create a conviction that such an organization, in a broader and longer perspective, is fully compatible with the economic interests of the firm and of society.

JOB CONTENT AND JOB SATISFACTION

Behavioral sciences since World War II have devoted much effort to developing firmly based and objective knowledge of the effects of highly rationalized production systems on people's general well-being and their job satisfaction. Special attention has been given to monotony, stress, and social isolation as consequences of the division and mechanization of labor. Other problems that have been considered are the relation between incentive pay, risk-taking, and accidents, and the consequences of shift work and irregular working hours for people's health, home life, and use of leisure time.

Similar research traditions exist in numerous industrial countries, in both the East and the West. Research has concentrated primarily on the relation between objective sociotechnical factors and people's perception and evaluation of their job content and working environment.

In many of these investigations the objective sociotechnical working conditions are reduced to two main dimensions: (1) the individual's ability to influence and control the organization of his work, work methods, work pace, and social contacts at work; (2) the qualification level required in order for work to be satisfactorily performed (qualification level refers to both theoretical and technical skills, initiative, the ability to initiate contacts, deal with unexpected situations, and so on). The assumption underlying many of these investigations is that working conditions that seriously constrain the individual's self-determination and his opportunities for using his creativity come in conflict with fundamental human needs related to the individual's self-esteem, need of varied stimulation, and need to control his environment. Tasks characterized by serious constraints in these respects are assumed to be harmful from both biological and social points of view.

We may sum up the findings of these investigations by saying that perceptions of monotony, coercion, mental strain, and social isolation are considerably more common and more intense among workers engaged in tasks that have been impoverished with respect to self-determination, variation, qualifications, and social contract. People feel powerless, often regard their job as meaningless, and see no value in their work other than the money it earns (Gardell, 1971). Similar findings are reported in studies carried out in various industrial societies, more or less independent of the differences in these societies' social and economic structures.

It is only when facts about low job satisfaction are combined with facts about personnel turnover, recruiting difficulties, and absenteeism that management finds this research worthy of attention. Consequently, most programs of reform in the field of working life that are initiated or supported by employers concentrate primarily on increasing motivation and productivity and thus gloss over the more profound psychological and social problems of modern working life. Hence it appears purposeless from a practical point of view to continue carrying out studies devoted merely to describing how specific sociotechnical conditions affect people's perception and evaluation of their jobs in terms of job satisfaction, and such. It might perhaps be more effective to formulate lines of research oriented toward other sets of values and address the question "What are the consequences of the demonstrated monotony, stress, and social isolation that follow from advanced division of labor and from systems control over working methods and work pace?"

We can distinguish two such lines of research today that are related to sets of values enjoying higher political priority, as illustrated in Figure 6.1. This research is still interested in the objective sociotechnical conditions and their significance for people's perceptions and feelings. The central questions that are put are concerned with the consequences of these perceptions and feelings. One line of research concentrates on the consequences for people's *health and well-being*, in both the short and the long term. In the long term, special interest is devoted to certain types of psychosomatic illness such as cardiovascular disease. The other line of research takes *activity level* as its central concept and sets out from questions connected with the workplace as an important field for social

Figure 6.1. Outline model of behavioral investigations of job satisfaction and its consequences for health and activity level

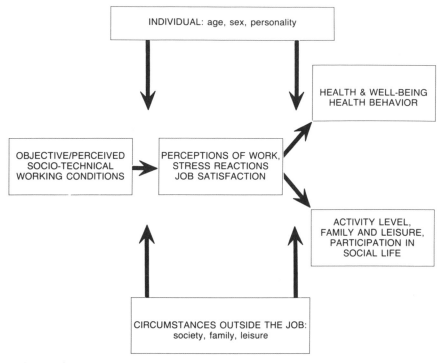

Source: Compiled by the author.

learning. The question is whether the experience of monotony, stress, and powerlessness results in a decline in the individual's activity level and thus affects his attitude not only to his job but also to his family, leisure, and participation in social life. The next sections review some of the main findings of these two lines of research.

HEALTH CONSEQUENCES OF PSYCHOSOCIAL WORK LOAD

The research that attempts to determine whether certain forms of job content and control are of any significance for people's health has devoted much attention to the question of how to identify long-term health hazards, both physical and mental, at an early stage. Symptoms that have been considered in various studies include neuroses, fatigue, and certain psychosomatic illnesses such as cardiovascular disease and stomach complaints. The relation between psychosocial factors and health is usually studied on a rather primitive theoretical level, where the most effort has gone into trying to determine whether significant statistical relations can be considered to exist at all. It was therefore an advance when Scandinavian scientists began using the results of psychobiological stress research to study various types of workplaces (Levi, 1972; Frankenhaeuser and Gardell, 1976). This psychobiological stress research has its theoretical foundation in the so-called activation theory, a theory of motivation based on the assumption of a systematic relation between physiological activation on the one hand and mental efficiency and well-being on the other hand (Frankenhaeuser and Johansson, 1974). Activation is defined as a state of alertness of the organism ranging from deep sleep to extreme excitation. The degree of activation can be assessed by a number of physiological functions, for example, hormonal and cardiovascular parameters. According to the theory, mental efficiency is greatest at a moderate level of physiological activation and declines progressively as activation increases or decreases. The level of activation varies with, *inter alia*, the amount and nature of stimulation in the environment. Both under experimental conditions in the laboratory and in field research on natural social situations it has been shown that the relation between stimulation and mental functions has the form of an inverted U: performance and well-being are both at a maximum under moderate stimulation and both decline in the presence of environmental understimulation and overstimulation. The control that the organism has over its environment also plays an important role for both physiological activation and emotional reactions.

Another important feature of Scandinavian research in this field has been the attempt to formulate research problems in such a way that the research performed will provide *general knowledge* about the influence of work organization on health and well-being. Generalizable knowledge about the effects of work organization on people is necessary for the research to be used for system-level changes in working life. This means that research must be formulated so that it does not merely give us explanations on the individual level by primarily emphasizing individual differences. It is self-evident that individual differences exist and must be taken into account—for example, differences in sex, age, and personality. The fundamental idea, however, is that psychological and medical data shall be usable for the purpose of identifying those aspects of job content and design that are critical for health. What we want to get at is the acute stress hazards and, ultimately, the long-term risks of physical and mental ill-health associated with the models that guide the forms of work organization today.

The findings in this area are not as extensive or as clear as those relating to job satisfaction. It can be claimed, however, that this research has shown the following features of job content and design to be critical from a health perspective:

- *Quantitative overload*: Too much to do, lack of time, repetitive work flow in combination with monotonous motor demands and the requirement of high superficial alertness. Factors of this kind are typical of mass production technology that is now in the process of taking over clerical work. It also seems as if a higher pace of work, with the aim of using time more efficiently, is one of the consequences of increased automation.

- *Qualitative underload*: Jobs that are excessively monotonous and restricted in content, lack variety of stimulation, and demand no creativity, problem-solving, or social interaction. Again, this type of task seems to become more common with increased automation, although contrary tendencies have also been shown. The manner in which new technologies are used plays a decisive role here.

- *Low degree of worker control*, particularly over work planning, pace, and methods. It is also important to observe the significance of the serious constraints on freedom of movement that characterize certain types of monotonous, machine-controlled jobs.

- *Poor social support* from fellow-workers and supervisors in case of difficulties in work. This lack of support appears to be especially critical from the point of view of stress in connection with conflicts and in jobs imposing a heavy load of responsibility for other people's safety. One should note here the tendency for person-person communication to be replaced with person-machine communication as a result of the increased use of computers at the workplace.

In practice one often finds a mixture of the above-mentioned critical factors in any given situation. Jobs characterized by qualitative understimulation are often also hectic and systems-controlled. Moreover, people in such situations have very little real opportunity to influence planning, internal work allocation, or methods, as these things are predetermined at a higher technical level and built into the system. Hence it is difficult—and sometimes meaningless—to try to deal with these factors in isolation. Instead we must adopt a scientific approach that accepts the fact that in any work environment there must be a mixture of stress factors—physical, chemical, and psychosocial—and that the study of working environments must take the whole picture into account.

The central problem for research is that of demonstrating in a sufficiently convincing manner that psychosocial conditions also have long-term consequences for health. The difficulties are numerous: it usually takes a long time for disease to manifest itself; people who feel that their work is adversely affecting their health try to find a new job, and those who stay are often the ones who enjoy their work or have escaped without serious health effects; working conditions are never static but are subject to continual change; people's conditions of life away from work influence their health and ill-health. Because of such considerations as these, it is difficult to link a certain type of ill-health conclusively with specific factors in the working environment.

One of the best investigations of psychosocial working conditions and health was performed a few years ago by a group of researchers at the Department of Psychology at the University of Stockholm (Johansson, Aronsson, and Lindström, 1978; Gardell, 1976). The investigation was an intensive study carried out within the framework of a broader survey of environmental conditions in the sawmill industry. In this survey certain relations had been demonstrated between job design and content, low job satisfaction, and self-reported medical symptoms. In order to clarify the mechanisms behind these findings and to make more precise the descriptions of the environmental conditions and of people's reactions to them, a study was performed in which psychophysiological stress research methods were used. Data extracted from questionnaire studies of job satisfaction were complemented by investigations in which job perceptions and feelings, expressed in psychosocial scale values, could be referred to the same working conditions and period of observation that were studied from the psychophysiological point of view. In addition, data on the nature of the work were collected from technical personnel and data on workers' health from a separate medical investigation. Some of the results in this study are presented in Figures 6.2 and 6.3.

The figures indicate the short-term physiological and emotional reaction to jobs ranging from monotonous to varied and to jobs in which the pace of work is determined by the production process and by the workers themselves. The figures show that both the physiological and the emotional stress reactions indicate greater stress the more monotonous the job is and the work pace is dictated by the production process. These findings are in line with the general pattern of results reported from research on job satisfaction. They directly contradict suppositions commonly entertained by production engineers and others that monotonous, mechanically controlled work involves less strain. On the contrary, individuals must mobilize more physiological resources in order to cope with the demands that such tasks make on them.

The findings of this investigation indicate that the prevailing efficiency models create jobs that cause a high degree of physiological activation combined with feelings of distaste. This combination of physiological activation and distaste, if very prolonged, may be assumed to have a general "wearing-down" effect on people and hence cause a higher risk of ill-health later in life. In one longitudinal field study with a risk group/control group design, we demonstrated that skilled, healthy workers can be broken down by the production system within a period of five to seven years. The results of the health study are presented in Table 6.1.

Factors in the physical environment, such as noise, sawdust, and other factors, obviously also play a major role, but the differences between the risk group and the control group in these respects are small compared with the differences in job content and job design. A factor that we believe to be

Figure 6.2. **Relation between variation in work tasks and psychological and physiological stress**

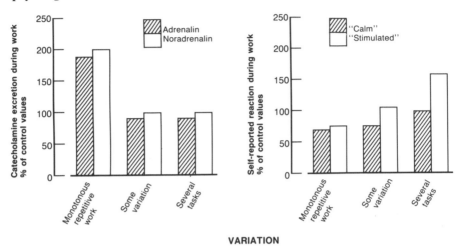

VARIATION

Source: Johansson et al., 1978.

Figure 6.3. **Relation between type of control over work pace and psychological and physiological stress**

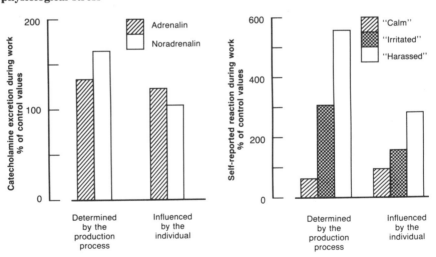

CONTROL OF WORK PACE

Source: Johansson et al., 1978

Table 6.1. Percentage of medical symptoms in workers with constrained and free job designs

Symptoms	Risk Group 38.4 Years	Control Group I 37.6 Years	Control Group II 38.3 Years
		Mean Age	
Hypertension	14	10	10
Headache	36	0	20
Nervous symtoms	36	0	0
Gastric ulcer, gastric catarrh	50	50	30
Back pain	43	10	10
Believe their health has suffered by their present working conditions	57	20	25
Thirty or more lost working days in past year	29	0	0
One or more absences because of stress or fatigue connected with present job	43	0	0

Source: Compiled by the authors.

especially critical for the health consequences is that people in the risk group have to make economically consequential decisions within extremely short times and that they have no influence at all over how, when, and where these decisions are to be made: They cannot influence the methods or the pace of work and they are physically tied to their work position throughout the working day. In other words, they have almost no opportunity to control and handle the demands of their job according to their own needs and resources.

Thus, extremely monotonous, systems-controlled tasks with little or no opportunity for the individual to control the pressure from the production process—by varying the work pace, "stretching ones legs," or taking on another task for a while—appear to be an unusually critical combination of job characteristics from the point of view of health. This hypothesis has been formulated for the analysis of large bodies of statistical material in a secondary analysis of the 1968 Low-Income Earners Report (Karasek, 1979, 1981). In this way the findings of individual case studies can be generalized. The model may be illustrated in a simplified form as shown in Figure 6.4.

Combining work load and self-determination we obtain four main categories of tasks. The most critical from the point of view of health is the combination of high work load and low self-determination, while the most favorable is a low work load with high self-determination. The model thus

Figure 6.4.   Ill-health as a function of work load and self-determination

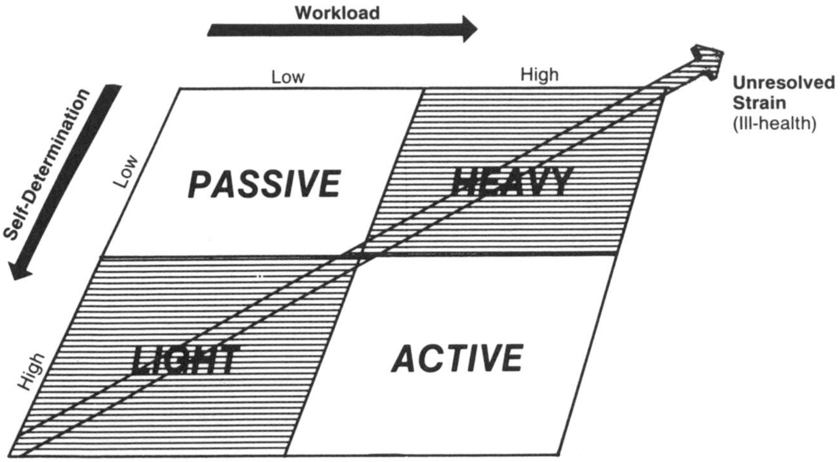

Source: Compiled by the author.

predicts that as we move along this diagonal, signs of ill-health become more numerous the closer we approach the corner representing high work load and low self-determination. The model also predicts that for any given work load, symptoms of ill-health will vary inversely with the individual's degree of self-determination.

Figure 6.5 illustrates an empirical test of this model on the Swedish Low-Income Earners Report and on a comparable American study. Both these studies are based on national random samples representing the entire workforce.

The figure shows that for the variables *nervous symptoms* and *fatigue* a pattern of symptoms appears that confirms the correctness of the model. Signs of psychosomatic ill-health are found most frequently in workers in jobs that can be described by the combination of high work load plus low self-determination. This group includes assembly-line workers, keypunch operators, and orderlies at large hosptials. We can also compare these groups with people having a high work load but different degrees of self-determination. People with a high work load and also high self-determination are often highly qualified persons employed as experts in various fields or in management. These people display far fewer nervous symptoms and symptoms of fatigue than those with high work load and low self-determination.

A follow-up study on the Swedish sample reviewed mortality from cardiovascular disease over the six-year period from 1968 to 1974 (Karasek et al., 1981). In other studies, people in jobs with varying degrees of work load and self-determination were tested with respect to a clinical risk scale for cardiovascular disease. These studies reported higher values among people with a high work load and low self-determination, that is, unskilled laborers and clerical workers with jobs of a routine, fragmented, monotonous nature, both with respect to risk as measured on the cardiovascular risk scale and with respect to·actual mortality. In highly qualified workers—in management positions—the frequency is considerably lower, though still high compared with groups with a low work load. Stress in managers is not a myth, but the problems appear to be still more

Figure 6.5.   Percentage of workers with nervous symptoms and fatigue for different combinations of work load and self-determination at work

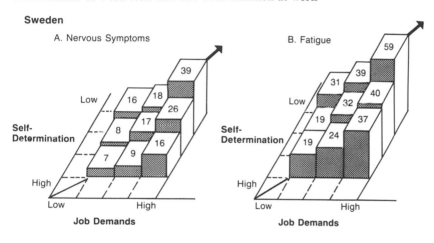

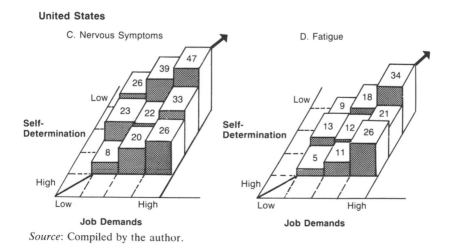

Source: Compiled by the author.

Figure 6.6.   Relation between time pressure and physiological stress in city bus drivers

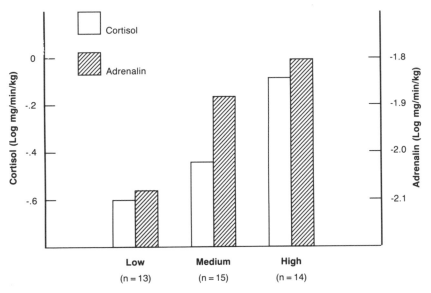

Source: Compiled by the author.

severe for groups with little or no opportunity to influence their own work situations.

Essentially the same model has been applied in a study of bus drivers in cities with one-man buses (Aronsson, Barklöf, and Gardell, 1980). The bus drivers show more signs of psychological and physiological stress the greater the time pressure under which they work. The time pressure is related to traffic factors over which the drivers have no control, for example, traffic density. An illustration of these results is given in Figure 6.6, which shows a very clear relation between perceived time pressure and cortisol and adrenalin excretion.

As a complement to these studies, an epidemiological study was carried out in Denmark in which bus drivers were compared with other age-matched occupational groups in the Copenhagen area with respect to cardiovascular disease and mortality. It was found that bus drivers in all age groups over 40 years have higher mortality than other occupational groups. They have significantly more cardiac infarctions than other groups, especially in the age range 50–59 years. Fatal cardiac infarctions are also more frequent in bus drivers than in other people, especially in the age range 40–55 years. The study also compared bus drivers in Copenhagen with bus drivers in two smaller towns. In the smaller towns there was no overmorbidity or overmortality in bus drivers. Thus the risk factors seem to be connected with the bus drivers' conditions of work in cities, which points to stress on the job as the cause of the increased risk of cardiac infarction (Laursen et al., 1980). This interpretation is supported by recent studies in both San Francisco and Moscow showing greater prevalence of hypertension in bus drivers.

It has been claimed, however, that the excess morbidity and mortality among bus drivers are not necessarily a result of mental stress, but might equally well be related to the lack of physical exercise in their job. The classical study in this field is an English investigation comparing bus drivers and conductors on London double-deckers (Morris et al., 1953). The study showed that mortality was higher among drivers than among conductors. This was interpreted by the authors in physiological terms as being related to the fact that the drivers sit still while the conductors move up and down between the two decks of the bus. The study was replicated in Rome, where single-decker buses are manned by a driver and a conductor (Berlinguer, 1962). This study also showed that the drivers have higher morbidity and mortality. However, since the conductors of these buses sit still, the physiological argument from the earlier English study does not apply. Instead the authors point to the stresses and mental strain involved in driving a bus in city traffic as the most probable explanation of the drivers' higher morbidity and mortality.

Thus an important conclusion that can be drawn from these studies is that job-related stress can cause morbidity and premature death. At the same time, this research shows that stress-conditioned ill-health cannot be related only to the strain to which people are subjected but to the many different kinds of resources they have at their disposal to cope with this strain. Management and the unions can do a great deal to build up cooperation and solidarity as a support for people engaged in hazardous and difficult tasks. Knowledge, information, and overview, as well as autonomy, are important resources that people need in order to meet the demands of modern working life.

As indicated above, another important strategy for handling stress on the job can be derived from the concept of "social support." A number of studies have shown that social support can function as a buffer between stress or strain at work and the health consequences of this strain (House, 1981). People who enjoy the strong support of workmates, management, or their family can cope with changes and other difficulties in their jobs better than those with weak support. Even in distressing situations of change, such as a shutdown, it has been shown that illness because of the strain connected with joblessness was considerably less common in persons with stable emotional support from family and friends (Cobb, 1976).

In Scandinavia the concept of social support has not been used in occupational research until quite recently. The concept of worker control has been considered more important and also easier to relate to

Figure 6.7.   Psychological working conditions and job dissatisfaction. Percentages with different combinations of self-determination, conflicts, and social support in problems at work

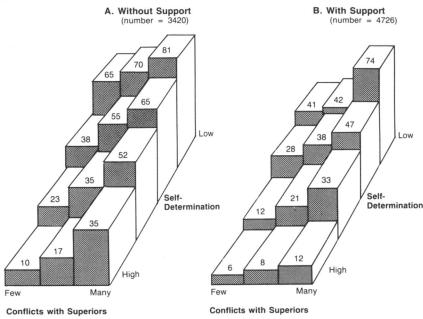

Source: Compiled by the author.

interventions in the working environment through statutes and collective agreements. Today, when such tools for intervention are in existence, interest in the concept of social support has grown. Both worker control and emotional support from others may suggest important lines of action in preventive psychosocial work. One might also imagine the two concepts interacting and reinforcing each other as resources for coping with strain; for example, in conflicts, in particularly responsible jobs, and so on. An illustration of this possibility can be found in a study of the working environment of clerical employees (Gardell, 1979). Figure 6.7 shows dissatisfaction in clerical employees as a function of strain (here, conflicts with superiors), self-determination at work, and support from colleagues. The figure shows, in the first place, that people with conflicts and with low self-determination are much more dissatisfied than those who have conflicts but are relatively autonomous in their job. In other words, it seems to be easier to live with conflicts with superiors if one has an independent job in which superiors cannot interfere.

In the second place, the figure shows that people who receive strong support from fellow workers also cope better with conflicts with superiors. This is true whatever the degree of self-determination in their job. Even with high self-determination, a sense of the support and solidarity of one's fellow workers in case of problems at work is not unimportant for job satisfaction.

Both worker control and social support are important ingredients in a democratic workplace organization where collective influence on strategic management decisions can be seen in connection with various forms of self-determination. If autonomous production groups—rather than the individual—are seen as the smallest unit of the organization, then the norms and values governing the group's behavior take on great importance. If the members of the group are to be able to support and help one another, all members must in theory be able to perform all the tasks involved in the group's work. Cooperation and mutual support must be extremely important elements of the group's system of values and norms and can be regarded as a precondition for the group's development toward increased autonomy and for its efficient functioning.

JOB CONTENT, ACTIVITY LEVEL, AND DEMOCRATIC PARTICIPATION

The other line of research that will be summarized here is related to the concept of activity level (see Figure 6.1). The question is whether impoverished job content and lack of participation in the processes of planning and control at the workplace can result in a general decline in people's activity level not only at work but also in their leisure time. Activity level is usually regarded as a dimension of behavior that is important for people's participation in society at large, in home life, and in various social and cultural activities. Activity level can also be seen as one of the resources that people need in order to give effective influence to various conditions in their workplace, in particular conditions related to working environment, health, and safety.

Within this line of research we can distinguish two different types of theory. The first refers to the concepts of overstimulation and understimulation. The assumption is that taxing jobs demanding a high degree of physiological mobilization require long periods for recovery: many leisure hours are spent merely "winding down." There is some support for this assumption in existing research. On the basis of national random samples, it has been shown that a higher percentage of people in monotonous, mentally taxing jobs need to rest longer hours after work before they can use their leisure for other activities, compared with people in less taxing jobs. In a study of the effects of prolonged periods of overtime work it has been shown that people are forced to mobilize physiological reserves in order to cope with the extra strain that overtime causes (Rissler and Elgerot, 1978). This physiological mobilization persists in the body and spills over into leisure time, not only for the duration of the overtime work but for several weeks afterward. These aftereffects of the physiological mobilization required to cope with job demands indicate the need for a lengthy period of recovery in mentally taxing work. Similar observations were made in the sawmill workers mentioned in an earlier section. In interviews several of them mentioned that they needed several hours' rest after work merely to be with their families in a normal way.

It is easy to see that shift work and other forms of abnormal working hours have effects on the use of leisure time. Disturbances of the circadian rhythm of certain body functions such as temperature, heart rate, and hormones regulating important mental functions have been found particularly frequently among rotating shift workers in a variety of occupations. It is also among rotating shift workers that insomnia and gastrointestinal symptoms are the most common. These facts are, of course, not merely of physiological and medical significance; ill-health also has deleterious effects on the use of leisure time and on people's opportunities to participate in various social and cultural functions (Magnusson and Nilsson, 1979).

The other assumption on which this line of research tries to shed light is concerned with the job as an important place for social learning. The question addressed is whether an impoverished, socially isolated job can lead to learned passivity or helplessness. If work is organized in such a way that people learn that others think and plan for them, that cooperation and social interaction are not necessary or even permitted, if suggestions and initiatives of various kinds are routinely ignored or rejected, people learn to be passive and to leave responsibility to others. Initiative and activity level decline. Since man is an indivisible whole, this learned passivity spills over into life outside work and people become "politically poor," that is, they display low participation in clubs and societies and in study activities, and they are less well-equipped to handle the various problems with which a complicated society confronts them.

One type of study addressing this question shows that when people's opportunities for self-determination and participation in various types of decision at the workplace are restricted by space, time, or the production process, their ability to develop active relations in their leisure time will also decline. These people, whose autonomy and social interaction at work are subject to real and strong constraints, take considerably less part in goal-directed activities outside work that require planning and cooperation with other people (Meissner, 1971; Gardell, 1976; Westlander, 1976).

In the 1968 Low-Income Earners Report, it was shown that workers in mentally taxing jobs participate far less than people in mentally nontaxing jobs in various organized activities in their leisure time. This is particularly true of cultural, political, and union activities requiring active participation and active communication with other people. Their leisure activities center on the nuclear family, sports events, outdoor activities, and television. They watch more television than other people, and the programs they watch are more likely to be of the light entertainment type. This study was repeated six years later, in 1974. In the latter study the same general tendencies in the relation between work and leisure were found as in 1968. A special analysis was carried out to follow up those people whose job content had changed in the course of the period with respect to autonomy and work-role complexity. Those whose job content had been enriched and who had gained greater self-determination at work by 1976 reported greater activity outside work, as in clubs and societies, union activity, and politics. Those whose jobs had been narrowed and impoverished—for example, by rationalization or automation, and whose degree of self-determination had thus declined, showed lower participation in nonwork activities in 1974 than in 1968 (Karasek, 1979).

A question of particular interest in connection with working environment is whether activity level related to their own job also affects people's interest in various types of health hazards at work. Karlsson et al. (1975) found that industrial safety work was most successful at workplaces where workers' activity level was generally high. The activity level was highest at workplaces with rich job content, where people were accustomed to self-determination and cooperation in order to get the work efficiently done. Similar experiences have been reported from case studies in which it was attempted to introduce greater autonomy and to increase demands on competence and interaction with others (Gardell and Svensson, 1981).

Perhaps the most convincing studies concerned with the relation between job design and workers' activity level outside work were those carried out at workplaces that participated in experiments with industrial democracy in the 1960s and 1970s. The Norwegian experiments have been followed up with respect to people's democratic participation in various types of organized activity outside work. In these studies it is known whether people have left their jobs in the meantime or if the data refer to the same people at different times. The Norwegian follow-up study indicates that the activity level outside work rose as a consequence of the democratization of the workplace. At the same time, a new "culture" has developed at the workplaces, with the result that new employees entering the environment learn to become more active and independent (Elden, 1981).

In Sweden we have detailed documentation of a very profound process of change that took place at a medium-sized engineering company (Gardell and Svensson, 1981). Here the workers themselves took the initiative for a democratization of the work organization, based on the active participation of the great majority of workers. This led to the democratization of the local union and a marked activation of workers in union work. From an attendance of only around 10 percent at union meetings, within a few years between 75 and 80 percent of the workers were regularly attending union meetings. After a few years an agreement was concluded with management to introduce a system of autonomous groups, within which the workers would undertake the organization and internal allocation of work and take collective responsibility for production within each group's field of operation. The traditional foreman was transferred and instead the groups elected a spokesman to be responsible for its transactions with the environment. Many of these spokesmen were union activists who subsequently represented the workers in the various codetermination arrangements that grew up in the 1970s. The relationship between codetermination on different levels of the company was thus simple and clear. A work organization was set up in which the workers are continually learning new things in their daily work, gaining a better overview of production and a better understanding of the relation between their own work and more general issues such as markets, economies, technical development, and so on. All this has led to a very marked activation of the workers. This heightened activity level, originating from a change in the organization of work, has spilled over into leisure time, leading to a heightened general interest in social questions.

Similar experiences have been reported from the Örebro Local Authority, where geriatric care and some of the recreation activities have been reorganized on similar principles (Svensson, 1984). There too the personnel involved work with a high degree of autonomy and take responsibility for the planning of the work and for maintaining the prescribed level of service. In these cases we have to deal with the same people who have changed in the course of time because they have been placed in new, more activating circumstances in their jobs. The changes have also led to a considerable gain in self-confidence, job satisfaction, and perception of the job as something meaningful. The psychological climate at the workplace is substantially improved and cooperation and solidarity have been strengthened. People generally feel better about the democratized work organization, a fact that is also noticeable in fewer working days being lost because of illness. Perhaps this may give us a hint of new models for work organization that combine efficiency with job satisfaction and mental health.

CONCLUSIONS FOR PREVENTIVE PSYCHOSOCIAL WORK

From the foregoing we may draw the conclusion that an unsuitable psychosocial working environment has two different types of effect on health. In the first place, there is a direct relation between certain objective working conditions and physical and mental stress and ill-health induced by these factors. In the second place, these taxing, distasteful jobs can cause fatigue or passivity, making people less inclined to involve themselves in processes of change at the workplace that might improve their working conditions.

What lessons for psychosocial work can be drawn from the investigations reported here? Preventive psychosocial work on the working environment must be concerned with several different planes—that is, with the individual level and the organizational level. Preventive work on the individual level is closely in line with traditional medical thinking. People can be counseled to live more healthily, stop smoking, take more exercise, eat better, and learn various types of relaxation exercises. Conversational therapy—individual or group—can also be regarded as an essential element in preventive psychosocial environmental work.

As we have already mentioned, however, it is not enough to work at the individual level only, since this would be transforming social problems in the working environment into the private problems of individuals. The pressure to change, to cope with problems, and so on, is directed only at the individual and not at the work organization that may be the basic cause of the problems revealed by individual-oriented health work. It is also necessary and perhaps in the long term even more important to try to counteract the continued impoverishment of job content and the coercion of the individual. Thus stress and stress-induced ill-health must be prevented by a different kind of work organization in which self-determination, social interaction, and professional responsibility are central concepts.

In Sweden, the development of work organization in this direction is encouraged by the Working Environment Act and the Codetermination Act. The Working Environment Act says that work shall be organized taking into account the individual's physical and mental resources and that work shall be arranged so that the individual can influence his own work situation. Obviously, individuals in isolation cannot gain adequate influence over their work. Collective action is necessary in order to achieve a good work organization. This is where the Codetermination Act comes in. The unions, too, have recently begun developing clear conceptions of what a good work organization should be like. These ideas are in essential agreement with the research findings I have described in this chapter. The demands for a kind of work organization that places self-determination, more complex work roles, and social support in the focus of attention can be expected to increase with the spread of new technologies. If we are to succeed in avoiding further job impoverishment, coercion, and social isolation of the individual, we must probably introduce working groups as the smallest unit of work individual. Individuals cannot by themselves fight the risks inherent in new technologies and cannot by themselves influence the conceptions held by those who decide on the application of these technologies. A group, on the other hand, can relate in a quite different way to new technologies, making them into a tool for competent, influential workers. The problem appears to be to convince management that this type of development is not only a good way to achieve better morale and better health in their personnel, but that a development along the lines suggested is also good for efficiency. What we need most today is not more research on the *principles* for this development, but *full-scale trials* in various parts of business and industry. Personally I consider that the research that has been presented makes it probable that these trials will also show that the working life of the future needs efficiency models that do not conflict with but promote people's involvement and health.

REFERENCES

Aronsson, G., Barklöf, K., and Gardell, B. 1980. Att arbeta inom lokaltrafiken. *Arbetsförhållanden—hälsa—fritid.* Forskargruppen för arbetslivets social-psykologi, Psykologiska Institutionen, Stockholms Universitet. Rapport No. 26.

Berlinguer, G. 1962. *Maladies and Industrial Health of Public-Transportation Workers.* Citta di Castello: Italian Institute of Social Medicine.

Cobb, S. 1976. Social support as a moderator of life stress. *Psychosomatic Medicine*, 38: 300–314.

Elden, M. 1981. Political efficacy at work: The connection between more autonomous forms of workplace organization and a more participatory politics. *The American Political Science Review*, 75(1): 43–58.

Frankenhaeuser, M. and Gardell, B. 1976. Underload and overload in working life: Outline of a multidisciplinary approach. *Journal of Human Stress*, 2: 35–46.

Frankenhaeuser, M. and Johansson, G. 1974. *On the Psycho-physiological Consequences of Understimulation and Overstimulation.* Reports from the Psychological Laboratories, The University of Stockholm. Supplement 25.

Gardell, B. 1971. *Produktionsteknik och arbetsglädje. En socialpsykologisk studie av industriellt arbete.* Personaladministrativa rådet. Stockholm.

————. 1976. *Arbetsinnehåll och livskvalitet.* Stockholm: Prisma.

————. 1979. *Tjänstemännens arbetsmiljöer: Psyko-social arbetsmiljö och hälsa.* Forskargruppen för arbetslivets socialpsykologi, Psykologiska Institutionen, Stockholms Universitet. Report No. 24.

Gardell, B. and Svensson, L. 1981. *Medbestämmande och självstyre. En lokal facklig strategi for demokratisering av arbetsplatsen.* Stockholm: Prisma.

House, J. S. 1981. *Work Stress and Social Support.* Reading, Mass.: Addison-Wesley.

Johansson, G., Aronsson, G., and Lindström, B. O. 1978. Social psychological and neuro-endocrine stress-reactions in highly mechanized work. *Ergonomics*, 21: 583–599.

Karasek, R. 1979. Job demands, job decision latitude, and mental health: Implications for job redesign. *Administrative Science Quarterly*, 24: 285–398.

————. 1981. Job socialization and job strain: The implications of two related psychosocial mechanisms for job design. In Gardell, B. and Johansson, G. (Eds.). *Working Life: A Social Science Contribution to Work Reform*,

75–94. London: John Wiley. (Also published in Swedish: *Arbetskrav och mansklig utveckling.* Stockholm: Prisma, 1983.)

Karasek, R., Baker, D., Marxer, F., Ahlbom, A., and Theorell, T. 1981. Job decision latitude, job demands, and cardiovascular disease: A Prospective study of Swedish men. *American Journal of Public Health*, 71(7): 694–705.

Karlsen, J. I., Naess, R., Ryste, O. Seierstad, S., and Sorensen, B. A. 1975. *Arbeidsmiljø og Vernearbeid.* Oslo: Tanum Forlag.

Laursen, P., Netterstrøm, B., Pedersen, T. K., and Whitta-Jørgensen, A. 1980. *Busschaufførers Arbejdsmiljø 1.* Institute for Social Medicine, Københavns Universitet, No. 11.

Levi, L. 1972. Stress and distress in response to psychosocial stimuli. *Acta Medica Scandinavica*, 191: supplement 528.

Magnusson, M. and Nilsson, C. 1979. *Att arbeta på obekväm arbetstid.* Stockholm: Prisma.

Meissner, M. 1971. The long arm of the job. *Industrial Relations*, 10: 238–260.

Morris, J. N., Heady, J. A., Raffle, P.A. B.,Roberts, C. G., and Parks, J. W. 1953. Coronary heart disease and physical activity of work. *Lancet*, 2: 1111–1113.

Rissler, A. and Elgerot, A. 1978. *Stressreaktioner vid overtidsarbete.* Report No. 23, Psykologiska institutionen, Stockholms Universitet.

Westlander, G. 1976. *Arbetets villkor och fritidens innehåll.* Stockholm: Personaladministrativa rådet.

7   Person–environment fit, Type A behavior, and work strain: the complexity of the process

R. Van Harrison, Gordon E. Moss,
T. E. Dielman, William J. Horvath,
and William R. Harlan

Attempts to understand stress at work often focus on demands of the job, such as work overload, competition, and alienating technologies. At other times the focus has been on characteristics of the worker, such as aptitudes, Type A behavior, and rigidity in dealing with problems. Over the years a great deal of information has been produced concerning many factors that appear to be relevant to job stress. However, most of the information is disconnected, sometimes contradictory, and often difficult to apply.

This chapter underscores the complexity of the processes associated with job stress and strain. It uses the framework of person-environment (P-E) fit theory to highlight the importance of taking into account characteristics of the job and characteristics of the worker not only separately, but also in relation to each other. The complexity of integrating information concerning job stress is illustrated by data relating two areas of research—P-E fit and Type A behavior—in predicting job strain. While these data are interesting in themselves, their additional purpose in this chapter is to demonstrate the complexity of the processes associated with job stress and strain.

The first part of the chapter provides a conceptual overview and background concerning person-environment theory and Type A behavior. The second part presents data concerning relationships between job demands, worker preferences, Type A behavior, and mental well-being in a representative community sample. The final part reviews the complexity of relationships and their implications for research and for interventions to reduce job stress.

BACKGROUND: JOB STRESS, PERSON-ENVIRONMENT FIT, AND TYPE A BEHAVIOR

A Broad Conceptual Model

A consistent problem in discussions concerning job stress is the lack of uniform definitions concerning the terms being used. The model in Figure

7.1 is similar to many models of stress and can be used to clarify terminology (Kahn et al., 1982). Box A represents social factors and circumstances reflecting the broad characteristics of the organizational and social environment according to which individuals can be grouped. Box B represents the job environment of the individual. Box C represents the psychological or subjective job environment of the individual. The individual then relates the perceived job demands to his or her own abilities and goals to determine their fit (see box D). If the environmental demands are perceived to threaten or frustrate important goals, then a number of short-term responses may occur (see box E). As the responses continue over a period of time, their repetitive and cumulative effects can lead to significant, long-term alteration in the individual's health (box F). Box G in Figure 7.1 represents a variety of personal characteristics and psychosocial resources that moderate relationships between variables in the other categories. For example, the individual's past experience, personality traits, or genetically determined biological predispositions may modify relationships.

The model has been presented without using the term "stress." Various researchers have used the term to refer to most of the boxes in the figure (Kasl, 1978). Indeed, even though only one or two of the boxes may be considered in a specific discussion, the overall process concerns job stress.

The primary focus of this chapter is on boxes C, D, E, and G—that is, the psychological job environment, the fit between the job and the person, responses to misfit, and other personal characteristics affecting this relationship. The perspective is drawn from social psychology, emphasizing the interface between the social environment and the person. With this perspective it is convenient to refer to demands of the job as stressors, perceived demands as perceived stressors, misfit between the person and the job as stress, and the psychological, physiological, and behavioral responses and subsequent health problems as strains.

Person-Environment Fit Theory

For several years researchers at the Institute for Social Research and elsewhere have been systematically developing a theory of the fit between the person and the environment and its relationships to job stress. Various aspects of the theory have been elaborated elsewhere (for example, French, Rogers, and Cobb, 1974; Caplan et al., 1980; French, Caplan, and Harrison, 1982; Caplan, 1983; Harrison, 1985). For the purposes of this chapter, the discussion will focus on the relationship between the individual's perception of the job, the individual's perception of himself or herself, and the relationship of these perceptions to strain. Of central concern is the individual's perception of the fit between the demands of the job and the individual's ability to meet them and the fit between the

Figure 7.1. A model of categories of variables reflecting job stress, health, and related variables. Examples of relevant variables are included in each category. Arrows representing feedback effects have been omitted.

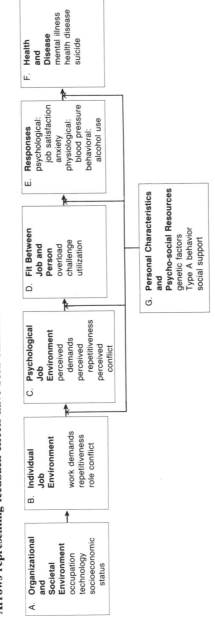

A. **Organizational and Societal Environment**
occupation
technology
socioeconomic status

B. **Individual Job Environment**
work demands
repetitiveness
role conflict

C. **Psychological Job Environment**
perceived demands
perceived repetitiveness
perceived conflict

D. **Fit Between Job and Person**
overload
challenge
utilization

E. **Responses**
psychological:
job satisfaction
anxiety
physiological:
blood pressure
behavioral:
alcohol use

F. **Health and Disease**
mental illness
health disease
suicide

G. **Personal Characteristics and Psycho-social Resources**
genetic factors
Type A behavior
social support

Source: Compiled by the author.

motives and goals of the individual and the rewards the job offers to meet
them.

P-E fit theory does not identify specific job demands or motives to be
studied. Investigators select demands or motives that appear to be most
relevant to the situation being studied. In the terms used by Campbell et al.
(1970), it is a "mechanical or process" theory. The basic process is that
strain should increase as P-E fit dimensions reflect increased insufficiency
of supplies for motives. To predict the type of strain that will occur, the
investigator usually considers additional factors such as the specific motives
that are not being met and the genetic and social background of the
individual. French et al. (1974) used the potential relationship between
P-E fit and strains to specify three differently shaped relationships that may
occur between a measure of P-E fit and a strain. These relationships are
presented in Figure 7.2. The vertical axis represents any strain that may
result from the sustained motive arousal. The horizontal axis is a scale of
P-E fit. The numbers on the scale are discrepancies between person scores
and environment scores on a dimension. The zero represents perfect fit

**Figure 7.2.   Three hypothetical shapes of the relationships between P-E fit on
demand-ability dimensions and strains**

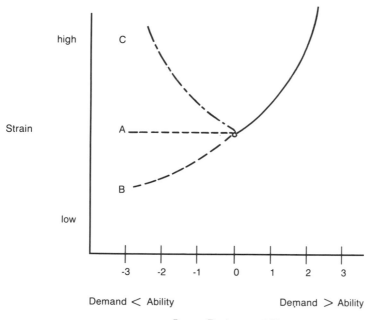

Source: Compiled by the author.

where the person score and the environment score are equal. The negative scores indicate the person scores increasingly larger than the environment score. The positive scores indicate the environment scores increasingly larger than the person score.

The solid line in Figure 7.2 illustrates the increase in strain that occurs as environmental demands become increasingly greater than an individual's abilities. This relationship applies to all demands that affect the rewards offered by the job (such as money, prestige, self-esteem). Job demands that are usually important include the amount of work to be performed and the performance of work at a particular level of complexity. Relevant demands may vary from job to job.

The relationship between P-E fit and strain is more complicated when the person's abilities exceed the demands of the job. House (1972) pointed out that excess abilities may have no further effect on strain so long as the lack of use of the abilities does not affect the individual. This relationship is described by line A in Figure 7.2. For example, when a person has completed the assigned work for the day, the person may simply leave. The ability to do more work will not reduce strain further.

The level of strain will continue to decrease when the excess abilities can be used to accomplish other valued goals. This relationship is represented by line B in Figure 7.2. For example, excess work time may be used to work for supplementary pay or to work on special projects of interest and value to the individual. The achievement of the additional goals because of excess work time could reduce strain below the level observed when abilities match demands on work load.

The final relationship between P-E fit and strain has the U-shape illustrated by curve C in Figure 7.2. French et al. (1974) suggest that excess abilities for a demand may be associated with insufficient opportunities to achieve valued goals. For example, individuals with training beyond that being used on a job may feel a loss of self-esteem or an individual without sufficient work may fear that the job will be eliminated.

The advance offered by P-E fit theory is that job demands may affect strain not simply through the level of demand, but also in relationship to the level preferred by the individual. Further, the crucial point in the interaction between the person and the environment is the point of perfect fit. At this point the relationship between P-E fit and strain may be altered.

Type A Behavior

In contrast to person-environment fit theory, Type A behavior is associated with a specific "content," a specific aspect of an individual's behavior that is related to strain. In the late 1950s, Rosenman and Friedman noted that their heart disease patients, particularly those under 60 years of age, exhibited a constellation of behaviors and emotional characteristics that was subsequently called a Type A behavior pattern. The absence of these characteristics was called the Type B behavior pattern. Friedman and Rosenman (1959) characterized Type A individuals as tending to be hostile, ambitious, competitive, and often preoccupied with deadlines and with work. Type A behavior was subsequently found to be associated with the doubling of the risk of coronary heart disease independent of the presence of other risk factors (Rosenman et al., 1976). The empirical evidence of this relationship and the general interest in psychosocial factors affecting health have resulted in a number of studies of this behavior pattern.

While the process relating Type A behavior to coronary heart disease is unclear, some aspects of the process have been suggested. Chesney and Rosenman (1980) reviewed much of the work concerning Type A behavior and work stress. Type As tend to describe their job as having more responsibility, longer hours, and heavier workloads than do Type Bs. However, Type As in general do not report more job dissatisfaction or other strains than do Type Bs.

The underlying mechanism appears not to be a general main effect of Type A behavior on strain, but an interaction between work stress and Type A behavior in affecting strain. Some evidence suggests that Type As have stronger physiological reactions to environmental stressors than do Type Bs (for example, Dembroski et al., 1979). Type A behavior may be viewed as a predisposing factor. When Type As are threatened, they may respond with a higher physiological arousal than Type Bs do. Over time this higher arousal may enhance processes associated with coronary atherosclerosis. Chesney and Rosenman (1980) review several studies showing that situational increases in work demands produce stronger relationships to strain (usually psychological responses) for Type As than for Type Bs. In discussing this interaction, they use the person-environment fit framework to characterize this interaction between environmental demands and individual preferences resulting in higher responses from Type As.

Across the studies of Type A behavior two methodological limitations are of note. One is the nonequivalence of commonly used measures of Type A behavior. The original measure is the Structured Interview, which involves an interview and subsequent rating of Type A behavior based primarily on the verbal and behavioral response style of the subject, with the content of the answers having less weight. The Structured Interview is the measure used in most predictive studies relating Type A behavior to disease (Matthews, 1982). Paper-and-pencil measures of Type A behavior such as the Jenkins Activity survey and the Framingham Type A questionnaire typically correlate only .25 to .40 with assessments based on the structured interview (Review Panel on Coronary-Prone Behavior and Coronary Heart Disease, 1981; Haynes, Feinleib, and Kannel, 1980;

Zyzanski, 1978; Dembroski et al., 1978; MacDougal, Dembroski, and Musante, 1979). The majority of the work on job stress and Type A behavior has used these less-expensive measures. The second problem concerns the focus of most studies of work stress on male white-collar workers. Much less information is available concerning the relationship between Type A behavior and work stress among blue-collar workers and women (Chesney and Rosenman, 1980).

Research formally linking P-E fit theory and Type A behavior is a natural consequence of the evidence suggesting interactions between work stress and Type A behavior produce strain. Of particular value would be data using the Structured Interview measure of Type A behavior along with measures of job stress collected across a representative sample of working people.

Hypotheses Concerning P-E Fit, Type A Behavior, and Strain

Several hypotheses have been presented or can be derived from the preceding discussion of P-E fit theory and Type A behavior:

- *P-E Fit theory and Type A behavior.* Type As should prefer higher levels of job demands than Type Bs. They should also have higher levels of demands placed on them in their work than Type Bs. It is possible that the preferences of Type As for higher levels of demands may lead them to seek situations where their fit is worse than that of Type Bs.

- *P-E fit and strain.* High demands should be related to strain. Preferences for high work demands may also be related to strain. Poor fit between demands and preferences should be related to strain. The relationship between poor fit and strain should be in addition to the independent relationships of demands and preferences with strains.

- *Type A behavior and strain.* Type As will not differ from Type Bs in overall levels of strain. Instead, Type A behavior will have an interactive relationship in predicting strain. Relationships between high demands and strain, between preferences for high demands and strain, and between poor fit and strain should be higher for Type As than for Type Bs.

These hypotheses were tested in a recent study conducted by the authors.

A STUDY OF PERSON-ENVIRONMENT FIT AND TYPE A BEHAVIOR

Methods

Sample The study consisted of a random sample of residents of Washtenaw County, Michigan. They were selected using a multistage probability sampling frame of households. This procedure yielded 902 respondents who completed the study. Of these respondents, 652 were working 20 or more hours per week. This subsample of working respondents was used for the analyses of Type A behavior and P-E fit on work demands. The sample included a wide distribution on sex, socioeconomic status, and other characteristics. The sample is further described by Moss et al. (1985).

Data Collection Instruments and Procedures. Respondents were initially interviewed in their homes by a member of the study staff using a survey interview protocol covering a number of aspects of the respondents' lives: demographic characteristics, work demands and preferences, health behaviors, mental and physical health problems, life events, social support, and marital relationships. Appointments were subsequently made for a second interviewer to come to the respondent's home to perform the Structured Interview of Type A behavior. These interviewers had been trained by a nationally recognized expert from SRI International. Data from both interviews were coded and entered onto computer files for analysis.

Measures. The assessment of Type A behavior was based on the Structured Interview performed by these interviewers. Respondents were rated on a six-point scale of Type A behavior (A1, A2, XA, XB, B3, and B4) that could also be collapsed to the more traditionally used four-point scale (A1, A2, X, and B). Checks on the interrater reliability of Type A assessments found the reliability to be high with an interclass correlation coefficient of .80.

The survey interview included six measures of P-E fit on work demands. However, the distribution of responses across levels of demands and across levels of preferences produced a good distribution across discrepancies between environmental demands and individual preferences on only three of the dimensions: work load, job complexity, and job competition. The measures of environmental demands and personal preferences on each of these three dimensions may be found in the original study. The responses to the items were averaged to produce the various indexes.

To produce measures of P-E fit the preference score was subtracted from the environmental score for each item. To simplify the analyses looking for the U-shaped relationship between P-E fit and strain, the P-E fit measure was transformed by taking the absolute value of the difference between the environmental demand and preference ($/E-P/$). This transformation ignores the sign of the discrepancy and presents a scale reflecting only the magnitude of discrepancy. It represents any underlying U-shaped relationship as an approximately linear relationship with a positive correlation reflecting higher levels of strain with increasing magnitudes of either "too much" or "too little" of the job characteristic. This transformation represents an interaction between the E and P measures and is of interest because it can account for variance in strain that is independent of the linear association between strain and the E and P component measures.

For this reason and to simplify the presentation of results, only this U-shaped relationship is presented in the results represented by the transformed "poor fit" measure (/E-P/).

Measures of strains included several reports of psychological and reported behavioral responses. As is usual in most survey studies, relationships between the measures of reported demands and the strains were very low or nonexistent. To simplify the presentation, results are presented only for the four measures with the strongest relationships to demands: job dissatisfaction, anxiety, irritation, and depression. The items were averaged to produce the index.

Results

Correlations within Categories of Measures. The sample size of 652 is sufficient to determine that correlations as low as .11 are statistically significant at the .01 level. The relationships among the E, P, and poor fit measures were examined first. Both the correlations between the E, P, and poor fit measures on each dimension and the correlations between dimensions on their E, P, and poor fit measures were examined. The three forms of measures (E, P, and poor fit) across three dimensions (work load, job complexity, and job competition) often have correlations ranging from .20 to .40. These modest relationships indicate that the various predictors are not highly confounded.

The correlations between the measures of strain were also examined. The reports of feelings of anxiety, irritation, and depression are fairly highly intercorrelated, ranging from .42 to .55. However, the correlations of these three measures with job dissatisfaction are never greater than .20, indicating that this evaluative response to the job is somewhat independent of the three affective responses.

Correlation between Type A Behavior and E, P, and Poor Fit. How is Type A related to environmental demands, individual preferences, and poor fit? The correlations between these measures are presented in Table 7.1. The first column shows low positive relationships with Type As reporting somewhat higher levels of work load, job complexity, and particularly job competition than Type Bs. The second column shows a similar pattern with Type As reporting a preference for somewhat higher levels of work load, job complexity, and job competition. However, the last column shows there is no difference between Type As and Type Bs in the magnitude of misfit on the three dimensions. Among Type As the higher reported levels of demands are evidently matched by the higher levels of preferences to the same extent that demands and preferences are matched among Type Bs.

The findings concerning demands and preferences fit the expected patterns. However, the results concerning poor fit measures suggest that even though Type As perceive themselves to be under more demands, they

Table 7.1.   Correlations between Type A behavior and E, P, and poor fit measures

Dimensions	Environmental Demand (E)	Preference (P)	Poor Fit (/E-P)
Work load	.10*	.11**	−.02
Job complexity	.16**	.22**	−.03
Job competition	.22**	.18**	.00

Source: Compiled by the authors.

Note: A positive correlation indicates Type As have higher scores on the measure than Type Bs have.

**p < .01

*p < .05

also prefer higher demands and therefore they are not experiencing increased misfit because of higher demands.

Relationships between Strains and Measures of E, P, and Poor Fit. These relationships are presented in Table 7.2. When the relationships between environmental demands and strains are examined, there is a low negative relationship between demands and job dissatisfaction. Individuals with higher levels of demands on all three measures report somewhat lower levels of dissatisfaction than do individuals with lower levels of demands. While this finding is counter to initial expectations, it conforms to results in earlier studies using these measures (for example, Caplan et al., 1980). Jobs with higher work load, higher job complexity, and higher job competition tend to be better paying and to offer higher levels of intrinsic rewards. This confounding of higher levels of rewards with higher levels of demands may account for the observed relationships with job dissatisfaction and the similar marginal relationship with depression.

None of the measures of preferences on work demands are related to strains. The strongest relationships are found between the measures of poor fit and strain. All three measures of poor fit are related to job dissatisfaction, indicating that higher levels of misfit are associated with high levels of dissatisfaction. Additionally, increasing misfit on job complexity is associated with somewhat higher levels of irritation and depression. These relationships fit the pattern expected between poor fit and strain.

To what extent does the interaction between environmental demands and individual preferences represented by poor fit account for variance in strains beyond that accounted for by the E and P measures? Stepwise multiple regression analyses were performed that initially fixed the E and P measures as predictors in the equation. If the interaction between E and P represented by the poor fit measure accounted for additional variance, it was then allowed to enter the equation. Later analyses were conducted

Table 7.2.   Correlations between strains and E, P, and poor fit measures

Predictor	Strains			
	Job Dissatis-faction	Anxi-ety	Irri-tation	Depres-sion
Environmental Demands (E)				
Work load	−.20**	−.01	−.03	−.09*
Job complexity	−.16**	.08	.02	−.08
Job competition	−.11**	.00	.00	−.04
Preferences				
Work load	−.08	.06	.02	−.02
Job complexity	−.01	.01	.02	−.03
Job competition	−.05	.00	.04	−.02
Poor Fit (/E-P/)				
Work load	.24**	.01	.04	.02
Job complexity	.26**	.03	.13**	.14**
Job competition	.10*	.04	.06	−.03

Source: Compiled by the authors.

**p < .01

*p .14 .05

utilizing either the E and P measures or E, P, and poor fit measures which account for significant amounts of variance. The first set of analyses contained E and P measures while the second group contained E, P, and poor fit measures. By comparing R^2 for E and P with additional variances accounted for by R^2 with E, P, and the poor fit measure, it became clear that poor fit measures (reflecting the U-shaped interactions between the person and the environment measures) generally account for as much variance in strain as linear relationships with E and P measures do. However, this pattern is not uniform. The amount of variance accounted for by the poor fit measure differs across the relationships and it does not account for any additional variance in the relationship between work load and depression.

Relationships between Type A Behavior and Strains. As expected, Type A behavior has little direct relationship to strain. Higher scores on Type A behavior are only marginally related to lower levels of job dissatisfaction ($r = -.10$, $p < .05$). Type A behavior is not related to anxiety, irritation, or depression (r's between −.04 and .03).

Does Type A behavior interact with work stress in producing strain? To test this hypothesis the Type A measure was used to group people into three categories: the A1s, the A2s, and the Xs and Bs combined. Analysis of covariance was used to see if the correlation between a measure of stress and a measure of strain was the same across each of the three groups of individuals that were low (Xs and Bs), moderate (A2s), and high (A1s) on Type A behavior. The analysis was repeated to check on the interaction between Type A and each of the three measures of environmental demands, each of the three measures of personal preferences, and each of the three measures of poor fit in predicting each of the four strains.

The main effects of the E, P, poor fit, and Type A measures on strains are reflected in the previous tables presenting the correlations between them. The instances where significant interactions were found are presented in Table 7.3. The first line in the table shows that job dissatisfaction has a moderate relationship with poor fit on job complexity among Bs and Xs, a weaker association among A2s, and no relationship among A1s. This finding is somewhat surprising in that it suggests that for this response, Type As are less sensitive than Type Bs. Evidently misfit on job complexity is less relevant to Type As when they evaluate their jobs and satisfaction with them.

The second line indicates that poor fit on job complexity interacts with Type A behavior in predicting anxiety. This instance fits the expected relationship with no association found for Type Bs and Xs or for A2s, but a

Table 7.3.   Interactions between Type A behavior and E, P, and poor fit measures in predicting strains

Strain	Predictor (E, P, or Poor Fit Measure)	Type A categories			Interaction p<
		B & X (n = 280)	A2 (n = 280)	A1 (n = 84)	
Job dissatisfaction	Job Complexity-Poor Fit	.38**	.23**	−.02	.002
Anxiety	Job Complexity-Poor Fit	−.07	.08	.28**	.02
	Job Competition-P	.06	.02	−.29**	.03
Irritation	Job Complexity-P	.10	−.02	−.25*	.02
Depression	Job Competition-P	.05	.01	−.27*	.04
	Job Complexity-P	.08	−.07	−.26*	.03
	Work Load-P	.09	.06	−.22*	.04

Source: Compiled by the authors.

Note: Entries are the correlations between the predictor measure and the strain for individuals within the category of Type A behavior.

**p < .01

*p < .05

modest relationship between increasing misfit and increasing anxiety for A1s.

The remaining five interactions are between Type A behavior and preferences for job demands in predicting strains. They all have a similar pattern with a relationship between preference level and affective response existing only for the A1 group. For this group, lower levels of preferences are associated with higher levels of affective responses. In other words, within this group of presumably hostile, ambitious, and competitive individuals, those who prefer lower levels of demands (whether they have them or not) tend to be somewhat more anxious, irritable, and depressed. The processes underlying this relationship are not clear at present. These individuals are evidently experiencing a "stressful" inconsistency between lower preferences and other aspects of their values and beliefs that are associated with Type A behavior. Fear of failure or feelings of low competence may be involved. Whatever the nature of process producing the underlying inconsistency, it may also be exacerbated by a second process: the potential for increased reactivity among extreme Type As.

DISCUSSION AND CONCLUSIONS

This chapter has two interrelated goals: (1) the exploration of the relationship between person-environment fit theory and Type A behavior in accounting for job stress, and (2) using these findings to illustrate the complexity of the processes that must be addressed by researchers and practitioners interested in understanding and reducing job "stress and strain." The first part of this section summarizes the results concerning hypotheses about P-E fit and Type A behavior. The second and concluding section considers implications of these results for the broader conceptualization of mechanisms of job stress and strain for both research and intervention.

Support for Hypotheses

P-E Fit and Type A Behavior. The results support previous studies in showing that Type As reported higher levels of job demands than did Type Bs. Further, they reported preferring higher levels of demands than did Type Bs. However, Type As did not differ from Type Bs in reporting poor fit. Type As appear to have sought out or created environments that matched their preferences just as well as did Type Bs.

P-E Fit and Strain. Higher levels of demands were not related to strain. In fact, higher levels of demands were associated with lower levels of job dissatisfaction. This may reflect a confounding between higher levels of demands and higher levels of rewards. Levels of preferences concerning job demands were not associated with the measures of strain. The measures of poor fit (that is, misfit of either too much demand or too little opportunity) had the strongest relationships to strains, particularly to job dissatisfaction. Adding the interaction represented by poor fit to the E and P component measures generally doubled the amount of explained variation in strain over that explained by linear relationships with the E and P component measures. However, this pattern was not uniform across all of the dimensions of job demands and strains.

Type A Behavior and Strain. Type A behavior had no appreciable direct relationship to the four strains. However, interactions between Type A behavior and other measures were found. The greatest number of interactions were found between measures of preferences and Type A behavior. For extreme Type As only, those who prefer lowered job demands were somewhat more anxious, irritated, and depressed. The mechanism underlying this relationship is not clear. It may reflect an inconsistency between the Type A orientation and the preferences concerning demands or it may be that these individuals actually have lower abilities and would prefer lower levels of demands in spite of (and in conflict with) their Type A behavior.

Two interactions were found between poor fit on job complexity and Type A behavior. For Type As only, increasing levels of misfit was related to increasing levels of anxiety. In contrast, there was no relationship between misfit on job complexity and job dissatisfaction for extreme Type As; however, this association increased among A2s and was strongest among Bs and Xs. This pattern suggests that there may be a response specificity associated with Type A behavior. They may use different dimensions in evaluating satisfaction with the job, while still being emotionally sensitive to the misfit and its potential threat.

Perhaps the most noteworthy result among the interactions between Type A behavior and the other measures was the absence of interaction between Type A behavior and environmental demands. This is at variance with some of the earlier studies reporting interactions with variables such as level of workload (Chesney and Rosenman, 1980). The results of the present study suggest that interactions may be more likely with measures of poor fit and more likely yet with measures of preferences concerning levels of job demands.

Limitations of the Study. The results summarized above necessarily have the limitations inherent in the study. The study was correlational and reflects associations, not necessarily causation. The advantage of the sample representing a wide variety of individuals also poses some methodological difficulties. Individuals and jobs may differ to such an extent that the meaning of the items on the questionnaire concerning work load, job complexity, and job competition may vary substantially for individuals in different occupations. Except for Type A behavior, the measures are based on self-reports rather than objective observations. The study was limited in the number of dimensions on which P-E fit was examined. It was also limited in that strain was represented only by cognitive responses with no actual measures of physiological responses or long-term health outcomes. However, compared to previous studies, the present one uses the best validated measure of Type A behavior in a more representative sample of the general population to perform the most systematic exploration of the relationship between P-E fit and Type A behavior.

Implications for the Study of Work Stress

Implications for Conceptualizing Work Stress. The results concerning relationships between P-E fit, Type A behavior, and work strain underscore the complexity associated with the topic of job stress. The relationships are not simple. In addition to main effects of characteristics of the job and of individuals, there are interactions between work demands and individual preferences, interactions between poor fit on demands and Type A behavior, and interactions between preferences and Type A behavior. Strain responses are often specific rather than general. Further, responses may be specific to a subgroup of individuals. The process is made even more complex by the simultaneous operation of a number of confounded factors, particularly the rewards often associated with demanding work.

The long-range challenge in the conceptualization of job stress is the integration required to reflect the processes operating across the several levels represented by boxes in Figure 7.1. For example, theories of social support can be integrated with P-E fit and Type A behavior, including measures of P-E fit on how much of various types of support is wanted and how much is available. Social support theory anticipates interactions with social support "buffering" relationships between stressors and strains. The addition of just this one set of variables can greatly increase the number and types of interactions, the number of unique relationships to specific strains, and confounding of factors that must be taken into account. The problems are only compounded with the inclusion of additional areas of interest such as differences between males and females, differences between specific occupations, and physiological responses and longer range problems with mental health, physical health, and behavior.

Implications for Research Concerning Work Stress. The study results suggest several specific lines of inquiry. For example, they support the use of P-E fit measures because of their additional explanatory power and the utility of P-E fit theory in conceptualizing relevant processes. Research is also needed to resolve a number of theoretical and operational issues including the relationships of various dimensions on which P-E fit is conceptualized, the stability of the meaning of dimensions across groups, and a resolution of issues concerning the association between an individual's perceptions and reports about contamination of environmental demands and individual preferences.

More systematic studies of the interaction between Type A behavior and characteristics of the job and of the individual are needed. The relationship between Type A behavior and strain is evidently not simple. Current work on the components underlying Type A behavior and the values and goals associated with Type A behavior provides some direction in understanding the specificity of relationships with particular types of strain. Also, consequences for positive responses (such as, self esteem, income) must be contrasted with negative health outcomes.

Much of the research on job stress in the next few years will necessarily be directed toward clarification of concepts and methodological issues within existing areas of inquiry. However, some integration should also be encouraged. The existing theoretical areas focus on limited domains concerning specific processes or content. The theories generally do not compete, but tend to complement each other. The simultaneous integration and testing of several theoretical areas is likely to be difficult, involving complex models, multivariate analyses, and designs constrained by factors in field settings. However, attempts should be made to bridge two or three areas whenever possible. The development of a broadly integrated conceptualization of job stress is most likely to evolve from these small integrative steps.

Implications for Conceptualizing Changes to Reduce Work Stress. The above discussion concerned the description of the processes associated with job stress. Attempts to modify these processes in real settings involve many additional considerations. How amenable to change are the various factors? What techniques can bring about change? What are their relative costs and effectiveness? What are the consequences of change beyond the reduction of job stress? What is the overall cost and benefit to the individual and to the organization?

Attempts to reduce job stress have generally been associated with one or both of two more general areas of inquiry and practice—one focusing on the functioning and well-being of the individual and the other focusing on the functioning and well-being of the organization. Several change efforts are directed toward the individual to detect problems resulting from job or other life stresses and to provide professional services to help individuals deal with these problems. The problems include clinical depression, marital difficulties, alcohol and drug abuse, and psychosomatic illness. Interventions directed toward the individual may also be more indirect, teaching individuals to identify their own problems and teaching them coping skills such as "assertiveness" training and stress management. By learning these skills individuals are more able to prevent problems and to resolve more problems without professional assistance.

Type A behavior is an example of a condition likely to be modified by individual-oriented approaches. Individuals high on Type A behavior may be identified by external evaluation and subsequently encouraged to modify the behavior by reevaluating goals and developing new response patterns. Alternatively, they can be advised of their heightened reactivity and encouraged to recognize and avoid unusually stressful situations. While some efforts are now being made to test these cognitive and behavioral modifications, the extent to which they will alter underlying physiological responses and disease is unclear.

Recognizing the overall theme of this book concerning the role of health care delivery systems, it is interesting to note that health care delivery systems traditionally direct their efforts toward the individual. The primary effort of health care delivery systems has been to provide professional services to help the individual deal with current emotional, behavioral, or physical problems. More recently an emphasis on preventive teaching has been added. The central focus of the health care delivery system has been the general well-being of the individual with relatively little attention directed toward modification of job demands as an etiological factor. The major innovations have been to increase access to health care services by bringing them into the workplace and to increase the social legitimacy of their use. In providing these services the health care delivery system plays an important role in helping individuals modify abilities and values that may contribute to job stress and in helping them cope with the consequences of job stress. However, the impact of the health care delivery system on jobs and organizational functionings is indirect (through some effects on individuals) and relatively weak. Aspects of job stress emerging from job demands and organizational functioning are currently more directly and effectively changed by means other than the health care delivery system.

The functioning and well-being of organizations has been a central interest of management and organizational behavior specialists. Setting aside general humanitarian concerns, the well-being of the individual is still important to the organization because the failure of individuals to perform their roles may threaten the well-being of the organization. Therefore, personnel management and other organizational specialists have developed a number of tools and strategies to ensure that work will be performed. They include procedures to select workers with appropriate skills, team-building to enhance the functioning of work groups, training programs for supervisors to help them better organize and direct the work of others, and the integration of technology and human factors in the development of efficient production and management roles. Many of these activities prevent or reduce stress on individuals as well as improve organizational functioning.

One of the useful applications of person-environment fit theory is the clarification of the potential relationship between stress experienced by the individual and functional difficulties occurring in the organization. Harrison (1985) examines the relationship in some detail using P-E fit theory to conceptualize the interface between individual and organizational functioning. Just as misfit between environmental supplies and on an individual's motives is fundamental to producing stress in an individual, misfit between organizational demands and an individual's abilities is fundamental to producing "stress" in organizational functioning. If the only misfit is between environmental supplies and an individual's motives,the individual is likely to initiate change. If the only misfit is between organizational demands and individual abilities, the organization is likely to initiate change. Misfit affecting both the fit between supplies and motives and the fit between demands and abilities is likely to motivate both the individual and the organization to seek remedies. The remedies may be attempts by either the individual or organization to modify individual values (for example, through counseling), individual abilities (through training), organizational demands (through job redesign), or rewards (changes in bonus schedules). These changes may be accomplished through cooperative collaboration between the worker and the organization ("quality circles") or through confrontation (strikes, lockouts).

Recent legal and social trends are linking the well-being of the company even more closely to the well-being of its employees. These trends include holding organizations legally and financially accountable for problems related to job stress experienced by employees and the expansion of company-paid health care benefits. Organizations are finding it to be in their best interest to commit resources to planning to reduce stress on the job; to handle acute, stressful events such as job loss; and to encourage general health promotion activities.

More extended applications of P-E fit theory in the systematic conceptualization of interventions to reduce job stress have been presented elsewhere (for example, Caplan et al., 1980; Harrison, 1985; French, Caplan, and Harrison, 1982; Caplan, 1983; Harrison, 1985). They consider changes to both the actual person and environment and to the individual's perception of self and of the environment. They emphasize the need for improving fit on an on-going basis: the initial matching between the person and the job at hiring, the adjustments as job demands and the individual's abilities and preferences change over time, and the planning and preparation for changes to different jobs across a work career. They highlight the importance of individual participation and control in the work setting as a particularly efficient and effective method to respond to changes in individual and job characteristics so that good fit is maintained. They also discuss various constraints imposed by technology, control, and reward systems in organizations, the need for some uniformity in spite of individual differences, and other factors that limit the extent to which misfit can be reduced.

Implications for Research on Prevention and Reduction of Work Stress.
Several potential directions for research follow from the limited discussion
of conceptual issues concerning change. Rather than discuss a few of the
many possible specific areas for research, these comments will focus on
some limitations holding back most current efforts at research on reduction
of job stress.

The first part of this section illustrated the complexity of the processes
underlying job stress. The section on conceptualizing change indicated the
added complexity when factors affecting intervention efforts are taken into
account. Given the lack of information integrating the many factors, most
current intervention efforts are simply trying to demonstrate that change
can be produced and that the effort involved is reasonably cost-effective.
The early stage of inquiry results in virtually no change projects
systematically comparing the effects of changing specific factors, using
various change technologies, changes in specific types of work settings, and
changes across various populations. When quantitative evaluations are
performed with any sophistication, they generally evaluate an intervention
that includes every reasonable action that could be included to increase the
probability of a successful intervention.

This assessment of research on the reduction of work stress has no
negative connotation. Given the knowledge base at this time, current
efforts are quite promising. The body of knowledge constituting the job
stress literature has many pieces with few interconnections. In the near
future most research concerning work stress is likely to continue the
description of underlying processes. Research concerning interventions to
reduce stress is likely to continue to be infrequent and to constitute the
evaluation component of demonstration programs. As the underlying
processes associated with job stress are defined and integrated, attention
increasingly will shift to the systematic study of change technology applied
to modify these processes in various settings, for various populations, and
for specific interfaces between settings and persons.

Acknowledgments: The research for this chapter was supported by Grant
No. HL 28094 from the National Heart, Lung, and Blood Institute.

REFERENCES

Campbell, J. P., Dunnette, M. D., Lawler, E. E., III, and Weick, K. E., Jr. 1970.
    Managerial Behavior, Performance, and Effectiveness. New York: McGraw-
    Hill.
Caplan, R. D. 1983. Person-environment fit: Past, present, and future. In Cooper,
    C. L. (Ed.). *Stress Research: Where Do We Go from Here?*: 35–77. London:
    John Wiley.
Caplan, R. D., Cobb, S., French, J. R. P., Jr., Harrison, R. V., and Pinneau, S.
    R., Jr. 1980. *Job Demands and Worker Health: Main Effects and
    Occupational Differences*. Ann Arbor, Mich.: Institute for Social Research.

Chesney, M. A. and Rosenman, R. H. 1980. Type A behavior in the work setting. In Cooper, C. L. and Payne, R. (Eds.). *Current Concerns in Occupational Stress*. New York: John Wiley.

Dembroski, T. M., Caffrey, B., Jenkins, C. D., Rosenman, R. H., Spielberger, C. D., and Tasto, D. L. 1978. Section summary: Assessment of coronary-prone behavior. In Dembroski, T. M., Weiss, S., Shields, J., Haynes, S., and Feinleib, M. (Eds.). *Coronary-prone Behavior*. New York: Springer-Verlag.

Dembroski, T. M., MacDougall, J. M., Herd, J. A., and Shields, J. L. 1979. Effect of level of challenge on pressor and heart-rate responses in Type A and Type B subjects. *Journal of Applied Social Psychology*, 9(3): 209–228.

French, J. R. P., Caplan, R. B., and Harrison, R. V. 1982. *The Mechanisms of Job Stress and Strain*. London: John Wiley.

French, J. R. P., Rogers, W., and Cobb, S. 1974. A model of person-environment fit. In Coelho, G. V., Hamburgh, D. A., and Adams, J. E. (Eds.). *Coping and Adaptation*. New York: Basic Books.

Friedman, M. and Rosenman, R. H. 1959. Association of specific overt behavior pattern with blood and cardiovascular findings—blood cholesterol level, blood clotting time, incidence of arcus senilis, and clinical coronary artery disease. *Journal of the American Medical Association*, 169(12): 1286–1296.

Harrison, R. V. 1985. The person-environment fit model and the study of job stress. In Beehr, T. A. and Bhagat, R. S. (Eds.) *Human Stress and Cognition in Organizations*. New York: John Wiley.

Haynes, S. G., Feinleib, M., and Kannel, W.B. 1980. The relationship of psychosocial factors to coronary heart disease in the Framingham Study: III. Eight-year incidence of coronary heart disease. *American Journal of Epidemiology*, 111: 37–58.

House, J. S. 1972. The relationship of intrinsic and extrinsic work motivations to occupational stress and coronary heart disease risk. Doctoral dissertation, University of Michigan. *Dissertation Abstracts International*, 33, 2514A. (University Microfilms No. 72–29094.)

Kahn, R., Hein, K., House, J., Kasl, S., and McLean, A. 1982. Report on stress in organizational settings. In Elliot, G. R. and Eisdorfer, C. (Eds.). *Stress and Human Health: Analysis and Implications for Research*. New York: Springer.

Kasl, S. V. 1978. Epidemiological contributions to the study of work stress. In Cooper, C. L. and Payne, R. (Eds.). *Stress at Work*. New York: John Wiley.

MacDougall, J. M., Dembroski, T. M., and Musante, L. 1979. The structured interview and questionnaire methods of assessing coronary-prone behavior in male and female college students. *Journal of Behavioral Medicine*, 2: 71–83.

Matthews, K. A. 1982. Psychological perspectives on the Type A behavior pattern. *Psychological Bulletin*, 91: 293–323.

Moss, G. E., Dielman, T. E., Leech, S. L., Harlan, W. R., Harrison, R. V., and Horvath, W. J. 1985. Demographic correlates of SI assessments of Type A behavior. *Psychosomatic Medicine*. Review Panel on Coronary-Prone Behavior and Coronary Heart Disease. 1981. Coronary-prone behavior and coronary heart disease: A critical review. *Circulation*, 63: 1199–1215.

Rosenman, R. H., Brand, R. H., Sholtz, R. I., and Friedman, M. 1976. Multivariate prediction of coronary heart disease during 8.5 year follow-up in the Western Collaborative Group Study. *American Journal of Cardiology*, 37: 903–910.

Zyzanski, S. J. 1978. Coronary-prone behavior pattern and coronary heart disease: Epidemiological evidence. In Dembroski, T. M., Weiss, S., Shields, J., Haynes, S., and Feinleib, M. (Eds.). *Coronary-prone Behavior*. New York: Springer-Verlag.

8 The effect of high job demands and low control on the health of employed women

Suzanne G. Haynes, Andrea Z. LaCroix, and Tobi Lippin

In the last decade, few studies have focused on the health of women in the workplace. Haw (1982) published a comprehensive review of women, work, and stress literature. Of the several questions that the review posed for future research, the following was of greatest interest to employers concerned with the health of women in the workplace:

What aspects of the job environment are responsible for the excess rates [of cardiovascular heart disease (CHD)] among high risk occupations in women, e.g., clerical work? Specifically, what effect does underutilization of skills, lack of autonomy and control, lack of recognition for accomplishment, presence of challenges,and excessive hours have on incidence rate of CHD? (Haw, 1982: 144)

This chapter will focus on the effect of high job demands and low control on the health of women in the workplace. Analyses from the Framingham Heart Study and the North Carolina Office Workers Stress Survey among communication workers will be presented.These studies suggest the need for surveillance and health care of visual display terminal (VDT) workers for ergonomic and stress-related symptoms. Potential benefit may be gained by conducting cardiovascular disease studies in the workplace for jobs characterized by high demands and low control.

OCCUPATIONAL FACTORS AND CARDIOVASCULAR DISEASE

The Framingham Heart Study (Haynes and Feinleib, 1980) was the first prospective study to examine the effect of employment, occupation, family responsibilities, and behavior on CHD incidence rates in women. After eight years of follow-up, no significant differences were observed between working women and housewives (7.8 versus 5.4 percent, respectively). However, CHD rates were twice as great among women holding clerical jobs (10.6 percent) as compared to housewives or other occupation groups. White-collar women, employed primarily as teachers, nurses, or librarians, had the lowest incidence rates of any occupational group studied (5.2 percent).

Both the work environment, and the family environment contributed to excessive coronary rates among clerical workers. One out of five (or 21.3 percent) of these workers developed coronary disease if they had raised children and were married to blue-collar husbands. The most significant work environment risk factors in this group of women were not discussing one's anger and having a nonsupportive boss. These findings were confirmed in both the eight- and ten-year follow-up studies (Haynes and Feinleib, 1980; Haynes, Eaker, and Feinleib, 1984).

The Framingham findings suggested that clerical workers may experience severe occupational stress, including a lack of autonomy and control over the work environment, underutilization of skills, and lack of recognition of accomplishments. The underlying thread linking clerical work to CHD was the issue of control.

Conceptually, work environment control has been broadly defined in previous research as summarized by Alcolay and Posick (1983: 1078):

An individual's level of control is equivalent to the extent to which she/he may determine how, where, why and when to act; the level of access to information necessary to make informed decisions, availability of resources for implementing choices, and the power to bring about desired choices.

Low job control is thought to be particularly stressful in combination with high job demands as suggested by Karasek's Job Strain Model (Karasek et al., 1982). The interaction of high psychological work load with inadequate resources for exerting control results in "High Strain" job situations. In contrast, jobs characterized by challenging high demands that provide sufficient control resources are thought to create an "Active" job situation that might actually be stimulating and health-promoting.

In fact, several investigators have shown that lack of control at work is related to systolic and diastolic blood pressure, excretion of catecholamines, hypertension, and prevalence and incidence of cardiovascular disease and mortality in men (Karasek, et al., 1981; Frankenhaeuser, 1979; Karasek et al., 1982, Karasek and Gardell, 1984; Alfredsson, Karasek, and Theorell, 1982; Chesney et al., 1981; Van Dijkhuizen and Reiche, 1980). A summary of these studies taken from LaCroix (1984) is shown in Table 8.1. In particular, the innovative work of Karasek and colleagues as reflected in Chapter 6 in this volume by Gardell, has consistently revealed that high demand/low control job situations are related to cardiovascular health.

Karasek and Gardell (1984) have recently reported on a second large Swedish data base (The Swedish White Collar Workers Labor Confederation, n = 8,700 men and women) with information on job characteristics

Table 8.1. Review of occupational stress and cardiovascular risk studies

Investigator	Country Year	Study Design	Variable(s) Studied	CHD Related Findings
Karasek and Gardell	Sweden/1984	Cross-sectional	Retrospective changes in Job control and demands as a result of forced job changes	Higher prevalence of CHD signs/symptoms
Alfredsson	Sweden/1982	Case-control (Incident M1 cases)	Hectic work Low control over work tempo/skill variety	Increased risk of myocardial infarction
Chesney	USA/1981	Cross-sectional	Perceived encouragement of autonomy	Lower SBP and DBP among Type As
M. van Dijkhuizen	Netherlands/1981	Cross-sectional	Role Ambiguity Work Load	Higher BP and cholesterol obesity, BP, smoking
Frankenhaeuser	Sweden/1979	Cross-sectional	"High Risk" sawmill conditions	Higher excretion of catecholamines
House	USA/1982	Cross-sectional	Work load Intrinsic rewards Control rewards Importance rewards	Medical evidence of hypertension, high CHD risk
Karasek	USA/1982	Cross-sectional	Decision latitude psychological work load	Prevalence of myocardial infarction

Source: LaCroix (1984).

and a heart disease signs/symptoms indicator. Of this sample, 2,500 workers had, in the previous two years, undergone a forced job change, with some workers taking new jobs characterized by more or less job control than their former jobs. In three out of four age-sex groups (for example, < 40 and > 40 years), Swedish workers who underwent job changes into situations of greater control had fewer coronary symptoms than those who changed into jobs having less control and those undergoing no job changes. However, since no information was available on symptoms or health status before the onset of job changes, this study is purely observational and cannot be considered as having a prospective, intervention design.

The introduction of computerized technology into office environments has created concern among occupational health researchers. Investigators at the National Institute of Occupational Safety and Health have studied the health effects of video display terminal use and likened machine-controlled clerical work to industrial assembly-line work (Smith et al., 1981a, b). A labor-union–initiated survey was conducted among volunteers in five worksites comparing three groups of workers: (1) VDT operators who were professionals (reporters, editors, and printers); (2) VDT operators who were clerical and office workers (data entry and retrieval); and (3) non-VDT operators who were also clerical workers. The clerical VDT operators reported less job autonomy and peer cohesion and greater work pressure and supervisory control than either professionals using VDTs or non-VDT clerical workers. The findings indicated that psychological stress and health complaints were highest among clerical VDT users. However, both VDT and non-VDT clerical workers had higher levels of stress and health complaints than professionals, suggesting that job content, not merely exposure to VDTs, was contributing to the higher levels of job stress in clerical VDT users. This was attributed to rigid work procedures, high workload demands, closeness of supervision, and, in general, little operator control over job tasks among clerical personnel. The authors conclude that for clerical VDT users,

the VDT was part of a new technology that took more and more meaning out of their work. . . .
    The inflexibility of this work system and the directive/corrective management style that it engenders seems to produce a feeling of loss of control over work activity (Smith et al., 1981a: 7).

These findings are also consistent with the Haynes and Feinleib (1980) study of Framingham women indicating that clerical workers had twice the incidence of CHD compared to housewives and other working women. Among clerical workers, the most significant predictors of CHD were having a nonsupportive boss, not changing jobs frequently during a previous ten-year period, and suppression of anger.

To explore the high demand/low control factor in more depth, a reanalysis of the Framingham data has recently been completed (LaCroix, 1984; LaCroix and Haynes, 1984). Clerical working women were stratified into four demand-control groups according to their perception of these job conditions: low-high, high-high, low-low, and high-low. The ten-year incidence rates of CHD in these groups were 2.4, 5.6, 13.6, and 31.3 percent, respectively. Overall, clerical workers with high demands were 5.2 times (p < .05) more likely to develop CHD than the other three groups combined, after controlling for the standard coronary risk factors.

The effect of high job demands and low control on the risk of a variety of diseases, including coronary disease, merited further attention. In order to carry the research one step further, occupations that fell in the category of high job demands and low control had to be identified. As seen in Figure 8.1 from LaCroix (1984), by using Karasek's scheme, it was possible to identify a number of occupations among working women in the United States that fell into the high demands/low control group.

Of the high-risk occupations listed in Figure 8.1 (bottom right-hand quadrant), communication workers seemed an interesting group for further study. Not only are these jobs characterized by rapid speed and pacing and constant demands, but they are also characterized by low control. Workers in the telecommunications industry seemed ideal for identifying a large number of "exposed" working women (high demand/ low control) for epidemiologic study. Interest in the study of telephone company clerical workers for stress-related disease gave birth to the North Carolina Office Workers Stress Survey, summarized below.

THE NORTH CAROLINA OFFICE WORKERS STRESS SURVEY

Purpose

In 1982 the North Carolina Occupational Safety and Health Project (NCOSH), a nonprofit organization of labor unions and health professionals, received an increasing number of health and stress complaints from office workers employed by telephone companies throughout the state (North Carolina Occupational Safety and Health Project, 1985). The health complaints included headaches, eyestrain, and backaches, while the stress-related complaints included anxiety, fatigue, and tension. Concerned by these complaints, NCOSH and the Communications Workers of America (CWA) developed and piloted a statewide survey of office workers employed within the telecommunications industry. The pilot survey was designed to address the following objectives:

1. Identify the nature and extent of health-related problems among CWA office workers in North Carolina, particularly those using VDTs.

2. Examine the relationships between reported health problems and working conditions.

3. Compare the types of problems (job design factors and health complaints) encountered in VDT operations and in general office environments in the telecommunications industry.

4. Provide documentation to aid in designing interventions and solutions to problems identified (Office Workers Stress Survey Results, 1985).

Figure 8.1.   Occupational distribution of QES women by mean Karasek job scores

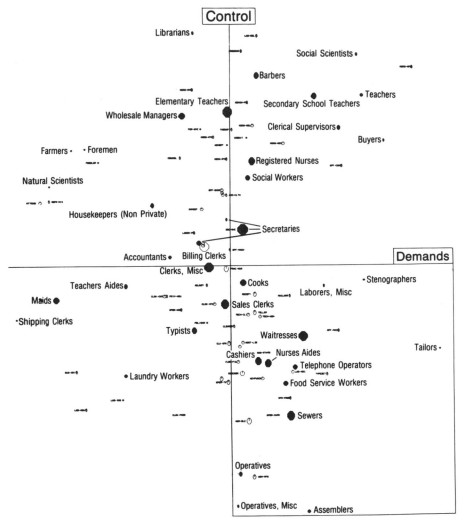

Source: LaCroix, 1984.

Because of the paucity of information on these workers, the study was exploratory in nature and was designed to generate hypotheses for testing in subsequent studies.

Population Studied and Methods

The study population included all active members of seven participating CWA local unions across North Carolina (NCOSH, 1985). Members of these unions were employed as office workers primarily by Southern Bell, American Telephone and Telegraph, Western Electric, and several independent phone companies. About 20 percent, or 2,478, of all CWA-represented employees in North Carolina were included in the pilot survey. Since only a proportion of local unions participated, the results do not represent all CWA workers in the state of North Carolina. The geographic areas represented do include major North Carolina cities, such as Raleigh, Fayetteville, Charlotte, Wilmington, Asheville, and Greensboro.

An extensive five-page questionnaire was mailed to the 2,478 CWA office workers included in the pilot study (NCOSH, 1985). It included about 250 items and assessed information on the office environment, job skills and responsibilities, acute and chronic symptoms and diseases, as well as coping skills and social support. The health effects examined included eyestrain, muscle strain (back, neck, arm, hand), headaches, fatigue, heart disease, ulcers, and tension. Questions for the survey were selected from multiple sources, including the Framingham Heart Study (Haynes et al., 1978), the 9-to-5 National Survey on Women and Stress, (NAWW, 1984), and the London School of Hygiene Cardiovascular Questionnaire (Rose and Blackburn, 1968). The questionnaire also included items related to job control and job demands, such that scales for these constructs were developed using factor analysis and inter-item reliability coefficients.

In order to assure the confidentiality of the responses, union locals mailed the questionnaire to their respective members between November 1983 and January 1984. The survey was carried out completely by the local unions. A more complete description of the method of study is published elsewhere (Paddock, 1984).

Of the 2,478 persons surveyed, completed responses (surveys or telephone follow-up interviews) were received from 966 office workers. Of these 966, approximately 75 percent completed the long form and 25 percent completed the short form of the questionnaire. Although the overall response rate of about 40 percent appears low, it is possible that some of the nonrespondents were ineligible for the study (that is, were not office workers) and did not fill out the questionnaire for that reason. Because of the necessity to use union membership lists for sample selection, this problem was unavoidable. Other reasons for nonresponse may include length of questionnaire, mode of administration (self versus interview), season of year, (November–December), or fear of reprisal from employers.

It is interesting to note that our response rate is comparable to response rates that NIOSH received in a study of health hazards from the use of video display terminals (VDTs) in three California Unions (Smith et al, 1981a, b). For all three unions combined, only 45 percent (412/923) of the VDT operators and non-operators responded to a health complaint and psychological status questionnaire. Responses were somewhat higher for VDT operators (50 percent) as compared to non-operators (37 percent) in that study. This suggests that new methods must be developed in future investigations of VDT operators to increase response rates. The pilot results presented in this paper, then, should be used for the purposes of generating questions to be addressed in future studies of office workers, particularly workers using VDTs.

Results

Of the 966 responses to the survey, 712 were office workers (640 women and 72 men). For analysis purposes, complete responses were available from 519 women, who serve as the focus of this report.

Based upon previous reports of health problems among VDT operators, we first divided the telecommunication office workers into two categories: those who reported they spent 50 percent or more of their working time on the VDT (VDT users) and those who spent less than 50 percent of their working time on the VDT (non-VDT users). We were initially interested in examining the effects of prolonged and intense use of VDTs by the telephone workers since many of them have jobs that are virtually completely machine-controlled. Subsequently, some analyses have also been performed using non-VDT, < 50 percent and ≥ 50 percent groupings in order to examine dose-response relationships. Table 8.2 summarizes selected demographic characteristics of the VDT users and nonusers in this study. As can be seen, the VDT users were, on average, about four years younger than the comparison group. This age difference most likely explains the slightly higher educational level, fewer years with the company (about two), and an average of one year less in current position. The VDT users were also more likely to be married than the non-VDT group. Because of the lower age of VDT users, all analyses were controlled for age using multiple regression techniques. Unadjusted prevalence estimates or age-specific comparisons will be presented in the text, when presenting rates among VDT and non-VDT users. Table 8.2 also shows the occupational distribution of the VDT and non-VDT groups. Most notable

Table 8.2.   Demographic characteristics of VDT and non-VDT telephone office workers among women aged 20–65 years

Selected Characteristics	VDT (n = 297)	Non-VDT (n = 238)
Mean age	34.8	38.4
Mean education	12.9	12.5
Mean years in company	11.8	13.8
Mean years in current position	6.0	7.2
Mean number of children	2.0	2.1
Mean number of children at home	1.6	1.5
Percent white	73.1	76.7
Percent married	68.0	61.9
Occupational title (in percents)		
Operators	12.4	36.0
Clerks and service reps	65.6	39.8
Records processing clerk	11.0	3.3
Secretaries, typists	.7	3.3
Sales representatives	.4	.8
Supervisors	3.9	.4
Material handling, and so on	6.0	16.3

Source: Compiled by the authors.

differences are the greater proportion of clerks and service representatives among VDT users and the greater proportion of operators among non-VDT users.

Table 8.3 presents prevalence rates of frequent health symptoms according to VDT use. VDT users were significantly more likely (about 1–5 times) to report eyestrain, headaches, fatigue, and tension often (2-3 times/week) or every day than non-VDT users. It is also notable that over one-half of all the VDT users surveyed reported eyestrain, headaches, and fatigue on a regular basis.

In the Chronic Medical Conditions section of Table 8.3, the only significant difference observed in chronic conditions between the VDT groups was in response to the Rose questionnaire items on angina (Rose and Blackburn, 1968). Twice as many VDT users reported angina symptoms as compared to non-VDT users (15.2 versus 7.7 percent, $p < .01$). The entire Rose questionnaire was administered to the workers, including a diagram to indicate the location of pain. Only pain experienced in the left-hand side (shoulder and midsection) and sternum (neck and midsection) areas of the chest were included in classifying women with

Table 8.3.   Prevalence of health conditions among women telephone office workers according to VDT exposure

Symptom/Condition	VDT Users		Non-VDT Users		p-value
	Percent	*Number*	*Percent*	*Number*	
	Frequent Health Symptoms				
Eyestrain	53.6	(278)	35.4	(226)	.0001
Headache	51.1	(276)	36.0	(228)	.0007
Insomnia	23.4	(273)	16.4	(219)	.06
Back/neck strain	41.3	(286)	34.1	(232)	.09
Arm/hand pain	16.4	(281)	17.8	(225)	.68
Fatigue	58.4	(281)	43.4	(226)	.0008
Tension	45.8	(286)	33.9	(224)	.007
	Chronic Medical Conditions				
High blood pressure	23.1	(286)	24.8	(226)	.65
Heart disease	2.6	(269)	2.3	(215)	.85
Angina pectoris	15.2	(283)	7.7	(221)	.01
Ulcer	10.2	(265)	14.5	(221)	.15

Source: Compiled by the authors.

angina. Since the angina symptoms were self-reported, further validation of these symptoms with a thorough medical evaluation (ECGs, angiography) would be required to confirm a diagnosis of angina pectoris.

Since the machine (the VDT) alone was thought unlikely to elicit these symptoms from women, working conditions associated with the use of the VDT were examined in an attempt to explain these findings. As discussed earlier, previous studies from the Framingham Heart Study had suggested that employment in occupations with high demands and low control was associated with the development of coronary heart disease. We were able to examine this dimension of work stress with questionnaire self-reports of job demands and control. Job demands included working fast, paying close attention to details, and meeting deadlines. Job control included making job decisions, monitoring of work, excessive pressure with no decision authority, monotonous work, and dealing with the public. Figure 8.2 shows the percentage of women employed in VDT and non-VDT work with high job demands or low job control, using median cutpoints for both scales to define high-low categories. As can be seen, VDT users were more likely to report high job demands and low job control in comparison to the non-VDT group.

Table 8.4 shows the prevalence of eyestrain, headaches, tension, fatigue, and Rose angina according to level of control on the job. In each case, the highest prevalence rates of symptoms were reported among VDT users with low control on the job, and the lowest rates were found among non-VDT users with high control. Similar, albeit weaker, findings were observed for the job demands scale and the combination of high demands with low control, with highest rates observed among VDT users with high job demands, or high demands and low control. In a multivariate analysis, lack of control proved to be the most significant correlate of symptoms when control, demands, and the combination were included in the analysis.

On the basis of these analyses, one might assume that lack of control on the job explained some of the associations of VDT use with symptomatology. In order to examine this possibility, multivariate analyses were performed for each outcome variable controlling for confounding variables. Logistic regression analysis was performed using the SAS Institute computer program LOGIST (SAS, 1983). Estimates of beta coefficients were calculated using unconditional maximum likelihood techniques as part of the LOGIST procedure (SAS, 1983). Odds ratios were calculated by taking e^B where B is the beta coefficient of a dichotomous exposure variable. The latter assumes that no interaction terms are present and that all other covariates are statistically controlled (Kleinbaum, Kupper, and

Figure 8.2.   High job demands and low job control

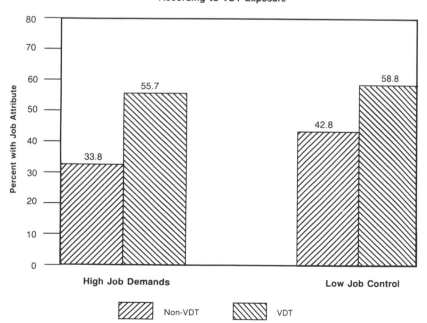

Table 8.4. Prevalence of frequent eyestrain, headaches, tension, fatigue, and Rose angina according to level of job control (in percent)

Symptoms	High Control		Low Control	
	Non-VDT (n = 127)	VDT (n = 121)	Non-VDT (n = 98)	VDT (n = 157)
Eyestrain	23.8	49.6	49.0	56.4
Headaches	24.4	39.8	51.0	59.2
Tension	19.7	29.5	52.8	57.7
Fatigue	30.1	45.4	59.2	67.7
Angina	4.0	14.9	13.2	15.5

Source: Compiled by the authors.

Morgenstern, 1982). The logistic models included age (20-year age groups), adequate chair (0 = yes, 1 = no), low job control (median split), and length of time spent at the VDT (long versus other).

Before presenting the multivariate analysis, reasons for the inclusion of adequate chair and length of time on VDT should be discussed. Having a chair with adequate back support was one of many environmental factors examined in relationship to symptoms. Others included temperature, supply of fresh air, unsafe working conditions, chairs with adjustable height, and chairs with adjustable back support. Of these, having a chair with adequate (not adjustable) back support, as judged by the worker, was significantly associated with eyestrain, headaches, tension, fatigue, back strain, arm/hand pain, and insomnia. The greatest odds of having symptoms were among working women with inadequate chairs. Use of a VDT coupled with inadequate chairs increased the risks of having eyestrain, headaches, insomnia, and fatigue, resulting in odds ratios of 5.29, 3.94, 4.27, and 4.40, respectively. Thus, VDT users with inadequate chairs were four to five times more likely to have these symptoms than non-VDT users with adequate chairs.

Length of time spent on the VDT was also significantly associated with several health outcomes among VDT users. The variable was recorded as follows: when you work on the VDT, what periods of time do you usually spend at the terminal?—short period (less than one hour), average periods (1–3 hours), or long periods (3 or more hours). The data from our study show that eyestrain, headaches, fatigue, tension, and Rose angina significantly increased as the length of time spent on the terminal increased. For all these symptoms, marked increases in prevalence are noted as one goes from short (< 1 hr) to average (1–3 hrs) periods, suggesting that more than one hour on the terminal a day is associated with increased symptoms.

Since most of the comparisons presented in this chapter are between VDT and non-VDT users, and the latter include both nonusers as well as < 50 percent users, it is important to note that the majority (62 percent) of users included in this category spent less than 25 percent of their time on the terminal.Table 8.5 also shows that the prevalence rates of symptoms associated with VDT use are generally less in the 25 percent and 25–49 percent groups as compared to 50 percent and above. From Table 8.5 it is difficult to argue that the association of VDT use with symptoms follows a steady linear dose-response curve. Rather, it appears that prevalence rates are about the same for < 25 percent and 25–49 percent time per day, with higher rates occuring thereafter as a greater proportion of time is spent on the VDT.

In general, the rates among women who spent no time on a VDT were sometimes higher than the rates among occasional users. For all symptoms, however, statistically significant differences ($p < .05$) were observed when comparing the 75–100 percent group with the "none" group for eyestrain and fatigue only. Likewise, among VDT users alone, statistically significant differences were observed among the four work time groups, for all health conditions in Table 8.5. For Rose angina, no significant difference was observed between the "none" and the 75–100 percent groups.

Comparison of the demographic characteristics of the "none" group showed that these women were slightly older (average age 39.5), had less education (12.3 years), and more years with the company (14.1) than VDT

Table 8.5.   Prevalence of selected health symptoms according to proportion of work time spent at the VDT (in percents)

Work Time Spent on VDT	(N)*	Health Symptom or Condition				
		Eye-strain	Head-ache	Fatigue	Tension	Angina Pectoris
None	(126)	39.2	42.3	43.7	40.7	12.0
< 25%	(64)	31.3	28.1	42.6	25.8	3.1
25–49%	(40)	32.5	30.8	42.1	23.7	2.6
50–74%	(32)	44.8	48.3	31.0	30.0	9.4
75–100%	(257)	54.2	51.0	61.7	47.9	15.8
P-Value (excluding none)		.002	.006	.0002	.002	.02

Source: Compiled by the author.

*Sample sizes may not sum to study population because of missing data on work-time variable.

users. Inclusion of the "none" group with the low VDT users is thus likely to make it more difficult to observe significant differences between regular VDT users and low VDT users. The results presented in this chapter are thus conservative estimates of the effect of VDT use on health symptomatology.

Summary of Results

1. VDT telephone office workers have jobs characterized by significantly higher job demands and lower job control than non-VDT telephone office workers.
2. VDT exposure among telephone office workers is associated with a higher prevalence of eyestrain, headaches, fatigue, tension, and Rose angina. These relationships appear to be worsened by low job control afforded by the work environment.
3. Ergonomic factors pertaining to the work station, in this case whether a chair provides adequate back support, were significantly associated with the five symptoms examined, after controlling for age, VDT exposure, and job control.
4. Psychosocial and work station factors appear to operate as intermediate modifying or conditioning variables that affect the quality of the worker-machine interface. These aspects of job design may either exacerbate the potential deleterious health effects of VDT exposure or, if designed taking human factors into consideration, they may optimize the beneficial effects of technology-assisted working roles.

Implications

The results presented in the North Carolina Office Workers Stress Survey must be considered preliminary until a comprehensive medical examination of a representative sample of office workers can be instituted. Implications of our research should be interpreted with caution unless similar evidence from other studies is available. This section is divided into two sets of implications: practical implications for work environment change and prospects for future research.

Given the overwhelming evidence for acute symptomatic eye problems with regular VDT use, several preventive measures should be considered for workplaces with high VDT use:

1. VDTs should be equipped with detachable or separate keyboards and, where needed, antiglare filters. In addition, VDTs should have adjustable contrast, brightness, and screen angle controls along with a nonglare mattefinish.
2. VDT users should be provided with magnifying lenses or special lenses upon request.
3. VDT operators should be provided with frequent, short rest breaks. Where this is not possible, rest breaks of ten minutes per hour should be provided.
4. VDT users should be provided with eye examinations at the company's expense upon beginning VDT use and annually thereafter.

Work Environment: Musculoskeletal Strain. In the North Carolina Office Workers Stress Survey, back/neck strain was five times more frequent among VDT users with inadequate back support from a chair as compared to non-VDT users with adequate back support. Based upon the findings from the North Carolina Survey, the following recommendations are suggested:

1. Adjustable chairs (if possible) with adequate back support should be provided to all VDT workers. Employees should be trained regarding the proper use and operation of adjustable features. The option to stand or stretch at the work station should be available to all workers.
2. VDT work should be structured so that no worker should spend more than three hours on the machine at a time.
3. As in the case for eyestrain, VDT operators should be provided with frequent, short rest breaks.

Work Environment: Stress-related Symptoms. Stress on the job has become a major concern for VDT operators. Although more research is needed to pinpoint the source of stressful reactions in particular industries, the following recommendations are suggested for consideration:

1. VDT users should have the opportunity to have meaningful input into how work is designed. This should include work load, work pace, monitoring practices, and supervisor attitudes and practices.
2. Quality rather than quantity of service should be emphasized, particularly in response time for handling customer contacts.
3. Jobs requiring constant VDT use should be redesigned to allow workers to perform non-VDT work for part of their work day.

Future Research: Rose Angina. The North Carolina Office Workers Stress Survey was the first epidemiologic study to examine and identify Rose angina as a problem for VDT users. The twofold risk of reporting symptoms of angina in the North Carolina workers is disturbing in light of the excess cardiovascular mortality that has been associated with Rose angina in women.

At first glance, the overall prevalence rates of angina symptoms in this study (11.9 percent) appeared much higher than expected. However, our rates fell within the range of other studies. For example, in an English study of women administered the Rose questionnaire, Campbell et al. (1984) reported angina prevalence rates between 10.4 and 14.9 percent for women aged 45 to 65 years. Surprisingly, in that study, the younger women (age 45 to 54 years) with angina had the highest mortality rates of any age group, with 20 percent dying over a 12-year follow-up period.

Based upon the North Carolina findings and the potential long-term health effects of angina symptoms in women, the following recommendation is made for future research:

Joint labor and management research should be initiated to further examine health effects specific to office work. In addition to studies of visual, musculoskeletal, and job stress-related symptoms, special emphasis should be placed on chronic diseases such as angina pectoris and heart disease.

CONCLUSION

This investigation was introduced on the premise that if psychosocial work environment hazards to cardiovascular health could be identified and understood, then intervention strategies aimed at the work environment could be adopted to abate these hazards. The purpose of human factors epidemiology is to protect worker health (Amick and Celantano, 1984). When the aggregate needs of human workers are compromised at the expense of their individual health states, the most efficient means for primary prevention are directed to changing aspects of job design and work structure to bring the worker back into balance with the environment. Future research should be directed to identifying specific strategies for adapting jobs to the specific human needs of workers. The results of this investigation lend support to a growing and impressive body of literature linking VDT use and worker control to psychological strain, cardiovascular reactivity, and ultimately manifestations of CHD.

Acknowledgments: Many people dedicated time and effort to ensure the successful outcome of this important project. Special mention goes to the CWA Team Leaders: Cindi Weeks, Barbara Sharpe, Jennie Sherill, Jean Walden, Marjorie Baldwin, Brenda Pyatt, Shirley Moore, and Heidi Newber; graduate students at the University of North Carolina School of Public Health: Patricia Paddock, Christine Branche, and Brenda Kurz; and David LeGrande, National CWA Health and Safety Representative. This study was funded in part from participating North Carolina CWA Unions, the National Institute of Occupational Safety and Health (Order No. 84–2022), and the North Carolina Occupational Safety and Health Project. Suzanne G. Haynes's participation was made available, in part, by an Established Investigator Award from the American Heart Association, 1982–84.

REFERENCES

Alcolay, R. and Pasick, R. J. 1983. Psychosocial factors and the technologies of work. *Social Science and Medicine*, 17: 1075–1084.
Alfredsson, L., Karasek, R., and Theorell, T. 1982. Myocardial infarction and

psychosocial work environment: An analysis of the male Swedish working force. *Social Science and Medicine*, 16: 463–467.

Amick, B. D. and Celentano, D. D. 1984. Human factors epidemiology: An integrated approach to the study of health issues in office work. In Cohen, B. G. F. (Ed.). *Human Aspects in Office Automation*. Amsterdam: Elsevier.

Campbell, J. J., Elwood, P. C., Abbas, S., Waters, W. E. 1984. Chest pain in women: A study of prevalence and mortality follow-up in South Wales. *Journal of Epidemiology and Community Health*, 38: 17–20.

Chesney, M. S., Sevelines, G., Black, G. W., Ward, M. M., Swan, G. E., and Rosenman, R. H. 1981. Work environment, Type A behavior, and coronary heart disease risk factors. *Journal of Occupational Medicine*, 23: 551–555.

Frankenhaeuser, M. 1979. Psychobiological aspects of life stress. In Levine, S. and Urgin, H. (Eds.). *Coping and Health*: 203–223. New York: Plenum Press.

Haw, M. A. 1982. Women, work and stress: A review and agenda for the future. *Journal of Health and Social Behavior*, 23: 132–144.

Haynes, S. G., Eaker, E. D., and Feinleib, M.1984. The effect of employment, family, and job stress on coronary heart disease pattern in women. In Gold, E. B. (Ed.). *The Changing Risk of Disease in Women: An Epidemiological Approach*: 37–48. Lexington, Massachusetts: The Collanne Press.

Haynes, S. G. and Feinleib, M. 1980. Women, work and coronary heart disease: Prospective findings from the Framingham Heart Study. *American Journal of Public Health*, 70: 133–141.

Haynes, S. G., Levine, S., Scotch, N., et al. 1978. The relationship of psychosocial factors to coronary heart disease in the Framingham Study, I. Methods and Risk Factors. *American Journal of Epidemiology*, 107: 362–383.

Karasek, R., Baker, D., Marxer, F., Ahlbom, A., and Theorell, T. 1981. Job decision latitude, job demands and cardiovascular disease: A prospective study of Swedish men. *American Journal of Public Health*, 71(7): 694–705.

Karasek, R. and Gardell, B. 1984. Managing job stress. Unpublished manuscript. Columbia University, Department of Industrial Engineering and Operations Research, New York.

Karasek, R., Theorell, T., Schwartz, J. E., Peiper, C., and Michael, J. E. 1982. Job characteristics of occupations in relation to the prevalence of myocardial infarction in the U.S. Health Examination Survey and U.S. Health and Nutrition Examination Survey. Unpublished manuscript. Columbia University, Department of Industrial Engineering and Operational Research, New York.

Kleinbaum, D. G., Kupper, L. L., and Morgenstern, H. 1982. *Epidemiologic Research, Principles, and Quantitative Methods*. Belmont, Calif. Lifetime Learning Publications.

LaCroix, A. 1984. Occupational exposure to high demand/low control work and coronary heart disease incidence in the Framingham cohort. Unpublished doctoral dissertation. University of North Carolina, Chapel Hill.

LaCroix, A. and Haynes, S. G. 1984. Occupational exposure to high demand/low control work and CHD incidence in the Framingham cohort. *American Journal of Epidemiology*, 120: 481.

National Association of Working Women (NAWW) 1984. The 9-to-5 National Survey on Women and Stress. Cleveland: NAWW.

North Carolina Occupational Safety and Health Project and North Carolina Communications Workers of America. 1985. Office Workers Stress Survey Results, Washington, D.C.

Paddock, P. 1984. Job demands and psychosocial stress among clerical video display terminal users in the communications industry: A preliminary study. Unpublished Masters Thesis, University of North Carolina, Chapel Hill.

Rose, G. A. and Blackburn, H. 1968. *Cardiovascular Survey Methods*. Monograph Series 56 1–88. Geneva: World Health Organization.

SAS Institute, Inc. 1983. *SUGI Supplemental Library User's Guide*, 1983 edition. Cary, N.C.: SAS Institute, Inc.

Smith, M. J., Cohen, B. G. F., Stammerjohn, L. W., and Happ. A. 1981a. *Potential Health Hazards of Video Display Terminals: Health Complaints*. DHHS (NCOSH) Publication No. 81–129. Cincinnati: DHHS.

———. 1981b. An investigation of health complaints and job stress in video display operators. *Human Factors*, 23: 387–400.

Van Dijkhuizen, N. and Reiche, H. 1980. Psychosocial stress in industry: A heartache for middle management. *Psychotherapy & Psychosomatics*, 34: 124–134.

9   *Behavioral factors in hypertension: lessons from the work setting*

Margaret A. Chesney

In the last decade, the workplace has become a focal point for hypertension control programs. Initially, high blood pressure screening, referral, and education efforts found their way into the workplace because the setting offered a number of advantages, including accessibility of employees, stability of populations for study, and availability of facilities, staff, and channels of communication for program implementation. It became apparent that the work setting was especially appropriate for hypertension control efforts when blood pressure was observed to increase in response to environmental stresses, including job stress and industrial noise (Cobb and Rose, 1973; Andren et al., 1980; Parvizpoor, 1976). Recently, ambulatory blood pressure monitoring in the work setting has confirmed that blood pressures of hypertensive patients taken at work are higher than blood pressures recorded in medical settings or at home (Harshfield et al., 1982; Pickering et al., 1982).

This chapter will review findings from worksite hypertension programs that have implications for future hypertension research and health promotion programs within and beyond the work setting. Two types of programs will be discussed. The first will be those that involved screening, referral, and follow-up of standard medical treatment for hypertension. The second will be those that involved behavioral intervention programs designed to reduce blood pressure.

SCREENING AND REFERRAL PROGRAMS

In the early 1970s it was shown that the medical community was successful in controlling blood pressure in no more than 30 percent of individuals who knew themselves to be hypertensive (Schoenberger et al., 1972; Shapiro et al., 1978). This finding prompted the National Heart, Lung, and Blood Institute to open a National Office of High Blood Pressure Education and to support a series of blood pressure screening, referral, and education projects. Among these projects were several conducted in the occupational setting. Industrial interest in hypertension was not surprising, given the belief that stress in the workplace is associated with elevated blood pressure and the fact that a major portion of the cost of uncontrolled hypertension is borne by employers through health benefits.

Predictors of Compliance with Referral

Model worksite hypertension programs showed that screening, pharmacological treatment, and follow-up led to substantial improvements in control among hypertensive employees (Alderman and Schoenbaum, 1975; Alderman and Davis, 1980; Logan et al., 1982; Baer, Parchment, and Kneeshaw, 1979). One worksite hypertension research program was conducted at a large California industrial facility by Stanford Research Institute to determine predictors of compliance (Chesney et al., 1978). In this program, 3,100 employees participated in a sequential screening procedure that was made highly convenient by taking blood pressure measurements at or near the worksite of each participant. That 97.5 percent of the targeted population consented to and completed the three-stage screening process was attributed to the program's convenience to the employees. As shown in Figure 9.1 of the subjects screened, 526 had elevated blood pressures. Of these, 281 were new referrals (employees who had not previously been told that they had high blood pressure) and 245 were hypertensives who had been currently under care for hypertension.

Subjects identified as hypertensive by the screening were given a letter referring them to their physicians for evaluation and blood pressure follow-up. Although the subjects had ready access to health care, only 54 percent of new referrals saw their physicians during the first four months following referral. Variables associated with blood pressure changes in and compliance by hypertensive employees were examined. Table 9.1 presents the seven variables found to discriminate significantly the new referrals who complied and saw their physicians from those who did not. The variable that most significantly discriminated between the two groups was the response to the question, "How long do you typically have to wait when you visit the physician?" This finding indicates that convenience had an important effect on compliance with referral in this sample. The average waiting time among those new referrals who saw their physicians was 17 minutes, while the average waiting time for those who did not comply was 28 minutes. Job stress was not related to adherence; however, the importance of convenience indicates that adherence is enhanced if the behaviors required do not add stress, as would be the case with long waiting times.

Significant reductions in blood pressures were observed over the follow-up period of four to six months. A surprising variable that predicted blood pressure reduction in this group of hypertensive employees involved "faith in physicians." There was a significant negative correlation between

Figure 9.1.   Incidence of hypertension and compliance to referral in a worksite hypertension screening program

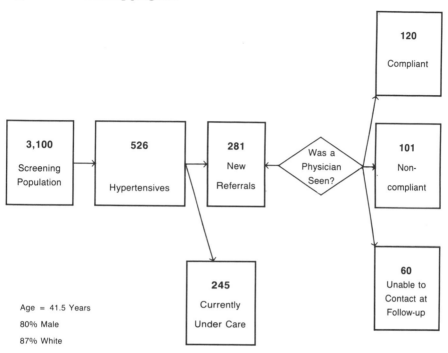

Source: Compiled by the author.

this variable and blood pressure change. This observation has been further studied and was interpreted as indicating that those persons who rely too heavily on health care professionals are *less* apt to change or adopt new personal health behaviors. In the subjects who were under care when screened but found to have uncontrolled blood pressure, faith in physicians was also found to be a significant predictor of poor blood pressure control at follow-up. Self-reports of stress on the job or in the home were not related to blood pressure change in either new referrals or hypertensives currently under care.

The questionnaire that provided data from which these predictive indexes were developed also included questions dealing with knowledge about blood pressure and its control. There was no relationship between knowledge of blood pressure or hypertension and blood pressure change at follow-up. Another significant variable found to predict blood pressure change in new referrals was the perception that one's risk of heart disease and stroke would be reduced by complying with the referral recommendation and the prescribed regimen. This variable measures a component of

Table 9.1.   Variables that significantly discriminated compliant from noncompliant new referrals

Variable	Compliant New Referrals	Noncompliant New Referrals
Length of wait at physician's office	17 min	28 min
Waiting time viewed as bothersome (percent agreeing)	19	35
High blood pressure viewed as limiting daily activities (percent agreeing)	23	0
High blood pressure viewed as interfering with sleep (percent agreeing)	14	4
Obtaining an annual medical examination (percent)	45	15
Spouse is concerned about subject's blood pressure (percent agreeing)	42	21
Subject's age (average)	51 years	45 years

Source: Compiled by the author.

what has been called self-efficacy (Bandura, 1977)—that is, the belief that engaging in a recommended behavior will be efficacious in achieving the desired results. In this situation, the perception that compliance reduces risk is related to knowledge about hypertension but is more directly associated with self-reliance (as contrasted with faith in physicians).

Worksite, Screening and Referral Trials

Two recent clinical trials (Logan et al., 1983; Foote and Erfurt, 1983) examined the relative efficacy of various approaches to screening, referral, and, in some cases, on-site treatment of hypertension in the work setting. Logan and his colleagues screened 9,743 employees at 38 businesses in metropolitan Toronto. Of these, 213 employees met the eligibility criteria for hypertension and were not already under treatment. Of the 194 who agreed to participate, 97 were randomly allocated to a group referred to their physicians for care (RC group), and 97 were randomly allocated to a group referred to their physicians and followed by an occupational health nurse (RC&F group). Employees assigned to the RC&F group participated in an intensive blood pressure control program, which included counseling on compliance and follow-up of missed appointments. In addition, if a subject had difficulty complying with medication regimens, the nurse introduced strategies found to be useful in other studies (NHLBI Working Group, 1982).

At the one-year follow-up, both groups showed significant decreases in blood pressure, but the difference between the two groups was not significant. In fact, of those in the RC&F group, only 41.8 percent were under good blood pressure control. This percentage does not compare favorably with the 60.7 percent observed in previous demonstration projects by these investigators (Logan et al., 1981) in patients treated by nurses and physicians at the worksite.

The investigators concluded from their trial that the addition of systematic monitoring and follow-up by the nurse was not associated with significantly greater improvement in blood pressure control over that achieved by employees referred for care in the community. Therefore, despite attention provided by intensive blood pressure monitoring and counseling to enhance compliance with the regimen prescribed by the physician, blood pressure control was notably low.

The previously described study by Chesney and associates (1978) may provide some insight into the disappointing results of the elegant clinical trial conducted by Logan and his colleagues. As discussed earlier, we found that the most significant predictor of blood pressure reduction and control was *less* faith in physicians. We interpreted this result as indicating that those employees who had considerably more faith in physicians relied on their doctors for treatment rather than engaging in health-enhancing behaviors. Inasmuch as achieving blood pressure control involved a number of specific behaviors—from taking medicines to keeping appointments—that are independent of the physician, those employees who were more self-reliant were more compliant. In the clinical trial just reviewed (Logan et al., 1983), it may have been that the efforts of the nurses rewarded and perhaps increased the subjects' reliance or dependence on the health care team, so that self-reliance and blood pressure control may have suffered.

Another major study of screening, referral, follow-up, and on-site treatment was conducted at four Ford Motor Company manufacturing plants in Michigan (Foote and Erfurt, 1983). Following screening, employees received various referral and follow-up interventions, depending on worksite. At Site 1, all identified hypertensives were referred to the physicians of their choice in the community. No further action was taken beyond the referral to care. At Site 2, hypertensives were followed semiannually by an on-site "blood pressure counselor" who monitored the employees' blood pressure, encouraged compliance, provided blood pressure information, and referred hypertensives back to their physicians whenever necessary. At Site 3, in addition to the Site 2 activities, the blood pressure counselor maintained contact with employees' physicians. At Site 4, hypertensives had the choice of receiving on-site treatment in the plant's medical department or of seeing their own physicians. Only 41 percent chose to be treated in the medical department of the plant.

Four years after the intervention, changes in subjects' blood pressures were examined. Employees who were not under care for hypertension at screening had significant reductions in both systolic and diastolic blood pressure at all four sites. Moreover, at all but Site 1 (the control site) the mean blood pressures were within the normal range at follow-up. At Site 1, the hypertensives' mean blood pressures were in the borderline range. Hypertensive employees at Sites 2, 3, and 4 who were under care but had uncontrolled blood pressure at screening also showed significant reductions in blood pressure resulting in levels in the normal range at follow-up. The mean blood pressure for this group of subjects at Site 1, on the other hand, did not decline to within normal levels. The greatest reductions for both new referrals and hypertensives under care were observed at Site 4 for those subjects who were treated by medical staff on-site. Subjects at Site 4 who were treated by their private physicians showed blood pressure changes similar to those achieved at Sites 2 and 3.

The authors concluded that screening, referral, and systematic follow-up of hypertensive employees resulted in significant decreases in blood pressure and significant increases in the proportion of employees with adequate blood pressure control, as found by Logan and his associates (1982, 1983). The highest level of control was achieved by on-site treatment (Site 4), but an analysis of costs indicated that such treatment was substantially more costly than the programs offered at Sites 2 and 3. Specifically, the annual cost of operating the program, excluding physician costs, per hypertensive at Site 4 was $96.19, compared with $26.26 and $35.00 at Sites 2 and 3, respectively. Furthermore, on-site treatment programs also represent a major break from the standard practice in occupational medicine of referral to community physicians and thus have not been widely accepted (Evans, Saidleman, and Daily, 1979). The similarity of the results observed at Sites 2 and 3 further indicates that effective blood pressure changes can be achieved by having a "blood pressure counselor" contact employees relatively infrequently (semi-annually), and that follow-up contacts with the employees' physicians do not result in larger group average blood pressure reductions.

Convenience and Self-Reliance

These results indicate the importance of convenience in effective worksite hypertension programs, a conclusion consistent with the findings of the screening and referral program conducted at the California plant. In the Ford program, convenience was maintained by providing blood pressure monitoring and information about hypertension, tailored to each employee's blood pressure level and treatment status, every six months at the worksite. The employee follow-up by the blood pressure counselor may have been particularly effective because convenience was offered but employees did not develop excessive reliance or dependence on blood pressure program staff.

Taken together, these selected studies of hypertensive screening, referral, treatment, and follow-up suggest that compliance with programs can be enhanced by increasing convenience for the subject. Indeed, the concept of conducting worksite hypertension programs was intended to capitalize on the importance of convenience in maintaining compliance with health care activities. When compliance is made convenient, the need to perform health-enhancing behaviors does not add to daily stress. These studies also indicate that self-reliance and self-efficacy are related to positive outcomes in persons with a health condition that is controlled, in many respects, by the patient's behavior. Conversely, if the concept of convenience is extended so far that health care staff take over health maintenance activities, such as direct setting of appointments, patients may become overly dependent or reliant on the health care providers, and such overreliance appears to reduce health-promoting changes in behavior.

The findings from the worksite hypertension screening, referral, treatment, and follow-up programs have implications for health promotion efforts in the work setting at both the organizational and employee levels. Specifically, health promotion, stress management, and illness prevention programs require adherence or compliance by the sponsoring organization and the participants. Program effectiveness will be enhanced if the program can be conveniently adopted and integrated into the organization's regular activities. Furthermore, a program is more likely to succeed when both the organization and the participants become actively involved and overreliance on providers is avoided.

BEHAVIORAL INTERVENTION PROGRAMS

Nonpharmacological treatments for hypertension have recently been evaluated in the work setting. Behavioral treatment approaches are currently recommended by the National Institutes of Health (NIH) as adjuncts to antihypertensive medications in patients with established hypertension and as an initial approach in the treatment of mild hypertension (Joint National Committee on Detection, Evaluation, and Treatment of High Blood Pressure, 1984). Specifically, the NIH Joint National Committee noted that

data concerning behavioral methods in hypertension management have demonstrated that various relaxation and biofeedback therapies (or combinations of such treatments) may consistently produce modest but significant blood pressure reduction in selected groups outside the laboratory for as long as one year. Such reductions are particularly relevant for the treatment of mild hypertension but may also be used in combination with pharmacologic therapy in patients with more severe hypertension (p. 14).

In response to the NIH recommendation, behavioral interventions are now being used to control blood pressure in both work and clinical settings. As was found with the screening and referral programs, behavioral interventions for hypertension control that are based on relaxation and other stress management approaches can be implemented effectively and evaluated in the work environment. In fact, prevention of the adverse health consequences of uncontrolled hypertension is one—if not the most demonstrable—benefit of stress management in the work setting.

Rationale for Worksite Stress Management Programs

Recent evidence from studies using ambulatory blood pressure (ABP) monitors provides a persuasive argument for stress management as a treatment for hypertension, and for the work setting as an appropriate site for these interventions. Ambulatory blood pressure monitors are devices that are worn by individuals and provide measurements of blood pressure in the natural environment. Using these monitors, investigators have shown that blood pressures taken at work are significantly higher than blood pressures taken in the home (Pickering et al., 1982; Harshfield et al., 1982). The higher work pressures were interpreted as a response to stress in the work environment (Harshfield et al., 1982). Similar differences also have been observed between home blood pressure measurements and those taken in physicians' offices, a phenomenon often ascribed to transient elevations because of the stress of visiting the physician (Pickering et al., 1982).

Worksite ABP also is generally higher than blood pressure taken in medical clinic settings, although the differences are not significant (Pickering et al., 1982; Harshfield et al., 1982). This is an important observation for two reasons. First, epidemiological data documenting the relationship of blood pressure to heart disease risk are based on measurements made in medical clinic settings. Therefore, the absence of a difference between the worksite and clinic pressures supports the clinical significance of worksite pressures. Second, ambulatory blood pressures in the work setting not only are as high as clinic measurements but are sustained throughout the working day. Given that transient pressure elevations in the clinic setting have been attributed to the patient's reaction to the stress of the physician visit (Pickering et al., 1982), ABPs taken at work may be indicative of the physiological effect of exposure to naturally occurring work stress and strain—an exposure that is not transient.

A further indication of the relevance of natural settings as primary sites of hypertension treatment is that ambulatory blood pressure elevations have been shown to correlate more closely with evidence of damage to the heart (Pickering et al., 1985), damage to peripheral blood vessels (Sokolow et al., 1966), and incidence of mortality from first myocardial infarction (Perloff, Sokolow, and Cowan, 1983).

The foregoing review provides a consistent picture of blood pressure being elevated in the work setting and these elevations being related to cardiovascular risk and damage. Therefore, the work setting may be the location of choice for treatment of hypertension and for the assessment of treatment outcome. Stress management approaches to treatment appear particularly appropriate, given that stress has been implicated as the source of blood pressure elevations observed at work.

Background and Early Evidence for Behavioral Interventions

The rationale for initiating treatment with behavioral approaches is twofold. First, clinical trials of pharmacological treatment of hypertensive patients, particularly the majority who have mild hypertension, have yielded mixed results, with two studies suggesting some benefit and three indicating no benefit. Moreover, the Oslo Study (Helgeland, 1980) and the Multiple Risk Factor Intervention Trial (1982) indicated that diuretic medications may be associated with increased risk of sudden death, particularly in hypertensive patients with abnormal electrocardiograms.

In the early 1970s, behavioral interventions based on relaxation, biofeedback, and related approaches were reported to result in significant blood pressure reduction in individual-case and small-group studies (Benson et al., 1971; Benson et al., 1974; Elder and Eustis, 1975; Blanchard, Young, and Haynes, 1975). These studies attracted interest but they suffered from numerous methodological weaknesses, including an absence of control groups, small sample sizes, confounding of behavioral and pharmacological treatments, statistical artifacts, and biased outcome measurements (Chesney and Black, 1986). Despite these weaknesses, the general conclusion to be drawn from these studies as an aggregate is that relaxation, biofeedback, and related approaches result in modest blood pressure reductions.

Controlled Studies of Behavioral Treatment

Following these initial studies, behavioral treatment was evaluated in more controlled investigations (Crowther, 1983; Seer and Raeburn, 1980; Jorgensen, Houston, and Zurawski, 1981; Frankel et al., 1978), including some conducted in work settings (Peters, Benson, and Peters, 1977; Southam et al., 1982; Charlesworth, Williams, and Baer, 1984). For example, Charlesworth and his colleagues (1984) found that 22 hypertensive employees showed significantly greater self-reported blood pressure reductions than did a waiting-list control group following a ten-week stress management program emphasizing relaxation, with additional sessions on cognitive restructuring and assertiveness training. Although studies such as this still suffered from one or more of the previously cited problems, the majority confirmed that behavioral treatments result in significantly greater reductions in blood pressure than no-treatment control conditions. These differences were shown to be maintained over time in some but not all studies.

Although most long-term studies have observed that treatment effects significant at posttreatment dissipated with follow-up of six months or longer (Frankel et al., 1978; Blanchard et al., 1979), Patel and her colleagues (1985) reported significant blood pressure differences between treatment and control groups of hypertensive employees at a four-year follow-up in a large worksite study conducted in England. In this study, 99 hypertensive employees of an electronics firm participated in an eight-week program that taught relaxation skills and their application for stress management. These employees were compared with 93 hypertensive employees assigned to the control condition and given brief health information.

Blood Pressure Reductions with Blood Pressure Monitoring

Not all studies have demonstrated that stress management or behavioral treatments result in greater blood pressure reductions than do control conditions involving blood pressure monitoring. Two recent large, controlled studies conducted in the work setting (Agras, 1985; Chesney and Black, 1983) indicate that, for mild hypertensives, systematic blood pressure monitoring results in blood pressure reductions equivalent to those observed in behavioral treatment groups. For more severe hypertensives, including those who have elevated blood pressure despite medication, behavioral treatments may prove to be more efficacious than blood pressure monitoring (Agras, 1985). The efficacy of systematic blood pressure monitoring, particularly in mild hypertensive patients, has also been reported by others (Goldstein et al., 1982; Jacob et al., 1985). However, the large, controlled worksite studies cited above draw particular attention to changes in the control groups that received only blood pressure monitoring. Two explanations for these similar effects in treatment and monitoring groups require consideration because they have implications for blood pressure reduction programs: the hypotensive effect of repeated measurement, and positive expectancy of blood pressure reduction.

Repeated blood pressure monitoring by the hypertensive patient or a professional has a modest hypotensive effect (Laughlin, Fisher, and Sherrard, 1979; Engel, Gaarder, and Glasgow, 1982; Goldstein, Shapiro, and Thananopavaran, 1984). The mechanism underlying this effect and the associated blood pressure reductions are not well understood. One possibility is that monitoring results in an increased awareness of blood pressure variability and a recognition of situational factors associated with elevations and declines. In this manner, monitoring may constitute a form of blood pressure biofeedback for the hypertensive.

A positive expectation regarding blood pressure reduction is sometimes given to control groups. In several of the controlled investigations in which relative efficacy of behavioral treatments was not demonstrated, subjects in the blood pressure monitoring groups were given the expectation that their participation in a program of repeated blood pressure assessment would lead to blood pressure reductions (Jacob et al., 1985; Goldstein et al., 1984). It may be that the positive mental set or expectancy given to these subjects was a sufficient condition for blood pressure reduction. Evidence of the importance of expectancy comes from the placebo-control studies of behavioral treatments. These studies have been reviewed by Wadden and his associates (1984), who concluded that "the more control conditions resembled actual treatment the greater the hypotensive effect." Consistent with this line of reasoning, studies that compared behavioral interventions with control conditions not conveying positive expectations, such as the waiting-list group in the Charlesworth et al. study (1984), generally found behavioral approaches to result in greater blood pressure reductions than the control conditions. However, a failure to find significant treatment effects is more common in those studies in which a greater number of nonspecific factors, such as contact with the therapists, are incorporated into the control condition.

The observation of blood pressure reductions in response to placebo conditions calls into question the importance of relaxation as an essential component in achieving blood pressure reduction. The role played by relaxation is further eroded by studies demonstrating no relationship between relaxation practice and blood pressure reductions (Taylor et al., 1983; Jacob, Beidel, and Shapiro, 1984). That significant blood pressure reductions are achieved by such means as repeated measurement, positive expectancy, and the support engendered by participating in studies regardless of assignment to the treatment or control group does not necessarily imply that hypertensive employees are not experiencing a reduction in stress. In fact, control group manipulations, and the support and attention they invariably involve, may be addressing stresses in the work setting as effectively as relaxation training.

Relative Efficacy of Behavioral Treatments

Investigations comparing behavioral strategies such as relaxation, meditation, blood pressure biofeedback, and electromyographic and temperature biofeedback have generally found few significant differences in the effectiveness of these strategies. From the studies conducted to date, the conclusion would be drawn that the two most thoroughly investigated strategies (relaxation and blood pressure biofeedback) are equally effective in achieving blood pressure reductions and that treatment combinations of biofeedback and relaxation are not significantly better than singular approaches.

The relative efficacy of behavioral and pharmacological treatments has been examined in only a few studies. Those that have made this comparison with newly referred hypertensive subjects indicate that pharmacological treatments are significantly more effective than behavioral interventions (Goldstein et al., 1982; Luborsky et al., 1982). An important issue is whether behavioral interventions are effective as an adjunct to pharmacological treatment when blood pressures remain elevated despite the use of medication. The studies investigating this issue have shown that patients with uncontrolled hypertension who receive behavioral interventions in combination with medication achieve better blood pressure control than patients receiving medication alone (Crowther, 1983; Southam et al., 1982; Agras, Southam, and Taylor, 1983).

The effectiveness of the combination of behavioral treatment and medication in lowering ABP has recently been demonstrated in a controlled worksite study (Agras, Southam, and Taylor, 1983). At a 15-month follow-up, subjects treated with medication and an 8-week relaxation training program showed persistent decreases in blood pressure, while employees in the measurement-only control group showed little change from baseline.

This study is of particular importance given the clinical significance of worksite blood pressure, as discussed previously in this chapter. Moreover, this study demonstrates the feasibility and the appropriateness of the work setting as the arena for stress management programs and for the evaluation of their effects.

A conceptual model showing the relationship between exposure of hypertensive individuals to work stress and cardiovascular disease risk is presented in Figure 9.2. Also shown is a summary of the elements of behavioral interventions and blood pressure monitoring discussed in the foregoing section. The figure indicates the point at which interventions or the simpler blood pressure monitoring can be introduced to reduce or block the capacity of work stresses and strains to increase blood pressure in hypertensive employees. By successfully blocking the impact of work stress and strain on blood pressure, these behavioral interventions may minimize the contribution of work stress to the development and progression of cardiovascular disease in hypertensive employees.

Implications for Worksite Hypertension Programs

The rationale for the use of behavioral interventions in the initial treatment of hypertensive employees presented at the beginning of this section remains unchanged despite the lack of conclusive evidence of the relative efficacy of specific nonpharmacologic interventions over blood pressure monitoring. Given the magnitude of the population with blood pressure in the mildly hypertensive range, coupled with evidence that blood pressure reduction in mild hypertension is associated with reduced

Figure 9.2.   Impact of blood pressure (BP) monitoring and behavioral interventions on the relationship between work stress and cardiovascular disease

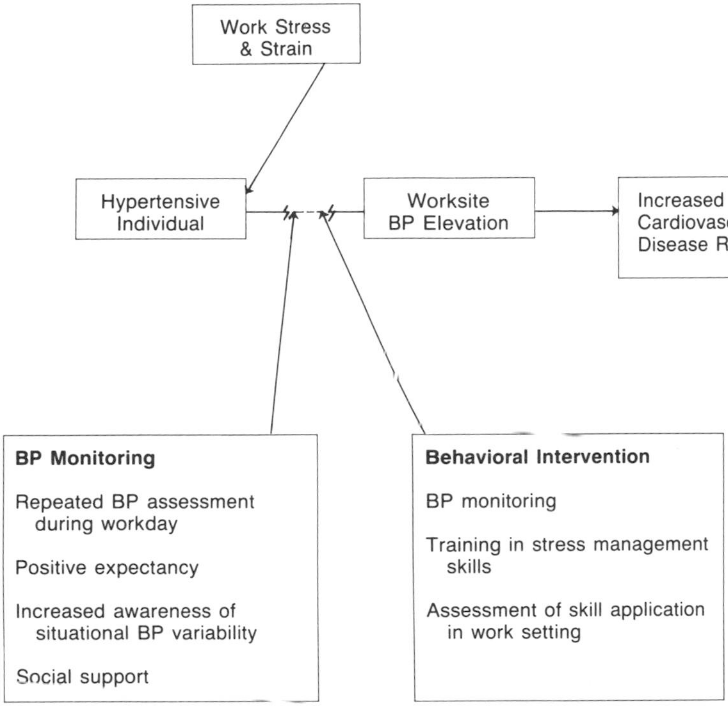

Source: Compiled by the author.

risk (Hypertension Detection and Follow-up Program Cooperative Group, 1979), systematic efforts to reduce blood pressure, particularly in this group, are needed.

The risk associated with hypertension, and the evidence of noncompliance with prescribed regimens among those who are aware of their hypertension status, points to the need for blood pressure screening, referral, and follow-up programs. The research on behavioral factors in hypertension control discussed in this chapter suggests a stepped approach that follows the process of screening, referral, and follow-up with behavioral interventions for treatment and control of hypertension.

Screening, Referral, and Systematic Monitoring. For newly screened employees, the first step could be repeated blood pressure measurement over a period of several months. Monitoring could be carried out by a nurse or allied health professional and should emphasize convenience for the employees. In light of the evidence for the effect of positive expectancy on blood pressure reduction, these individuals should be given the expectation that this monitoring may result in blood pressure decreases.

The monitoring might include elements such as self-assessment of blood pressure in order to foster the employees' taking an active role in monitoring and to avoid developing an overreliance on health care professionals. As noted previously, research has demonstrated that a substantial number of employees will show marked blood pressure decreases during this monitoring period.

From an organizational perspective, employee participation in and compliance with program recommendations will be enhanced if the screening, referral, and monitoring activities are made convenient and the results are clearly designated as confidential. Employees should be informed about blood pressure variability and encouraged to keep a personal record of their blood pressures along with their observations of possible factors that might be associated with stress (such as vacations, report writing under deadline). The employees are likely to examine these records for possible associations between their blood pressures and events, and to initiate personal health behavior changes. They could be given general guidelines to assist them in this examination and to avoid premature conclusions.

Similarly, while protecting the privacy of the employees, the organization could keep an anonymous record of blood pressures by major organizational units and by events (such as work cutbacks). Should a relationship be observed from this organizational monitoring, the organization could consider making changes that might reduce the stresses and strains and, by doing so, prevent or minimize blood pressure elevations.

In this and the subsequent stages of blood pressure control, the organization can promote hypertension control by providing an environment that is supportive to the concept of health promotion and conducive to employee involvement in health promotion programs.

Behavioral Interventions. For employees whose blood pressure remains in the mild range after monitoring, specific stress management interventions could be introduced as a second step. In addition to the interventions based on relaxation and biofeedback that were the focus here, other behavioral approaches such as sodium restriction and weight reduction could also be considered in light of patient characteristics.

The organization could enhance the effectiveness of these programs by making them convenient to the employees. For example, a facility in a convenient location could be made available, and employees could be given time off for participation in the interventions. Certain materials and equipment (such as recorders for tape-recorded relaxation exercises) could be made available on loan to participants. For other behavioral approaches, healthful low-sodium foods could be made available in vending machines and cafeterias, and the sodium content of foods could be listed on menus. Scales for monitoring weight could be located conveniently throughout the worksite.

Combined Behavioral and Pharmacological Interventions. When behavioral approaches do not achieve adequate blood pressure control, pharmacological interventions could be added as a third step. Behavioral interventions should be continued when pharmacotherapy is introduced, in light of the additive effects and reduced need for medication when used in conjunction with nonpharmacological therapy. The organization could enhance the effect of combined pharmacological and nonpharmacological treatment by continuing the blood pressure assessment and follow-up, and by offering counseling for compliance in a manner that is convenient for subjects and that fosters self-efficacy and self-reliance.

CONCLUSION

The work setting has provided an ideal, naturalistic laboratory for research on hypertension and for the development and testing of programs directed toward its control. The accessibility of employees, the stability of the work force for long-term studies, and the availability of medical facilities, occupational health nurses, and other resources have enabled the behavioral medicine research community to make significant progress in the areas of hypertension screening, referral, treatment, and follow-up. Worksite hypertension screening, referral, and follow-up programs have served as the primary source for much of our current knowledge about compliance, including the importance of convenience, avoiding dependency, and engendering self-efficacy.

More recently, in the area of behavioral interventions for hypertension treatment, the advantages of conducting research in the work setting have made it possible to conduct large-scale controlled studies to test the efficacy of behavioral interventions that had appeared promising in smaller, clinical studies. The results of these studies suggested a stepped approach to hypertension control that is particularly applicable to the work setting. In the future, this stepped approach undoubtedly will be evaluated and refined, tailoring treatment strategies to individual differences determined in part by dynamic patterns of blood pressures, as recorded by ambulatory monitors in response to environmental stressors. In all likelihood, the work setting will remain a primary "laboratory" for this research and for the trials to evaluate the next generation of biobehavioral interventions for hypertension control.

REFERENCES

Agras, W. S. 1985. Behavioral interventions in hypertension. Paper presented at the Annual Meeting of the American Psychological Association, Los Angeles, August 23–27.

Agras, W. S., Southam, M. A., and Taylor, C. B. 1983. Long-term persistence of relaxation-induced blood pressure lowering during the working day. *Journal of Consulting and Clinical Psychology*, 51: 792–794.

Alderman, M. H. and Davis, T. K. 1980. Blood pressure control programs on and off the worksite. *Journal of Occupational Medicine*, 22: 167–170.

Alderman, M. H. and Schoenbaum, E.E. 1975. Hypertension control at the worksite. *New England Journal of Medicine*, 2: 65–68.

Andren, L., Hansson, L., Bjorkman, M., and Jonsson, A. 1980. Noise as a contributory factor in the development of elevated arterial pressure. *Acta Medica Scandinavica*, 207: 493–498.

Baer, L., Parchment, Y., and Kneeshaw, M. F. 1979. Hypertension in health care providers and effectiveness of worksite treatment. *Preventive Medicine*, 8: 125.

Bandura, A. 1977. Self-efficacy: Towards a unifying theory of behavioral change. *Psychological Review*, 84: 191–215.

Benson, H., Rosner, B. A., Marzetta, B. R., and Klemchuk, H. M. 1974. Decreased blood pressure in pharmacologically treated hypertensive patients who regularly elicited the relaxation response. *Lancet*, 1: 289–291.

Benson, H., Shapiro, D., Tursky, B., and Schwartz, G. E. 1971. Decreased systolic blood pressure through operant conditioning techniques in patients with essential hypertension. *Science,* 173: 740–742.

Blanchard, E. B., Miller, S. T., Abel, G.G., Haynes, M. R., and Wicker, R. 1979. Evaluation of biofeedback in the treatment of essential hypertension. *Journal of Applied Behavior Analysis*, 12: 99–109.

Blanchard, E.B., Young, L. D., and Haynes, M. R. 1975. A simple feedback system for the treatment of elevated blood pressure. *Behavior Therapy*, 6: 241–245.

Charlesworth, E. A., Williams, B. J., and Baer, P. E. 1984. Stress management at the worksite for hypertension: Compliance, cost-benefit, health care and hypertension-related variables. *Psychosomatic Medicine*, 46: 387–397.

Chesney, M. A. and Black, G. W. 1983. Hypertension: Biobehavioral influences and implications for treatment. Paper presented at the Meeting on Biobehavioral Factors in Coronary Heart Disease. Wintersheid, West Germany, June.

———. 1986. Behavioral treatment of borderline hypertension: An overview of results. *Journal of Cardiovascular Pharmacology*, 8 (Suppl. 5): S57–S63.

Chesney, M.A., Black, G. W., Jordan, S., and Sevelius, G. G. 1978. Unexpected predictors of compliance among newly referred hypertensives. Paper presented at the National Conference on High Blood Pressure Control, Los Angeles, April 2–4.

Cobb, S. and Rose, R. M. 1973. Hypertension, peptic ulcer, and diabetes in air traffic controllers. *Journal of the American Medical Association*, 224: 489–492.

Crowther, J. H. 1983. Stress management training and relaxation imagery in the treatment of essential hypertension. *Journal of Behavioral Medicine*, 6: 169–187.

Elder, S. T. and Eustis, N. K. 1975. Instrumental blood pressure conditioning in outpatient essential hypertension. *Behavior Research and Therapy*, 13: 185–188.

Engel, B. T., Gaarder, K. R., and Glasgow, M. S. 1982. Behavioral treatment of high blood pressure. I. Analyses of intra- and interdaily variations of blood pressure during a one-month baseline period. *Psychosomatic Medicine*, 43: 255–270.

Evans, W., Saidleman, M., and Daily, N. H. 1979. Obstacles to worksite hypertension programs. *Preventive Medicine*, 8: 158.

Foote, A. and Erfurt, J. C. 1983. Hypertension control at the worksite: Comparison of screening and referral alone, referral and follow-up, and on-site treatment. *New England Journal of Medicine*, 308: 809–813.

Frankel, B. I., Patel, D. J., Horowitz, D., Friedwald, W. T., and Gaarder, K. 1978. Treatment of hypertension with biofeedback and relaxation techniques. *Psychosomatic Medicine*, 40: 276–293.

Goldstein, I. B., Shapiro, D., and Thananopavaran, C. 1984. Home relaxation techniques for essential hypertension. *Psychosomatic Medicine*, 46: 398–414.

Goldstein, I. B., Shapiro, D., Thananopavaran, C., and Sambhi, M. P. 1982. Comparison of drug and behavioral treatments of essential hypertension. *Health Psychology*, 1: 7–26.

Harshfield, G. A., Pickering, T. G., Kleinert, H. D., Blank, S., and Laragh, J. H. 1982. Situational variations of blood pressure in ambulatory hypertensive patients. *Psychosomatic Medicine*, 44: 237–245.

Helgeland, A. 1980. Treatment of mild hypertension: A five-year controlled drug trial. *American Journal of Medicine*, 69: 725–732.

Hypertension Detection and Follow-up Program Cooperative Group. 1979. Five-year findings of the Hypertension Detection and Follow-up Program: II. Mortality by race, sex, and age. *Journal of the American Medical Association*, 242: 2572–2577.

Jacob, R. G., Beidel, D. C., and Shapiro, A. P. 1984. The relaxation word of the day: A simple technique to measure adherence to relaxation. *Journal of Behavioral Assessment*, 6: 159–165.

Jacob, R. G., Fortmann, S. P., Kraemer, H. C., Farquhar, J. W., and Agras, W. S. 1985. Combining behavioral treatments to reduce blood pressure: A controlled outcome study. *Behavior Modification*, 9: 32–54.

Joint National Committee on Detection, Evaluation, and Treatment of High Blood Pressure. 1984. The 1984 Report of the Joint National Committee on Detection, Evaluation, and Treatment of High Blood Pressure. *Archives of Internal Medicine*, 144: 1045–1057.

Jorgensen, R. S., Houston, B. K., and Zurawski, R. M. 1981. Anxiety management training in the treatment of essential hypertension. *Behavior Research and Therapy*, 19: 467–474.

Laughlin, K. D., Fisher, L., and Sherrard, D. J. 1979. Blood pressure reductions during self-recording of home blood pressure. *American Heart Journal*, 98: 629–634.

Logan, A. G., Milne, B. J., Achber, C., Campbell, W. P., and Haynes, R. B. 1981. Cost-effectiveness of a worksite hypertension treatment program. *Hypertension*, 3: 211–218.

Logan, A. G., Milne, B. J., Campbell, W. A., and Haynes, R. B. 1982. A comparison of community and occupationally-provided antihypertensive care. *Journal of Occupational Medicine*, 24: 901.

Logan, A. G., Milne, B. J., Flanagan, P. T., and Haynes, R. B. 1983. Clinical effectiveness and cost-effectiveness of monitoring blood pressure in hypertensive employees at work. *Hypertension*, 5: 828–836.

Luborsky, L., Crits-Christoph, P., Brady, J. P., Kron, R. E., Weiss, T., Cohen, M., and Levy, L. 1982. Behavioral versus pharmacological treatments for essential hypertension: A needed comparison. *Psychosomatic Medicine*, 44: 203–213.

Multiple Risk Factor Intervention Trial Research Group. 1982. Multiple risk factor interventional trial: Risk factor changes and mortality results. *Journal of American Medical Association*, 248: 1465–1477.

NHLBI Working Group. 1982. Management of patient compliance in the treatment of hypertension. 4: 415–423.

Parvizpoor, D. 1976. Noise exposure and prevalence of high blood pressure among weavers in Iran. *Journal of Occupational Medicine*, 18: 730–731.

Patel, C., Marmot, M. G., Terry, D. J., Carruthers, M., Hunt, B., and Patel, M. 1985. Trial of relaxation in reducing coronary risk: Four-year follow-up. *British Medical Journal*, 290: 1103–1106.

Perloff, D., Sokolow, M., and Cowan, R. 1983. The prognostic value of ambulatory blood pressures. *Journal of the American Medical Association*, 249: 2792–2798.

Peters, R.K., Benson, H., and Peters, J. M. 1977. Daily relaxation response breaks in a working population: II. Effects on blood pressure. *American Journal of Public Health*, 67(10): 954–959.

Pickering, T. G., Harshfield, G. A., Devereux, R. B., and Laragh, J. H. 1985. What is the role of ambulatory blood pressure monitoring in the management of hypertensive patients? *Hypertension*, 7: 171–177.

Pickering, T. G., Harshfield, G. A., Kleinert, H. D., Blank, S., and Laragh, J. 1982. Blood pressure during normal daily activities, sleep, and exercise. *Journal of the American Medical Association*, 247: 992–996.

Schoenberger, J. A., Stamler, J., Shekelle, R. B., and Shekelle, S. 1972. Current status of hypertension control in industrial populations. *Journal of the American Medical Association*, 222: 559.

Seer, P. and Raeburn, J. M. 1980. Medication training and essential hypertension: A methodological study. *Journal of Behavioral Medicine*, 3: 59–71.

Shapiro, M., Bleho, J., Curran, M., Farrell, K., Klein, D., Weigensberg, A., and Weil, K. 1978. Problems in the control of hypertension in the community. *Canadian Medical Association Journal*, 118: 37.

Sokolow, M., Werdegar, D., Kain, H. K., and Hinman, A.T. 1966. Relationships between level of blood pressure measured casually and by portable recorders and severity of complications in essential hypertension. *Circulation*, 34: 279–298.

Southam, M. A., Agras, W. S., Taylor, C. B., and Kraemer, H. C. 1982. Relaxation training: Blood pressure lowering during the working day. *Archives of General Psychiatry*, 39: 715–717.

Taylor, C. B., Agras, W. S., Schneider, J. A., and Allen, R. A. 1983. Adherence to instructions to practice relaxation exercises. *Journal of Consulting and Clinical Psychology*, 51: 952–953.

Wadden, R. A., Luborsky, L., Greer, S., and Crits-Christoph, P. 1984. The behavioral treatment of essential hypertension: An update and comparison with pharmacological treatment. *Clinical Psychology Review*, 4: 403–429.

10 *Neuroendocrine effects of work stress*

Robert M. Rose

INTRODUCTION

Over the past quarter of a century there has been increasing interest in what might be referred to as the psychoendocrinology of everyday life. It is now well established that the psychological and social environment of individuals not only can function to stress the individual's adaptive capacity, but also in this context provokes a variety of changes in endocrine secretion. Before embarking on a review of the endocrine effects of work stress, it is important to attempt to clarify two areas. The first relates to operational definitions of stress. The second relates to clarifying and reviewing some of our knowledge relating to the effects of stress in general on endocrine function. It is then possible to focus more specifically on how stress at work may function to alter endocrine activity.

Although many workers in the field have attempted to review the physiology of stress without using the word "stress," it turns out that this is even more cumbersome than the various definitions that abound regarding stress. Stress as a word is used essentially in three overlapping connotations. The first relates to the characteristics of the environment as in speaking of "a stressful event" or "stressful environment." In Selye's (1976) terms, these are referred to as *stressors*. The second definition relates to the use of the word "stress" to define the responses of the individual—either endocrine, cardiovascular, other physiological or psychological responses. This is in the context of the individual being *stressed*. Those workers who consider the fit of an individual in his environment refer to these responses as the individual being under *strain* rather than being stressed. The third definition of stress, and the one that I prefer, refers to the field of stress research in general. It encompasses the characteristics of the environment, the responses of the individual, and those factors that mediate or modify those responses—all subsumed under the concept of stress. The difficulties or confusion relating to stress often arise because we refer to the individual being stressed or the environment being stressful, without really knowing if this is so. Thus we confuse by failing to ask the question; instead we just claim that it is indeed a fact. For a more detailed and in-depth discussion of these definitional issues of stress, especially as related to its possible importance as risk for illness, the reader is referred to a recent review by Martin (1984).

For the purposes of this chapter, it will be important for us to attempt to clarify what aspects of the work environment may potentially function as specific stressors as measured by endocrine responses (Szabo, Maull, and Pirie, 1983). Although we do have some information about this, it is far from clear in many situations what are the most difficult aspects of the work environment or that which is most stressful.

It is not possible to provide a comprehensive overview on the endocrinology of stress. The reader is referred to two recent reviews that attempt to summarize the available information (Rose, 1980; Rose, 1984).

One major conclusion from stress research in both animals and man is that our knowledge is most complete about the endocrine responses to *acute* or *novel* events. Most experiments have focused on what happens when individuals are exposed to events that are unfamiliar, usually involving some aspect of threat or challenge and in which they are obliged to participate or perform. What emerges is that much of the stressor effect of these stimuli relates to these characteristics of novelty or unfamiliarity. What appears less relevant is the nature of specific task and, more relevant, the degree to which it has been encountered previously. Thus we find that when individuals are required to perform physical exercise that is unfamiliar to them, it exerts a more provocative effect on a number of endocrine systems, compared to the effect seen in experienced athletes.

One of the most impressive phenomena that emerge from study of individuals who are exposed initially to various challenging stimuli is that there is generally an adaptation of the endocrine response. This adaptation is not a product of the inability of the endocrine system to respond because of exhaustion or fatigue, but rather the stimulus loses its novel, threatening, or challenging characteristics. If a new stimulus is substituted or the endocrine system is stimulated directly by the appropriate hormones controlling the secretion of peripheral endocrine organs (upstream in the chain of control), the endocrine gland is capable of responding. Thus it is not physiological adaptation or inability to respond further, but rather the consequence of a change in perception in altering the endocrine responses to repeated stimuli. These issues have great relevance in attempting to understand the potential effects of work stress on endocrine systems. Therefore it is crucial to understand the degree to which a stimulus is novel in assessing its potential stressful qualities as opposed to more specific aspects of work itself; for example, increased energy expenditure relating to changes in tasks or increased demand for performance as a potential stressor. One exception to this may relate to the effects of *chronic* stressors, which have not been well studied and will be discussed later in this chapter. However, novelty has been demonstrated to be such an important factor in any given stimulus that it must be kept constantly in mind when evaluating putative work stress.

There is now ample evidence that many endocrine systems are capable of being stimulated and affected by various psychosocial stressors. We now know that there are a number of specific peptides elaborated in the brain that control the secretion of hormones from the pituitary gland. These changes in the pituitary secretion also lead to changes in the other endocrine glands such as the thyroid, gonads, adrenal cortex, and so on. Most psychoendocrine research, until most recently, and certainly most research on the endocrine effects of work stress, have focused primarily on two major systems. One relates to the hypothalamic-pituitary-adrenal cortical system evaluated by the changes in cortisol in humans and other primates or in corticosterone in rodents. The other system relates to the changes in the catecholamines or epinephrine and norepinephrine, also known as adrenaline and noradrenaline. The adrenal medulla secretes most of the epinephrine that circulates in the body, while most norepinephrine comes from the sympathetic nerve endings located throughout the body. Both epinephrine and norepinephrine are potent hormones and it has been known for a long time that they exert a major influence on a variety of bodily functions such as heart rate and blood pressure, and induce sensations of anxiety or discomfort. Although there have been an increasing number of reports of the changes in other hormones such as growth hormone or prolactin, there is relatively little research available on the effect of work on these or other endocrine products. Also, although stress has been clearly shown to effect gonadal hormones (in males, testosterone, and in females, estrogen and progesterone), there are very few reports in the literature on the effects of potential work stress on these gonadal steroids. There is also a recent and growing literature on the effects of stress on various peptides found in the brain known as endorphins and enkephalins, but these also have yet to be studied systematically in individuals subjected to various changes in their work environment. Consequently, this chapter will focus primarily on the collected data that have been studying either the pituitary adrenal cortical system or the catecholamine system measuring epinephrine and norepinephrine.

CATECHOLAMINES

Psychoendocrinology really began with Cannon's investigations of the changes in catecholamines in animals exposed to a variety of stressful stimuli. Catecholamines change very rapidly and very significant elevations, up to tenfold increases, can be observed within a few minutes following exposure to provocative stimuli. It is a very easily perturbed system and responds to a large variety of stimuli, in addition to stressful events, including changes in posture when individuals stand from the lying or sitting position. Also changes in catecholamines appear to be relatively nonspecific. That is to say, a large number of changes in the environment seem to be capable of provoking changes in catecholamines. Thus we know that playing a card game, watching an interesting movie, carrying out mental arithmetic tasks, being bored, or having to do repetitive tasks have been shown to be provocative of catecholamine changes (Frankenhaeuser, 1980). Catecholamines are thus easily perturbed and can be found to change rapidly even with pleasurable stimuli (certainly with intense pleasurable stimuli as has been observed during sexual intercourse and orgasm) (Weideking, Lake, and Zeigler, 1977). Catecholamines may be viewed as hormones of vigilance, attention, or involvement. When individuals are *interacting* more intensely with their environment, either positively or negatively, there seems to be an increase in catecholamines.

Early research relied primarily on measuring urinary catecholamines by relatively difficult fluorometric techniques. More recent research involving the use of newer assay techniques has permitted the measurement of catecholamines in the plasma rather than in the urine. Urinary catecholamines are difficult to interpret because individuals differ in how they metabolize the hormone in the blood. Therefore, a given level of epinephrine in the urine may reflect varying blood levels.

Frankenhaeuser and her colleagues at the Karolinska Institute have been pioneers in the study of catecholamine responses in individuals exposed to a wide variety of tasks, work conditions, and other psychological manipulations (Frankenhaeuser, 1979; Frobert et al., 1970). They have concluded that conditions that are characterized by novelty or unpredictability are usually associated with rises in epinephrine and norepinephrine. When the individuals were observed to gain control over a particular task, epinephrine levels fell, but norepinephrine appears still to remain elevated. This is consistent with the explanation that norepinephrine secretion appears more related to paying attention, the necessity for vigilance, or whether or not the individual anticipates that significant effort be expended in performing any given task. These conclusions are also certainly consistent with our understanding of the autonomic sympathetic nervous system being involved in regulating the degree of preparation or need for preparedness, priming the organism to act, so to speak.

Epinephrine appears to be a relatively sensitive index of the degree of discomfort that individuals experience independent of work output. It has been recorded that when passengers had to crowd on a train car at a time when there was a gasoline shortage, there was a relatively close correspondence between their epinephrine level and the total number of passengers per car (Lundberg, 1976). A similar finding was made in individuals who were asked to perform tasks in the context of loud distracting noises. They had significantly elevated adrenaline and noradrenaline excretion when the noise was louder (Lundberg and Frankenhaeuser, 1978).

When individuals are asked to work for a prolonged period of time without sleep, there is also evidence that they have increased levels of adrenaline and noradrenaline excretion following their period of sleeplessness. Sleeplessness itself also appears to be associated with increased catecholamine excretion. These findings could be explained by both the influence of novelty or unfamiliarity combined with the phenomena of having to perform work following the period of sleeplessness (Kalimo et al., 1980).

Paramedics were studied on the days that they had to work compared to the days they stayed at home (Dutton et al., 1978). Although there were no differences in cortisol, which we will discuss later, there were statistically different higher levels of epinephrine on the day that they were working compared to the day that they were off. Similarly, it has also been reported (Frankenhaeuser, 1979) that when Scandinavian workers were asked to work overtime, there was a significant increase of adrenaline excretion in the evening, which rose progressively as the number of the weeks of overtime grew toward ten. Again this is a combination of some novelty as well as increased work demand. The Scandinavian workers also report that when workers have to deal with significant repetitiveness of work tasks, increased amount of physical constraint while working, or loss of control of the pace of work there is an associated increase in both adrenaline and noradrenaline excretion. There also appears to be an increased catecholamine excretion when job demands are high and reported feelings of well-being are low.

Consequences of work also have been shown to affect urinary adrenaline and noradrenaline. Timio and Gentili (1976) showed that both these catecholamines were significantly elevated when the method of pay for work was changed. When individuals were paid by piecework compared to salary, there was a significant increase in adrenaline and noradrenaline excretion. This was regardless of whether or not they started out with piecework and went to salary or started at salary and went to piecework. The study would argue that it was not just the novelty of changing but rather the consequences of the change—that is, the means by which they were paid for their work. It also, however, must be pointed out that there might be some uncertainty as to whether or not they would receive adequate compensation when they had to be paid for piecework as opposed to by salary, along with the accompanying distress of the change in means of being paid for their efforts.

Urinary excretions of catecholamines have also been shown to correlate significantly with energy output. In a careful study of 14 fishermen engaged in offshore fishing, Astrand et al. (1973) reported that the fishermen's working daily average energy expenditure was about 40 percent of the maximum with peaks up to 80 percent. They found that on the average there was a tenfold increase in epinephrine and a fourfold increase in norepinephrine observed during work as compared with resting values.

In summary, it appears that catecholamines are a rather sensitive index to potential work stress. However, although they are quite sensitive, they are relatively nonspecific in nature. That is to say, a variety of conditions appear to be able to perturb the catecholamine system. These include feelings of irritation, increased physical expenditure of work, uncertainty, increased boredom, increased expectation, or arousal. They may be considered as indexes of both engagement and involvement in tasks, the amount of vigilance or connectedness experienced, as well as reflecting feelings of any distress or dysphoria. It is not clear from the studies that have been done whether or not chronic work stress leads to any alterations in catecholamines as opposed to acute work stress. For example, we do not know whether or not individuals who are exposed to discomforting or unpleasant work environments, or ones in which individuals would describe themselves as chronically hassled, are associated with continued elevations of catecholamines.

CORTISOL

Our appreciation of the sensitivity of the hypothalamic pituitary adrenal cortical system to changes in the environment had its origins with Hans Selye, who was one of the first investigators to show that adrenal cortical activity increased significantly with a variety of stressors. Subsequently, Mason (1975) in reviewing Selye's work has pointed out that much of the similarity of cortisol responsiveness relates to the *psychological* aspects of a variety of stressors, such as heat, cold, hunger, and such. When appropriate controls are utilized, it is apparent that the major stimulating effect on cortisol secretion is the magnitude of discomfiture, novelty, or threat, which animals or humans experience in responding to stressful events.

Early research in studying cortisol responses to stress, similar to catecholamines, focused on a wide variety of stiuations including surgery, examinations, and exercise (Rose, 1980). Although not as liable as catecholamines, cortisol was found to be responsive to a variety of different environmental challenges. However, it became clear that individuals differed significantly in terms of their responses to these potentially stressful events. It was possible, therefore, to predict which parents of children dying from leukemia had increased cortisol activity during the course of the child's often terminal illness (Wolff et al., 1964). It was also possible to predict which young men inducted into the army and undergoing basic combat training had increased levels of adrenal cortical activity during this experience by observing and talking with the men (Rose, Poe, and Mason, 1968). What emerged from these studies in which individual responses were predicted was that the individual's appraisal of the degree of novelty, threat, or discomfiture was the major factor of determining their cortisol levels. It also is apparent from studies over the last several years that an individual's *anticipation* of difficult events can be as stressful or provocative a stimulus as the event itself. Thus Czeisler et al. (1976) studied plasma cortisol every 20 minutes in patients the day prior to their elective coronary-artery bypass surgery. When patients were undergoing preoperative surgical preparation, when their chest was scrubbed in the evening prior to their surgery when cortisol is usually low, there were huge increases during this period of time, secondary to the anticipatory response this preparation evoked.

As noted earlier, prolonged exercise is also associated with increased cortisol levels, similar to that found for catecholamines. However, individuals anticipating exhausting exercise showed significant rises in cortisol, many with levels comparable to that seen actually during the exercise itself. Individuals anticipating the fact that they had to move from where they were living were also found to have increased cortisol levels prior to the move (Kral, Grad, and Berenson, 1968), thus reinforcing the importance of anticipation as a stressful stimulus. Despite the fact that individuals may have significant anticipatory responses to a negative or feared event, and despite the fact that individuals have significantly different responses to a potential stressor like being inducted into the Army, it is clear that individuals *adapt* to stressful events.

An event as potentially stressful as learning how to parachute jump is associated with rapid adaptation. By the third or fourth jump, cortisol levels are back to normal (Ursin, Baade, and Levine, 1978). Parenthetically, catecholamines, as one might expect, tend to remain elevated for a longer time.

In general, when individuals have been studied following repeated exposure to a once-stressful stimulus, it is interesting how rapidly adaptation occurs. This was the case, for example, with students taking examinations (Bridges and Jones, 1967), or pilots landing on an aircraft carrier as part of a training course (Miller et al., 1970). It also was found to develop in helicopter medics in Viet Nam when one compared their flying days to nonflying days. These individuals had been flying, picking up wounded men, for many months at the time they were studied (Bourne, Rose, and Mason, 1967). Cullen, Fuller, and Dolphin (1979) found no increase in cortisol in experienced truck drivers when they had a particularly hard driving day of over 11 hours compared to a day of less time and less difficulty. Paramedics who showed increased epinephrine activities on the day worked compared to the days off failed to show increased cortisol activities on the work days (Dutton et al., 1978).

Because of the importance of work stress in altering endocrine activity and the possibility of endocrine activity reflecting significant individual differences in response to potential work stress, we had the opportunity to follow a group of 400 air traffic controllers over several years at work. The next section of this chapter discusses the nature of this research and the findings that were made.

AIR TRAFFIC CONTROLLER STUDY

The Air Traffic Controller Health Change Study was a five-year project sponsored by the Federal Aviation Administration to study a group of approximately 400 air traffic controllers (Rose, Jenkins, and Hurst, 1978). A large number of variables were included, including changes in physical health, psychological well-being, as well as psychiatric symptomatology. A number of predictor or independent variables were also assessed including years of experience, type of facility worked, attitude toward work, ratings of competence as an air traffic controller, family supports, and blood pressure and endocrine responses at work.

The endocrine responses at work were performed by observing men on several different days for a five-hour period of time while they had a blood-collecting device attached. Blood samples were collected every 20 minutes, and cortisol values were measured in these samples (Rose et al., 1982a). At the same time the blood samples were collected, the technicians recorded the amount of work they were performing, including the number of planes with which they were working, whether the planes were descending or climbing, the nature of the sector where the air traffic controller worked, his behavior at the time of the sample, and so on (Hurst and Rose, 1978). Other measures included assessment of mood when they came to work as well as any subjected difficulties they experienced during the course of their day at work. This was a comprehensive study and when one counts observations also performed when blood pressure was measured, more than 40,000 observations were made.

The analyses of the endocrine responses to work were based primarily on 201 men who were studied three or more days during a three-year period. The cortisol values were measured in 20-minute integrated samples. Total area was calculated for the entire period of time. Peak episodes were calculated when the cortisol increased more than 2 μg/dl (Rose et al., 1982a).

We were interested in evaluating which work-related variables were significantly changed when the individual had a high cortisol day versus a low cortisol day (Rose et al., 1982b). Each man was compared with himself (ipsative). The results are shown in Table 10.1. Low and high cortisol day were defined in terms of the average cortisol for that day, controlling for time of day the diurinal samples were collected—that is, the tendency for cortisol to fall during the day as a result of diurinal variation.

It is clear that the amount of work performed as defined by manwork, a variable incorporating the time spent on position, amount of work, and so on, was not very much higher on the high cortisol day (494.4 versus 502.2). There was a significant difference in the average behavior ratings between the high and low day. Although elevated on the high day, it was only a small change (2.6 versus 2.7). Individuals who had a recent change in sleep had significantly different cortisol levels replicating the well-known

Table 10.1. Objective work-related variables during high versus low days ordered by cortisol secretion comparing each man with himself (ipsative)

	n	Low Day	High Day	t	p
Average cortisol-defining variable	201	92.1	108.9	27.90	0.0001*
Work Variable					
Manwork	195	494.4	502.2	1.70	0.05*
Paceload	195	44.3	47.3	1.57	0.05 < p 10*
Total times on position	195	9.00	9.04	0.20	NS
Average behavior rating	195	2.6	2.7	2.60	0.005*
Days since midnight shift	90	6.0	5.9	0.62	NS
Days since sleep cycle change	89	3.4	2.9	2.29	0.02**
Days off ≥ 48 hr	86	2.7	2.3	2.41	0.02**
Cortisol peak area-defining variable	201	92.0	109.6	26.7	0.0001*
Work Variable					
Manwork	196	492.2	502.8	2.38	0.01*
Paceload	196	44.6	47.3	1.56	0.05 < p 01*

Source: Compiled by the author.

*p value by directional test.

**p value by nondirectional test.

Note. The values expressed for cortisol are residual scores, adjusted for time of day, rescaled to a mean of 100 with a standard deviation of 10.

observation of changes in sleep on cortisol secretion. Similar findings were found for cortisol peak area as were found for cortisol area.

Figure 10.1 shows the relationship of work to plasma cortisol. Although on the average plasma cortisol clearly increases with increasing work, it is not true that those with the largest increase in work showed the largest increase in cortisol. In the bottom panel of the figure, the men were divided into three groups; those with a small, middle, or large increase in work. Average cortisol values for each group are shown on the top panel. Those who had a moderate increase in work had the largest increase in cortisol.

Figure 10.1. Relationship of work to plasma cortisol. Although cortisol increases with increasing work on the average, those with the largest increase in work do not show the largest increase in cortisol

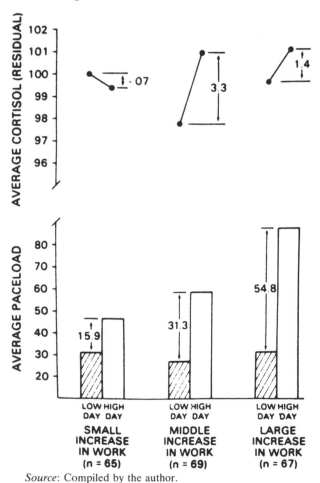

We were also interested in observing whether subjective work-related variables were changed when individuals had higher cortisol levels. These results are shown in Table 10.2.

Scores on the subjective difficulty questionnaire, which asked men about any difficulties with mechanical equipment, or difficulties in communicating with pilots, and so on, were significantly higher on the high cortisol day than the low cortisol day. The psychological response to work, which is based on the subjective difficulty questionnaire, but factoring out the amount of work, is also higher on the high cortisol day. Individuals also tended to report more frequent feelings of being blue or down, that is, on the Profile of Mood States (POMS) depression scale, on the high cortisol day.

We also utilized one final strategy to analyze the relationship between cortisol and work. In this analysis we selected only men who had experienced a substantial change in work over the three times they were studied. The previous analyses could be criticized in that although men were studied three times, this was really not often enough to evaluate any effect of substantial increases in the work load. For this analysis, we selected 75 men out of the larger sample of 201 only if on one of the three days work increased by at least 70 percent over the average of the other two days. The 75 men who fulfilled this criterion were divided into three groups of 25 each based on the relationship between their cortisol levels and work load. A responder group was defined as those who showed a parallel increase in cortisol when work increased. The two other groups showed either no change in cortisol or an actual fall in cortisol when work increased. We again looked for variables that would discriminate these responders from the other two groups. Neither years of experience as a controller nor age discriminated between the three groups, nor did the responders perform more or less work over the course of the entire three years. The responders did not show more behavior arousal at work nor did they report more subjective difficulty.

However, we did find that there were several psychological variables that did discriminate this responder group from the other two. Responders were judged to be more *technically competent* by their peers. The responders were nominated a total of 2.3 times compared to being nominated only 1.4 times for individuals in the other two groups, ANOVA, F = 6.5, p < .01. Responders also reported greater work satisfaction and less frequent life change events. They also claimed their supervisor provided them more freedom at work.

Thus, the men who showed an *increase* in cortisol to increasing work appeared to be psychologically different from the others, but not in the direction we anticipated. Rather than being more dissatisfied or less competent, they reported themselves as more satisfied and regarded by their peers as more competent.

Table 10.2.   Subjective work-related variables during high versus low days ordered by cortisol responses comparing each man with himself (ipsative)

	n	Low Day	High Day	t	p
Average cortisol-defining variable	201	92.1	108.9	27.90	0.0001*
Work Variable					
Subjective difficulty	195	21.2	22.8	2.60	0.01*
Psychological response to work	195	99.8	101.6	1.94	0.05*
Total personal comments	201	0.06	0.19	1.80	0.05*
POMS depression	200	39.8	40.5	2.48	0.02**
POMS fatigue	200	39.4	40.5	1.89	0.10**
POMS vigor	198	50.4	48.9	1.86	0.10**

Source: Compiled by the author.
*p value by directional test.
**p value by nondirectional test.
Note. The values expressed for cortisol are residual scores, adjusted for time of day, rescaled to a mean of 100 with a standard deviation of 10.

Table 10.3. Average endocrine activity comparing men with varying frequencies of physical illness

	Total n	<1 Episode Per Year	1–2.5 Episodes Per Year	2.6–4.9 Episodes Per Year	5+ Episodes Per Year	F	p
Average annual illness							
Average cortisol	197	101.5 (42)*	101.5 (55)	100.0 (61)	96.7 (34)	4.69	.0039
Any average cortisol	327	102.2 (68)	101.2 (98)	99.8 (106)	97.3 (55)	5.95	.0009
Average growth hormone	243	101.6 (53)	99.6 (68)	99.5 (79)	99.6 (43)	0.85	NS

	Total n	0 Episodes Per Year	<1 Episode Per Year	1–1.9 Episodes Per Year	2+ Episodes Per Year	F	p
Acute respiratory							
Average cortisol	197	101.6 (43)	100.8 (62)	99.2 (39)	98.8 (53)	1.75	NS
Any average cortisol	327	102.1 (78)	101.0 (97)	99.3 (72)	98.6 (80)	4.16	.0068
Injuries							
Average cortisol	197	100.9 (128)	99.5 (40)	97.2 (29)	—	3.66	.0267
Any average cortisol	327	101.0 (214)	99.4 (65)	98.5 (48)	—	3.10	.0451
Acute GI							
Average cortisol	197	100.8 (88)	100.2 (71)	98.2 (38)	—	1.86	NS
Any average cortisol	327	101.3 (164)	100.3 (108)	97.3 (55)	—	6.96	.0015

Source: Compiled by the author.

*Parenthetical values are sample size.

Note. The values expressed for cortisol and growth hormone are residual scores, adjusting for time of day, rescaled to a mean of 100 and show a standard deviation of 10.

As a part of the Air Traffic Controller Health Change Study, we measured health changes, assessed by monthly diaries as well as by the individuals coming for physical and laboratory examinations on the average of every nine months, a total of five times during the course of the study. We were interested in determining if there was any relationship between cortisol responses to work and the frequency of health problems among the air traffic controllers.

As has often been observed in groups of generally healthy men (ATC's are screened yearly for health problems), the most prevalent illness episodes relate to upper respiratory infections. However, we did measure all episodes of physical illness throughout the course of the study (Rose et al., 1982c). The relationship between average cortisol and frequency of physical illness is shown in Table 10.3. The men are divided into four groups: those with infrequent episodes (less than 1 per year), those with intermediate numbers of episodes (two groups—1–2.5 per year and 2.6–4.9 per year), and those with the greatest number of episodes (5 or more). Of the 201 men who were studied three or more times, we had frequency of illness data for 197. These are shown in the first line in the table. It is apparent from this that those with the most frequent episodes had the *lowest* amount of cortisol. When we looked at the larger sample of men—the 327 on whom we measured cortisol at work at least once—the same findings were obtained. Those with the lowest cortisol tended to have the most frequent illness episodes. This relationship appears to hold for various kinds of illness episodes, including acute respiratory illnesses, injuries, and acute gastrointestinal disturbances. We also looked at whether the individuals who were defined as responders also showed any differences with respect to illness frequency. The findings were consistent. Individuals whose cortisol decreased when work increased had the highest amount of health episodes compared to the others (4.22 annual events versus 2.82 for those whose cortisol increased or stayed the same when work increased, $F = 4.65$, $p < .01$).

DISCUSSION

Our findings strongly support the interpretation that the hypothalamic pituitary adrenal cortical system does adapt to stressful stimuli and, therefore, we found that most of the time cortisol increased only slightly with increasing work load. We also found that men who showed a significant increase in cortisol as work increased (the responders) were not more distressed, less competent, or more dissatisfied. The responders were judged by their peers to be more competent; they described themselves as more satisfied with their jobs. The responders also interestingly enough did not show more health change, but less frequent illness episodes. It is also true that those who had higher cortisols at work did not show more health change, but those who had the lowest cortisol for any given level of work tended to have more minor health problems. It is noted that these findings are somewhat opposite than expectation. That is, those with higher cortisol levels at work might be interpreted as being chronically stressed, which would lead to greater frequency of illnesses.

One interpretation of the unexpected findings is that these responders were men who when subjected to greater work load remained more engaged or involved in their work. This increased engagement, as described by Singer (1974), occurs in individuals who are more highly invested in what they do. This enhanced investment might be associated with higher cortisol levels. It should be noted that while we are talking about higher versus lower cortisols, we are talking about relatively small differences and these are not levels of hormonal increase we see when people are exposed to very intense, threatening, or challenging situations (Rose et al., 1982a). It is as if the individuals with higher cortisol levels tended to be somewhat more aroused or connected compared to the others, and this arousal may exert a positive effect on health.

These findings have been partially replicated recently in another population in which endocrine samples were taken from a group of surgeons while they were performing cardiothoracic surgery. Payne et al., (1984) have found that on the days individuals reported experiencing more stress their cortisol was elevated, but this was not accounted for by differences in the level of experience. Rather, the investigators found that those surgeons who had the greatest length of experience had the highest cortisol level ($r = .96$, $p < .005$). The authors concluded that those who were highly trained, had a demanding job, but were very invested and liked what they did had higher cortisol. They hypothesized that perhaps the high cortisol was reflective of an increased physiological toll. However, at least if one can extrapolate from the air traffic controller studies, higher cortisol at work did not necessarily predict increased amounts of health change.

CONCLUSIONS

The results suggest that there are no simple or obvious conclusions about the neuroendocrine effects of work stress. It is likely that challenging work situations, especially those that demand that when work load is externally placed, and one has little control over the work environment, there is more evidence of job stress. From the measurements of catecholamines, it is apparent that a wide number of variables that include not only novelty but also vigilance and arousal in general are associated with increased levels of epinephrine and norepinephrine. Cortisol tends to adapt rapidly to changes in the work situation as it does to other potential stressors.

Earlier workers believed that the amount of physiological cost of work could be measured by assessing the classical stress hormones, cortisol and catecholamines. Our results with air traffic controllers indicated that higher cortisol is not necessarily associated with increased amounts of illness. Indeed, individuals who tended to have higher cortisol levels in a work situation to which they were well adapted appeared to have been more invested and involved in work and had more positive attitudes toward work than those who had lower levels. Whether this will be replicated by other studies is not clear, but it raises some interesting questions.

It may well be that a certain amount of challenge or stimulation is important at work, and this may be reflected by higher levels of cortisol or catecholamines. Too much stimulation or too much challenge obviously is disruptive of behavior. We do not know what the best measures of the long-term physiological cost of work stress are, as the studies in the literature do not provide us information about this. We have no "stress hormone" that provides us insight in terms of the amount of wear and tear from work stress and from which we can infer that when levels go up the individual has a higher risk for future illness.

Our results suggest that individuals who were active and busily engaged in work and who report a challenge but not a sense of being threatened or overwhelmed are better described as *engaged* rather than *stressed* and this appears to reflect a desirable state of affairs.

REFERENCES

Astrand, I., Fugelli, P., Karlsson, C.G., Rodahl, K., and Vokac, Z. 1973. Energy output and work stress in coastal fishing. *Scandinavian Journal of Clinical Laboratory Investigation*, 31 (1): 105–113.

Bourne, P.G., Rose, R. M., and Mason, J. W. 1967. Urinary 17–OHCS levels. Data on seven helicopter ambulance medics in combat. *Archives of General Psychiatry*, 17: 104–110.

Bridges, P. K. and Jones, M. T. 1967. Personality, physique and the adrenocortical response to a psychological stress. *British Journal of Psychiatry*, 113: 601–605.

Cullen, J., Fuller, R., and Dolphin, C. 1979. Endocrine stress responses of drivers in a "real-life" heavy-goods vehicle driving task. *Psychoneuroendocrinology*, 4: 107–115.

Czeisler, C. A., Moore Ede, M. C., Regestein, Q. R., Kisch, E. S., Fang, V.S., and Ehrlich, E. N. 1976. Episodic 24-hour cortisol secretory patterns in patients awaiting elective cardiac surgery. *Journal of Clinical Endocrinology and Metabolism*, 42 (2): 273–283.

Dutton, L. M., Smokensky, M. H., Leach, C.S., Lorimor, R., and Hsi, B. P. 1978. Stress levels of ambulance paramedics and fire fighters. *Journal of Occupational Medicine*, 20 (2): 111–115.

Frankenhaeuser, M. 1979. Psychoneuroendocrine approaches to the study of emotion as related to stress and coping. In H. E. Howe and R. A.

Dienstbier (Eds.). *Nebraska Symposium on Motivation 1978*: 123–161. Lincoln: University of Nebraska Press.

―――. 1980. Psychobiological aspects of life stress. In S. Levine and H. Ursin (Eds.). *Coping and Health*. New York: Plenum Press.

Froberg, J., Karlsson, C. G., Levi, L., Lidberg, L., and Seeman, K. 1970. Conditions of work: psychological and endocrine stress reactions. *Archives of Environmental Health*, 21: 789–797.

Hurst, M. W. and Rose, R. M. 1978. Objective workload and behavioral response in airport radar control rooms. *Ergonomics* 21 (7): 559–565.

Kalimo, R., Lehtonen, A., Daleva, M., and Kuorinka, I. 1980. Psychological and biochemical strain in firemen's work. *Scandinavian Journal of Work and Environmental Health*, 6: 179–187.

Kral, V. A., Grad, B., and Berenson, J. 1968. Stress reactions resulting from the relocation of an aged population. *Canadian Psychiatric Association Journal*, 13 (3): 201–209.

Lundberg, U. 1976. Urban commuting: crowdedness and catecholamine excretion. *Journal of Human Stress*, 2: 26–32.

Lundberg, U. and Frankenhaeuser, M. 1978. Psychophysiological reactions to noise as modified by personal control over noise intensity. *Biological Psychology*, 6: 51–59.

Martin, R. D. 1984. A critical review of the concept of stress in psychosomatic medicine. *Perspectives in Biology and Medicine*, 27 (3): 443–464.

Mason, J. W. 1975. A historical view of the stress field: part one. *Journal of Human Stress*, 1 (1): 6–12.

Miller, R. G., Rubin, R. T., Clark, B. R., Crawford, W. R., and Arthur, R. J. 1970. The stress of aircraft carrier landings. I. Corticosteroid responses in naval aviators. *Psychosomatic Medicine*, 32: 581–588.

Payne, R. L., Rick, T., Smith, G. H., and Cooper, R. G. 1984. Multiple indicators of stress in an 'active' job—cardiothoracic surgery. *Journal of Occupational Medicine*, 26 (11): 805–808.

Rose, R. M. 1980. Endocrine responses to stressful psychological events. *Psychiatric Clinics of North America*, 3 (2): 251–276.

―――. 1984. Overview of endocrinology of Stress. In S. H. Koslow and S. Reichlin (Eds.). *Neuroendocrinology and Psychiatric Disorder*: 95–122. New York: Raven Press.

Rose, R. M., Jenkins, C.D., and Hurst, M. W. 1978. *Air Traffic Controller Health Change Study*. Galveston: University of Texas Medical Branch Press.

Rose, R. M., Jenkins, C. D., Hurst, M., Livingston, L., and Hall, R. P. 1982a. Endocrine activity in air traffic controllers at work. I. Characterization of cortisol and growth hormone levels during the day. *Psychoneuroendocrinology,* 7 (2/3): 101–111.

Rose, R. M., Jenkins, C. D., Hurst, M., Herd, J. A., and Hall, R. P. 1982b. Endocrine activity in air traffic controllers at work. II. Biological, psychological and work correlates. *Psychoneuroendocrinology*, 7 (2/3): 113–123.

Rose, R. M., Jenkins, C. D., Hurst, M., Kreger, B. E., Barrett, J., and Hall, R. P. 1982c. Endocrine activity in air traffic controllers at work. III. Relationship to physical and psychiatric morbidity. *Psychoneuroendocrinology*, 7 (2/3): 125–134.

Rose, R. M., Poe, R. O., and Mason, J. W. 1968. Psychological state and body size as determinants of 17–OHCS excretion. *Archives of Internal Medicine*, 121: 406–413.

Selye, H. 1976. *The Stress of Life*, 2nd ed. New York: McGraw-Hill.

Singer, M. T. 1974. Engagement-involvement: a central phenomenon in psychophysiological research. *Psychosomatic Medicine*, 36: 1–17.

Szabo, S., Maull, E. A., and Pirie, J. 1983. Occupational stress: understanding, recognition and prevention. *Experientia*, 39 (10): 1057–1180.

Timio, M. and Gentili, S. 1976. Adrenosympathetic overactivity under conditions of work stress. *British Journal of Preventive and Social Medicine*, 30: 262–265.

Ursin, H., Baade, E., and Levine, S. 1978. *Psychobiology of Stress*. New York: Academic Press.

Wiedeking, C., Lake, C. R., and Ziegler, M. 1977. Plasma noradrenaline and dopamine-beta-hydroxylase during sexual activity. *Psychosomatic Medicine*, 39 (2): 143–148.

Wolff, C. T., Friedman, S. B., Hofer, M. A., and Mason, J. W. 1964. Relationship between psychological defenses and mean urinary 17–OHCS excretion rates: I. A predictive study of parents of fatally ill children. *Psychosomatic Medicine*, 26: 576.

III   *Prevention and intervention*

11 *Preventive stress intervention: a challenging area for researchers*

John M. Ivancevich

Stress has become a fashionable "buzz" word in the past decade, its popularity extending from press news releases to television documentaries to scientifically oriented books. Society in general has become increasingly concerned about the potential role of stress as it affects health, productivity, and the standard of living. Furthermore, stress has become recognized as a contributor in the pathogenesis of cardiovascular disorders and has been implicated in such work behaviors as absenteeism, accident frequency, tardiness, and sabotage. It is estimated that stress-related factors result in a productivity loss of over $100 billion annually in the United States. Although this productivity loss estimate has not been validated, there are few individuals who would claim that excessive and chronic stress is not costly. Furthermore, some experts suggest that up to 80 percent of all illness seen in physicians' offices is related to psychosocial stress (Suls and Sanders, 1982).

IMPLEMENTING STRESS MANAGEMENT INTERVENTIONS

Although there is general acknowledgement that stress plays a major role in everyday life, there is considerable debate and controversy when one attempts to obtain agreement on adopting an appropriate intervention strategy to manage stress within tolerable limits (Murphy, 1984; Sharit and Salvendy, 1982). Today neither researchers nor practitioners are able to establish a particular or universally applicable intervention approach that has a positive and lasting effect. Furthermore, there is little agreement on who is responsible for intervention—the company, the employee, the government, the union? There is also the issue of whether minimization or the reduction in stress can be quantified.

These and similar questions suggest that selecting and implementing stress management intervention programs is not yet based on a sound theoretical and empirical base. Therefore, stress intervention programs, although they are intuitively appealing, need to be subjected to rigorous empirical testing before they are embraced as a viable approach to improving the health and quality of life of Americans.

Preventive stress interventions are defined as a set of theoretically and empirically grounded activities and programs that are designed and implemented for the purpose of minimizing individual and organizational distress and its consequences. Certainly we know that there is such a phenomenon as "good" stress. However, in Part III we will direct our attention toward negative or what we assume to be "bad" stress. The notion of preventive intervention suggests that action can be taken to minimize the negative consequences of stress. The key initiators of action in organizational settings are managers and union leaders. From a managerial perspective, an organization has a responsibility for minimizing stress and contributing to employees' well being. Humanitarian responsibility for one's employees is a worthy endeavor that contemporary managers are beginning to accept and endorse publicly. Of course, another reason for management's interest in initiating prevention activities involves economic concerns. Sick, disabled, or expired employees cost money, training replacement time, and lost performance (Matteson and Ivancevich, 1982).

The union, in its role as the representative of members, has a responsibility to attempt to have working conditions, management practices, and collective bargaining agreements tailored to enhance the well-being of employees. Union leadership has accepted the responsibility of protecting members from exposure to the causes of disease, disability, or injury. Since stress has been implicated in such exposures, union leaders have openly raised questions about programs that must be implemented to control stress within tolerable limits.

OVERVIEW OF PREVENTIVE STRESS INTERVENTION CHAPTERS

Preventive stress intervention practices and responsibilities are highlighted in the six chapters in Part III. It is obvious that there is no one best preventive intervention that works in every situation, with all employees, and for extended periods of time (Davis et al., 1984; Fielding, 1984). In fact, there is no one theoretical framework that categorizes preventive stress intervention programs on the basis of costs, length of time, training methods, structural changes, and sampling procedures.

The one theme suggested by the six authors was that there is little research on which kind of intervention is effective. The lack of research is the result of (1) short-term views of a program; (2) constituencies who promote a particular intervention have a natural bias in favor of one particular approach; (3) poor company records of objective data that could be used to track the impact of preventive intervention over time; and (4) logistical and methodological difficulties in conducting valid research. These are not excuses that were used in the six chapters, but these are limiting facts that apply to each of the preventive interventions introduced by the experts. In straightforward terms, today we do not have enough well-grounded research evidence to indicate the strengths and weaknesses or the superiority of one preventive stress intervention program over another.

In Part III Rita Numerof presents team building as a viable intervention (Chapter 13). She offers team building as a way of improving relationships within and between groups so that the intensity of stressors can be reduced. A significant outcome of effective team building could be the creation of positively cohesive work groups that provide supportive reinforcement for members. Unfortunately, as is the case with most interventions, there is no empirical evidence that can be provided to accept or reject Dr. Numerof's suggestion. Since team building can be implemented with naturally occurring work groups, it should be tested as a viable intervention in field settings using repeated measures and time series research designs.

Richard S. DeFrank and Judith Pliner discuss the issues of job loss and outplacement services in Chapter 14. The notion that job loss can have lasting and short-term health, emotional, and psychological effects has been studied in numerous samples. As an attempt to buffer the potential effects of job loss, some organizations have implemented outplacement programs. The authors portray the steps and the process as well as the potential benefits of outplacement. Drs. DeFrank and Pliner indicate that potential benefits of outplacement have not been subjected to empirical testing.

Chapter 12 is by Michael T. Matteson. He calls attention to the importance of individual-organizational relationships in terms of health, psychological, and organizational consequences. Preventive actions are described that reduce the likelihood of negative stress and burnout that can result from poor individual-organizational relationships. Included in the suggestions are more effective socialization techniques and better recruit-ment–selection matching, providing realistic job previews. Unfortunately, the preventive measures for improving individual-organizational rela-tionships have not been comparatively or singularly tested. There are available, however, empirical studies on the effects of realistic job previews that offer implications for reducing stress (Wanous, 1980; Popovich and Wanous, 1982).

William W. Winpisinger presents a union leader's viewpoint of managing stress in Chapter 15. Environmental stressors that can disable and injure union members have been identified as being particularly troublesome by union researchers. Becoming aware of and doing something about the stress-health-environmental interaction is what the union will continue to investigate. Winpisinger emphasizes that the union and management need to become fully aware of the severity of stress so that negotiations and grievances can be settled in a way that makes the work environment safer for employees.

William B. Baum, E. J. Bernacki, and J. Alan Herd report on studies conducted in the firm that examined the relationship of job performance to exercise adherence (Chapter 16). The Tenneco-based studies include four job categories: management, professional, clerical, and other. These groups were placed in five exercise adherence groups: exercised more than two times per week, exercised one to two times per week, exercised less than one time per week, nonexerciser, and nonmember in the corporate fitness program. It was determined that a strong association was found between better-than-average performance and increasing exercise adherence. This type of evaluative research over a long time span is what is needed with any preventive intervention program.

Gilbert T. Adams, Jr. discusses the trends in compensation awards for stress disabled workers in Chapter 17. Claims for psychiatric injuries are increasing dramatically. These claims have for the most part implicated job stress as a contributor to health and quality of life problems. The potential sources of stress claimed in legal cases include requirements of the job, the organizational structure, nonwork factors, and career opportunities. The legal community is now asking managers to illustrate how they address dysfunctional stress at the workplace. Each jurisdiction interprets job stress a little differently and this has added to the confusion of attempting to develop a clear picture of the role stress plays. However, the message emanating from the courts is that some type of preventive program initiated by management would be a welcome step in the direction of correcting job stress problems.

CONCLUSION

In sum, the six chapters in Part III demonstrate that programmatic research efforts are badly needed to understand what benefits, if any, accrue from preventive actions. Preventive interventions have intuitive potential to reduce stress and its consequences. However, intuition is not acceptable when one is dealing with the career, the health, or the employment of individuals. More tightly crafted research should provide management, unions, individuals, and society with a clearer understanding of what preventive interventions can and cannot accomplish. It is hoped that the call for evaluative research on preventive stress intervention programs will stimulate significant research involvement.

REFERENCES

Davis, M. F., Rosenberg, K., Iverson, D. C., Vernon, T. M., and Bauer, J. 1984. Worksite health promotion in Colorado. *Public Health Reports*, 99: 538–543.

Fielding, J. E. 1984. Health promotion and disease prevention at the worksite. *Annual Review of Public Health*, 5: 237–265.

Matteson, M. T. and Ivancevich, J. M. 1982. *Managing Job Stress and Health*. New York: The Free Press.

Murphy, L. R. 1984. Occupational stress management: A review and appraisal. *Journal of Occupational Psychology*, 57: 1–15.

Popovich, P. and Wanous, J. P. 1982. The realistic job preview is a persuasive communication. *Academy of Management Review*, 7: 570–578.

Sharit, J. and Salvendy, G. 1982. Occupational stress: Review and appraisal. *Human Factors*, 24: 129–162.

Suls, J. and Sanders, G. (Eds.) 1982. *Social Psychology of Health and Illness*. Hinsdale, N.J.: Erlbaum.

Wanous, J. P. 1980. *Organizational Entry: Recruitment, Selection, and Socialization of Newcomers*. Reading, Mass.: Addison-Wesley.

12 Individual–organizational relationships: implications for preventing job stress and burnout

Michael T. Matteson

It has been suggested that the most remarkable fact about the word "stress" is that it has persisted and grown into such wide usage, although there is almost no agreement as to what it means (Ivancevich and Matteson, 1980). While what constitutes a proper definition of the term may be the subject of considerable debate, that stress is *real, pandemic* in nature, and exceedingly *costly* in both human and material terms is generally not seriously questioned by the growing number of professionals working in the area.

The distinction that is frequently made between work- and nonwork-related stress is, at best, an artificial one. Nonetheless, it is a distinction that will be made here because it allows us to focus on an extremely important area of human activity: work and work organizations. It is a fact of life that for the overwhelming majority of employed persons in this country, no other single activity or interest commands more of their time and energy than their work. Most of us, in fact, spend over 60 percent of our waking hours in some combination of getting ready for work, commuting to and from work, at work, and/or thinking about work. Not only do we spend a great deal of time at work, many of us find a substantial portion of our satisfaction and identity in our work. It is therefore not surprising that for many of us a substantial portion of the stress we experience in our lives is work-related.

SOME DEFINITIONS

It is the thesis of this chapter that much of the dysfunctional stress outcomes that are job- and work-environment–related can be prevented, minimized, or delayed, with the proper understanding of their etiology, coupled with judicious preventive maintenance on the part of both individuals and organizations. Before pursuing this, however, there are three key terms used in the chapter title that need to be operationally defined: stress, burnout, and individual-organizational relationships.

While there are a multitude of ways in which stress may be defined (see, for example, Lazarus, 1966; Weitz, 1970; Selye, 1974; and Cox, 1978), most definitions fall into one of three categories: stimulus definitions,

156

response definitions, or stimulus–response interaction definitions. Defining stress as the result of an interaction between the stimulus and response, between the environment and the person, would seem to offer the most realistic view of the dynamic nature of stress. It is such an interactional definition, or what is sometimes called a transactional view (Cox and Mackay, 1981), that will be used here. Thus, *stress is an adaptive response, mediated by individual characteristics, that is a consequence of any external action or event that places special demands upon a person.*

To only a slightly lesser extent than stress, the term "burnout" has been defined in many different ways. To some, in fact, the terms "stress" and "burnout" are interchangeable. To others, burnout is used to describe a condition of excessive or accumulated stress. That is, if stress is intensive enough, or of sufficient duration, burnout is what follows. Much of the research that has been done on burnout has focused on individuals in the human service professions, such as social workers, teachers, parole officers, physicians, and nurses (see, for example, Perlman and Hartman, 1982, for a review). This is probably a reflection of a definition of burnout that considers it to be a unique type of stress reaction experienced by people whose work requires extensive contact with other people (Jackson, 1984). Maslach (1976) identifies three basic aspects or stages of burnout: emotional exhaustion, feelings of depersonalization, and apathy or reduced personal accomplishment. For our purposes here, *burnout will be viewed as a possible response to prolonged stress, particularly likely to occur when the individual experiences a significant loss of satisfaction previously experienced or anticipated from the work situation.* While recognizing the role extensive human contact may play in the development of burnout, this is not viewed as a necessary condition for an individual to burn out.

If stress is defined in terms of a relationship between an individual and the environment, then work stress may be viewed as a consequence of the relationship between an individual and the work environment. Seen from this perspective, the concept of individual-organizational relationships is central to examining virtually any aspect of work related stress. *An individual-organizational relationship exists when there is any association or interaction between any aspect of the work environment and any aspect of the individual.* A central premise here is that this individual-organizational interaction is a major determinant of, among other outcomes, stress and that the quality of this relationship can be improved to the benefit of all concerned.

CONCEPTUALIZING INDIVIDUAL–ORGANIZATIONAL RELATIONSHIPS

There are numerous ways of conceptualizing an interactionist view of work stress. Perhaps the most frequently used and most fully developed is the notion of person-environment congruence or fit. Person-environment fit (P-E fit) theory has been developed over a number of years by several investigators associated directly or otherwise with the Institute for Social Research at the University of Michigan (see French, Rogers, and Cobb, 1974; Harrison, 1978, 1985; Caplan et al., 1980; Caplan, 1983). The foundation of the P-E fit model rests on descriptions of motivation offered by Lewin (1951) and Murray (1959).

The model makes a real distinction between *objective* P-E fit, which is the result of the degree of congruence between the work environment as it exists and the person as he or she really is, and *subjective* P-E fit, which is a function of how the person sees the objective environment and how they see themselves. According to P-E fit theory, it is subjective fit (or lack thereof) that is the major cause of dysfunctional stress reactions or strains.

The Michigan person-environment fit model focuses on two dimensions or types of fit. One type is the extent to which the work provides rewards that meet or match the person's needs. Rewards include both formal and informal, tangible and intangible. Misfit on this dimension reflects stress. For example, the job may provide too little security, insufficient money, or not enough recognition to meet the individual's needs or preferences. Presumably, the rewards may be in excessive supply as well, resulting in a mismatch. The second type of fit that is part of this model deals with the extent to which the individual's skills, abilities, and expertise match with the demands and requirements of the job. To the extent the individual's talents are insufficient for job demands or are underutilized by job requirements, the model predicts a state of stress, followed by strain and even illness. It should be noted that these two types of fit—needs-rewards and capabilities-requirements—are often related.

Another interactionist approach similar to the P-E fit model is that of Cox (1978) and Cox and MacKay (1981). They see stress as the result of a transaction between the individual and the environment. Specifically, stress arises when there is an imbalance between perceived demand and the person's perception of his or her ability to meet that demand. The model stresses the perceptual part of that process, emphasizing that the balance or imbalance that is important is not between actual demand and capability to meet it, but rather the balance or imbalance that results from the individual's cognitive appraisal of the demand-ability relationship. This is consistent with the emphasis placed in the Michigan model upon subjective fit.

While some of the components of the models are different and different terminology is applied, both the P-E fit model and the transactional model are similar in some very important aspects. Both see the important variables in stress to be the individual and the environment; both see stress as a function of the interaction of the two; and both view the key to stress control as being the improvement in the quality of that interaction, one by improving fit and the other by reducing imbalance.

Empirical support for this type of approach is not difficult to come by. Caplan and his associates (1980) looked at goodness of fit between people and their work environments along several dimensions, including the complexity of the work, the work load, and the amount of responsibility for other people. Not surprisingly, they found that not everyone experiences the same amount of stress with respect to these variables. What is of particular interest, however, is the manner in which these factors contribute to the individual's stress. For example, with respect to the amount of work load, people were asked to indicate how heavy their work load was (an organizational factor) as well as how heavy a work load they would personally prefer (an individual factor). Responses to neither of these questions were related to stress as strongly as was the difference, or lack of fit, between the two (how heavy was actual load versus how heavy was preferred load).

Findings such as these offer strong support for the notion that stress prevention efforts in organizations focusing on either individuals or environmental conditions are less effective than they might otherwise be if they looked at improving the quality of the interaction that takes place between the individual and the environment. Perhaps even more importantly, they suggest that a number of environment improvement programs that have been and still are touted as positive (that is, increasing satisfaction, and thus, by implication, reducing stress) are not necessarily going to have universal stress reduction effects. Job enlargement and job enrichment programs that increase job scope, and thus job complexity for all effected workers, will certainly change the degree of fit each worker experiences on this variable. No doubt the effect will be to improve fit for many; just as certainly, however, for others the level of fit will be reduced. The lesson here is that improvement of fit requires an individualized program.

While the person-environment fit model is a good one, reflecting a great deal of careful theory building and much empirical support, the idea of individual-organizational relationships may also offer a useful way of thinking about stress sources in organizations, and thus in implementing preventive actions and programs. The concept of individual-organizational relationships is broader than the P-E fit model, and includes a number of types of interaction between the person and the environment that fall outside those considered in traditional P-E fit theory. As one example, consider the notion of organizational climate or personality (Forehand and Gilmer, 1964), which relates to certain characteristics of the organization's philosophy or operating style and which may be observed in the way that an organization interacts with its employees. In this manner, organizations have been described as authoritarian, conservative, creative, supportive, and so on, in much the same way as individuals are frequently described. Thus the nature of the interplay between individual and organizational "personality" is a potentially important aspect of the overall individual-organizational relationship that may either contribute to or lessen employee stress.

Consideration of individual-organizational relationships is important when one considers the possible consequences of poor relationships, whether they be reflected in lack of fit, imbalance, or any other type of incongruency. The cost of ignoring poor relationships can be expressed in terms of physiological, behavioral, cognitive, or organizational effects. Before turning to a consideration of possible preventive actions to minimize these effects of poor relationships, two further examples of potentially important dimensions of individual-organizational relationships are worth noting.

Type A Individuals and Organizations

One of the more widely discussed and researched concepts relating to work, stress, and health is that of the coronary-prone or Type A behavior pattern (TABP). The TABP, first identified and described by a pair of cardiologists (Friedman and Rosenman, 1959, 1978) characterizes individuals who are hard-driving, competitive, striving to accomplish more and more in less and less time, and who exhibit a chronic impatience with people and situations they perceive as thwarting their attempts to maintain high levels of goal achievement. Type Bs, on the other hand, exhibit few, if any, of these characteristics. The TABP has been associated with a variety of negative consequences, foremost among them being an increased likelihood of developing coronary heart disease (see, for example, Friedman and Ulmer, 1984).

It has been suggested that just as individuals may be characterized as Type A or B, so also may organizations (Matteson and Ivancevich, 1982; Ivancevich and Matteson, 1984). Here, then we have a dimension along which both the individual and the organizational setting or environment may be described. There are several perspectives from which this aspect of the person-environment relationship may be viewed. One way would be to focus on the match between the person and the environment. Thus a Type A person would "match" or fit a Type A environment, as would a Type B person fit a Type B environment. Type A individuals in Type B environments and Type Bs in Type A environments would be mismatched or show lack of fit.

Another way would be to ask the individual to describe what his or her environment was like (in A and B terms) and then indicate what they would like it to be. The resulting difference would be the degree of fit, with the assumption being that no difference represented good fit, presumably a positive or desired state.

Both of these perspectives would result in less-than-desirable conclusions, however. In the first case it would be concluded, for example, that being a Type A in a Type A organization is better than being a Type A in a Type B organization. Based on a large sample of medical laboratory professionals, however, just the opposite is in fact the case. Type As in Type A environments, relative to those in Type B environments, report a significantly greater frequency of health complaints, higher stress levels, greater levels of job dissatisfaction, more work disruption because of health problems, and a greater number of psychiatric symptoms (Matteson and Ivancevich, 1982).

The foregoing points out the need (1) to broaden the scope of variables that are considered in looking at person-work interactions, and specifically to include the category of so-called personality variables; and (2) to think in terms of the quality of the relationship that exists between the person and the work situation, rather than more narrowly in terms of simple fit alone.

Expectations versus Reality

The second example of an important dimension of individual-organizational relationships deals with the issue of individual needs, values, and perception and the extent to which the job and larger work setting are consistent with these. An important part of virtually any person-environment fit model is the degree of congruence between a wide variety of individual needs and the organization's reward system. Similarly, the match between individual capabilities and job requirements is an equally important consideration in P-E fit models. What is being addressed here, however, is a particular set of need-reward and capability demand relationships that have to do with the extent that an individual's expectations regarding the job, the work environment, extrinsic and intrinsic payoffs, career and professional development and progression, and a host of related concerns match the actual reality of the chosen job and work situation.

The issue of the gap between a job holder's expectancies and the reality of the situation is not one of presence or absence, but of degree. It is unlikely that anyone has experienced complete congruence over a typical working life of 40 or more years. Rather, the issue relates to the depth and range of the disparity. Gaps of sufficient magnitude lead to what Kramer (1974) calls "reality shock" and may be associated with a variety of stress reactions and burnout. While reality shock may be a problem in virtually any profession/career/occupation to which the individual brings preconceived notions regarding roles, appropriate values and behavior, and anticipated sources of satisfaction, Kramer's focus was upon nurses and, specifically, why nurses leave the nursing profession. Jackson (1984: 98) summarizes the problem succinctly:

Nurses and others who enter human service professions are often strongly motivated by a concern for humanity and a desire to help people. Upon beginning their first job, they anticipate being able to make visible improvements in other people's lives and ... they also expect their contributions to be recognized as valuable. As any seasoned human service worker has discovered, the lofty expectations and goals they had as a novice were unrealistic. From the beginning they were doomed to failure if success meant achieving those naive goals.

As Appelbaum (1981) points out, reality shock is very real and will take its toll because of those who leave a profession as well as those who decide to retire on the job. The individuals experiencing reality shock, the organizations of which they are a part, and the client or customer they serve are all adversely affected by the situation.

In summary, the notion of individual-organizational relationships is offered as a way of viewing potential precursors of work-related stress and burnout. The individual-organizational relationship concept is somewhat broader than the more traditional person-environment fit models in that it includes a greater range of variables and does not necessitate measuring both the person variable and the work variable along the same dimension. The remainder of the chapter will focus on examples of what organizations can do to improve the quality of individual-organizational relationships. In so doing, emphasis will be placed upon actions to prevent poor relationships from developing, rather than healing current problems. Whether it be medicine or management, prevention is almost always easier, less costly, and more rewarding than a cure.

IMPROVING INDIVIDUAL–ORGANIZATIONAL RELATIONSHIPS

Preventive actions to reduce the likelihood of negative stress and burnout through improving individual-organizational relationships could be undertaken even prior to the individual joining the organization. The processes of recruitment and selection, for example, offer an early basis for maximizing the likelihood of obtaining positive relationships.

Recruitment Considerations

For a great many individuals the first few months in a new job with a new organization are particularly stressful as they struggle to learn the ropes, become accepted by others, make a positive contribution to organizational goals and objectives, and, very importantly, come to grips with the inevitable disappointments and gaps between personal expectations and organizational realities. The number and magnitude of such gaps, as well as the individual's ability to adapt, determine in large part the extent to which the individual-organization marriage will be a successful one or will be marked by frustration and conflict and ultimately divorce. The greater this gap, previously referred to as reality shock, the greater the likelihood of disenchantment, frustration, stress, lost potential, and turnover. Katz (1985) very perceptively argues that if organizational newcomers are given more accurate information about their prospective jobs, they would be in a better position to make informed choices as to the appropriate course of action for them to take. They would be, in Katz's words, "better innoculated against the idealistic hopes and expectations that so many young employees form about their upcoming organizational involvement" (p. 118). The place to begin this process is prior to employment, during the recruiting process. Presumably for competitive reasons, many organizations tend to showcase the positive, glamorous aspects of a job to prospective recruits, while downplaying or even ignoring possible unpleasant or negative aspects. It can be argued that while there may be some short-term payoffs to the organization in this strategy (they fill their positions, for example), the long-run costs in disenchantment, performance degradation, and turnover tip the scales in the other direction.

Wanous (1980) identifies as important the two types of matchings common to most person-environment fit models: individual abilities and organizational job requirements, on the one hand, and individual needs and organizational climates, on the other. (Wanous's use of "climates" rather than the usual "rewards" represents an important and positive deviation from most P-E Fit approaches.) He suggests that *selection* has its greatest effect on the first matching, while *recruitment* has its greatest effect on the second matching. One step in the right direction with respect to recruitment is the use of realistic job previews, or what McGuire (1964) calls a "vaccination."

In a medical context vaccination refers to the process of injecting an individual with a small amount of a disease-causing virus with the expectation that the body will develop a resistance to the virus, thus protecting the individual from contracting the disease caused by the virus. Used in the context of realistic job previews, vaccination consists of giving the job applicant a dose of organization reality to assist the individual in building a resistance to unrealistic high expectations. "Telling it like it is" is certainly not a new or innovative suggestion, but it does represent a philosophy that hasn't frequently been applied to organizational recruiting efforts.

In addition to the vaccination concept, Wanous (1980) suggests two other ways in which recruitment realism can lead to better matchings or higher quality individual-organizational relationships. One is the self-selection, matching effect and the other is the personal commitment effect. The first suggests that since people want to be satisfied, they choose jobs and organizations they believe will maximize personal satisfaction levels. The better (more realistic) the information the job candidate has, the more effective his or her organizational choice will be. In the second case, when individuals believe that they themselves have made a decision, free from strong influence or inducements from others, they tend to be more committed to that decision. Thus, if a job candidate accepts a position because of strong external inducements, the candidate may not feel the same level of internal commitment to that decision that would come from a "free choice." Consequently, less effort might be expended to "making it work."

Selection Considerations

The purpose of any organization's selection program is to obtain the optimal human resources for the organization in a manner that is not disproportionate in costs to the return on the individuals ultimately hired. Traditionally this has meant organizational attempts to insure that job candidates possessed the requisite skills, knowledge, experience, or abilities for the job. Frequently an attempt is also made to ascertain motivation, that is, assess "will do" as well as "can do." To this might profitably be added assessment of individual characteristics and values that would assist improving individual-organizational relationships.

As Brousseau (1983) suggests, individual-organizational relationships may be improved by more closely linking specific characteristics of jobs to corresponding qualities in individuals that may be related to determining their responses to those job characteristics. Examples cited include a case where a job involves complex information processing, a corresponding individual characteristic might be the complexity of an individual's decision style. Or, if a job requires significant cooperation/collaboration with others, corresponding personal qualities that may influence an individual's responses to the job might be sociability and self-esteem.

Closely related to this concept is that of meshing personal predispositions or "personality traits" to relevant aspects of the organizational environment. An example may serve to illustrate the point. Some individuals require a great deal of structure. They have a strong need to have all aspects of their work environment well defined: exactly what they are to do, in what order they should proceed on various tasks, how the tasks should be accomplished, and so on. These individuals are generally very reluctant to make decisions, preferring to have supervisors make them and then inform them of what to do. Other people, on the other hand, have no reluctance to make decisions or operate without the detailed information required by the first group. This first group is said to have a low tolerance for ambiguity; the second group, a high tolerance (even preference for).

Individuals with a low tolerance for ambiguity who find themselves in jobs or organizational environments where there is little structure will very likely find that stressors are more likely to result in unwanted dysfunctional stress outcomes. The individual with low tolerance, for example, will find conditions of role ambiguity much more stressful than someone with a higher tolerance. It makes sense to place individuals with a high need for structure in a more structured environment or to place in or out in the selection process those individuals whose personal predispositions with respect to structure matched or didn't match organizational realities. In many instances an emphasis on placement within the organization rather than on selection per se would accomplish the desired outcomes.

Earlier, in developing the notion of individual-organizational relationships, the idea of Type A and B individuals and organizations was introduced. Knowledge of the tendency of the organization (or specific units therein) to exhibit Type A or B characteristics could be coupled with individual behavior tendencies to make higher quality selection or placement decisions. Maximizing, for example, the number of Type B employees selected for a Type A area within the organization is likely to result in fewer stress and burnout-related problems than selecting Type A individuals for those same positions. An additional benefit of such a strategy would be the probable longer run effect of making that environment less Type A in nature, which has further individual and organizational benefits.

There are of course many, many other dimensions that may be relevant to improving some important aspect of individual-organizational relationships. Many that would be important in one job or type of organization may not be of significance in another. The contention here is not that there are some finite number that should always be considered, but rather that this is a relevant dimension and each organization can profit from determining what is important to its individual-organizational relationships and taking these into some degree of account in its selection and placement processes.

Socialization Programs

Of critical importance in minimizing the likelihood of dysfunctional stress and burnout is a successful period of individual-organizational adaptation once selection and placement decisions have been made. Porter, Lawler, and Hackman (1975: 160) describe it this way:

Once the individual and the organization have chosen each other ... the usually complex and often difficult adaptation period begins. The new employee and the organization must mutually learn to adjust to each other. In some instances, the "marriage" settles down into an easy complete relationship. In others there is an abrupt separation that leaves scars with both parties. In between these two extremes are the remaining majority of cases of individual-organizational adaptation: flexible accommodations that result in a never-ending series of compromises— the individual never completely obtaining all he wants from the organization, and the latter never fully utilizing him for its own purposes.

Socialization, as it relates to organizations, refers to the process by which this individual-organizational adaptation is facilitated. That is, it is the process by which the individual learns and internalizes the values, abilities, expected behaviors, and social knowledge that are important for becoming an effective organizational member. A variety of activities, such as orientation programs, are designed to hasten this process for new organizational members.

As a preventive strategy, socialization may be effective by formalizing and structuring a large part of the process that in many organizations occurs informally. The advantage in this is that broader coverage of relevant factors can be better assured than if the process was left to chance; additionally, much of the process could be completed in a shorter period of time, thus minimizing a great deal of the distress experienced by unsocialized organizational members. In reference to time savings, it should be noted that in some respects socialization is an on-going process, continuing for as long as the individual is an organizational member. Nonetheless, most of the process tends to be compressed in a relatively short period of time.

Many models of organizational socialization are stage models. That is, they view socialization as occurring in several different stages, and for most models the final stage begins very early in the life of the individual-organizational relationship. Even a cursory examination of the titles or labels given the different stages in the various models explains why proper socialization is such an important aspect of improving individual-organizational relationships. Thus, for example, there is "getting in," "breaking in," and "settling in" (Feldman, 1976); prearrival, encounter, change, and acquisition (Porter, Lawler, and Hackman, 1975); entry, socialization, and mutual acceptance (Schein, 1978); and confronting and accepting organizational reality, achieving role clarity, locating oneself in the organizational context, and detecting signposts of successful socialization (Wanous, 1980).

All of these above-mentioned models include a preentry stage. The preentry aspect of socialization deserves special mention. While realistically much of the preentry phase is beyond the direct control of the organization, it nonetheless can play a crucial role in reducing the gap between expectations and reality. Kramer (1974) argues that an important contributor to stress in general and burnout specifically among members of human service professions (specifically, nurses) is this expectations-reality gap. The novice enters with lofty expectations and goals based upon an incomplete and frequently incorrect perception of job reality and is thus doomed to failure. These feelings of failure lead to dissatisfaction and stress and hasten the onset of burnout.

Kramer builds a case for the use of anticipatory socialization programs to decrease the magnitude of reality shock and its negative consequences. The underlying assumption behind anticipatory socialization programs is that any gap between expectations and reality should be experienced prior to the time the individual begins a job and that it should be confronted in a context that allows for and even encourages the development of coping strategies for dealing with the unexpected realities one is about to face. There are several important features of anticipatory socialization programs. First, the major goals of such programs are to give individuals realistic pictures of jobs they are about to assume, and to provide skills for coping effectively with reality shock. Second, since these programs are aimed primarily at burnout prevention, they are most applicable to new members of a profession or occupational group. Last, it should be understood that such programs are not designed to change reality in any way, but merely to provide an advance exposure to it in the hope that it will lead to better preparation for it. The anticipatory socialization program developed by Kramer (1974) was targeted specifically for nurses. Using a control group design, it was possible to compare nursing groups who went through the program with those who did not. In summarizing the results she reports the program was quite effective:

The nurses who had the program seemed to experience less reality shock. They seemed happier and more content in their jobs. They definitely remained in their initial jobs longer, did less job hopping, remained in hospital nursing longer [and] . . . retained their professional beliefs . . . to a greater degree than were the nurses who had not had the program (p. 218).

Additional Preventive Actions

There are, of course, a multitude of activities, programs, and strategies that may be used to minimize or prevent dysfunctional stress among organizational participants. Increasing participation opportunities is an example. The emphasis here is on increasing opportunities for participation, rather than increasing participation per se. There will always be some individuals who do not wish participation and thus will experience greater stress levels if placed in situations where participation is mandated. Providing opportunities for increased participation, however, permits individuals who so wish to increase their involvement. Recent studies in the health professions suggest that increasing participation can lead to increasing the amount of control employees have, which in turn decreases burnout (Maslach and Jackson, 1982).

Jackson (1984) identifies three ways in which increased participation can reduce stress and burnout: (1) by giving individuals an opportunity to influence how others define their roles, thus minimizing role conflict; (2) by providing information about formal and informal policies and procedures, thereby reducing role ambiguity and improving the individual's ability to work within the constraints of the organization; and (3) by facilitating the development and maintenance of a supportive social network among employees. Indeed, while it is certainly not being recommended here, Levi (1984) reports that participation has been virtually legislated in two countries through the Working Environment Acts of Sweden and Norway.

Role analysis and clarification (RAC) programs are another example of an organizational strategy that can be stress-preventive. RAC programs are designed to provide answers to such employee questions as "Is my job clear? Is it consistent with my expectations? With my career plans? Are organizational performance standards clear?" Information from answers to these and similar questions can be assembled to help the employee know more about the job and the nature of job relationships and thus reduce conflict and ambiguity. Or, in some cases, the answers will reveal that changes need to be made in job descriptions, divisions of labor, structural reporting relationships, or similar aspects of the job and its environment. In any case, the objective is the same: improve the quality of the existing individual-organizational relationships and, consequently, minimize the amount, severity, and duration of dysfunctional stress.

SUMMARY

In summary, if prevention (rather than treatment) of stress and burnout in organizational settings is the primary objective, the earlier preventive measures are taken the better. For this reason, emphasis has been placed here on actions taken early on in the individual-organizational relationship. Anticipatory socialization programs, realistic job previews, matching of personality characteristics during employee selection and placement, and providing "innoculations" for new employees are all examples of preventive actions. While these might seem to be primarily organizational and management issues, they should be health care provision issues as well. Stress and burnout are clearly health issues; so also should their prevention be. Health care providers, whether internal or external to the organization, have a stake in minimizing dysfunctional stress and burnout. Working with management in an external consultant capacity, as part of an organizational employee assistance program unit, or in any other role, health care providers along with corporate management and the individual employee have an important function to perform in stress prevention.

REFERENCES

Appelbaum, S. H. 1981. *Stress Management for Health Care Professionals.* Rockville, MD: Aspen Systems.

Brousseau, K. R. 1983. Toward a dynamic model of job-person relationships: Findings, research questions, and implications for work system design. *Academy of Management Review*, 8: 33–45.

Caplan, R. D. 1983. Person-environment fit: Past, present and future. In Cooper, C. L. (Ed.). *Stress Research: Where Do We Go from Here?* London: John Wiley.

Caplan, R. D., Cobb, S., French, J. R. P., Harrison, R. V., and Pinneau, S.R., Jr. 1980. *Job Demands and Worker Health: Main Effects and Occupational Differences.* Ann Arbor, Mich.: Institute for Social Research.

Cox, T. 1978. *Stress.* Baltimore: University Park Press.

Cox, T. and Mackay, C. 1981. A transactional approach to occupational stress. In Corlett, E. W. and Richardson, J. (Eds.). *Stress, Work Design, and Productivity.* New York: John Wiley.

Feldman, D. C. 1976. A contingency theory of socialization. *Administrative Science Quarterly,* 21: 433–452.

Forehand, G. A. and Gilmer, B. V. H. 1964. Environmental variation in studies of organizational behavior. *Psychological Bulletin*, 67: 361–382.

French, J. R. P., Rogers, W., and Cobb, S. 1974. A model of person environment fit. In Coelho, G. V., Hamburgh, D. A., and Adams, J. E. (Eds.). *Coping and Adaptation.* New York: Basic Books.

Friedman, M. and Rosenman, R. H. 1959. Voice analysis test for detections of behavior pattern. *Journal of American Mental Association*, 188: 1286–1296.

————. 1978. *Type A Behavior and Your Heart.* New York: Knopf.

Friedman, M. and Ulmer,D. 1984. *Treating Type A Behavior and Your Heart.* New York: Knopf.

Harrison, R. V. 1978. Person-environment fit and job stress. In Cooper, C. L. and Payne, R. (Eds.). *Stress at Work.* London: John Wiley.

————. 1985. The person-environment fit model and the study of job stress. In Beehr, T.A., and Bhagat, R.S. (Eds.). *Human Stress and Cognition in Organizations.* New York: John Wiley.

Ivancevich, J. M. and Matteson, M. T. 1980. *Stress and Work: A Managerial Perspective.* Glenview, Ill.: Scott, Foresman.

————. 1984. A Type A-B Person-Work Environment Interaction Model for examining occupational stress and consequences. *Human Relations.* 37: 491–513.

Jackson, S. E. 1984. Organizational practices for preventing burnout. In Sethi, A. S. and Schuler, R. S. (Eds.). *Handbook of Organizational Stress Coping Strategies.* Cambridge, Mass: Ballinger.

Katz, R. 1985. Organizational stress and early socialization experiences. In Beehr, T.A. and Bhagat, R. S. (Eds.). *Human Stress and Cognition in Organizations*. New York: John Wiley.

Kramer, M. 1974. *Reality Shock: Why Nurses Leave Nursing*. St. Louis: Mosby Press.

Lazarus, R. 1966. *Psychological Stress and the Coping Process*. New York: McGraw-Hill.

Levi, L. 1984. *Stress in Industry.* Geneva: International Labour Office.

Lewin, K. 1951. *Field Theory in Social Science*. New York: Harper.

Maslach, C. 1976. Burned-out. *Human Behavior*, 5: 16–22.

Maslach, C. and Jackson, S.E. 1982. Burnout in health professions: A social psychological analysis. In Sanders, G. and Suls, J. (Eds.). *Social Psychology of Health and Illness*. Hillsdale, N.J.: Erlbaum.

Matteson, M. T. and Ivancevich, J. M. 1982. Type A and B behavior patterns and self-reported health symptoms and stress: Examining individual and organizational fit. *Journal of Occupational Medicine, 24.*

McGuire, W. J. 1964. Inducing resistance to persuasion. In Berkowitz, L. (Ed.). *Advances in Experimental Social Psychology*. New York: Academic Press.

Murray, H. 1959. *Explorations in Personality*. New York: Oxford University Press.

Perlman, B. and Hartman, E. A. 1982. Burnout: summary and future research. *Human Relations*, 35: 283–305.

Porter, L. W., Lawler, E.E., and Hackman, J. R. 1975. *Behavior in Organizations*. New York: McGraw-Hill.

Schein, E. H. 1978. *Career Dynamics: Matching Individual and Organizational Needs*. Reading, Mass.: Addison-Wesley.

Selye, H. 1974. *Stress Without Distress*. New York: J. B. Lippincott.

Wanous, J. P. 1980. *Organizational Entry*. Reading, Mass.: Addison-Wesley.

Weitz, J. 1970. Psychological research needs on the problems of human stress. In McGrath, J. E. (Ed.). *Social and Psychological Factors in Stress*. New York: Holt, Rinehart and Winston.

13   *Team-building interventions: an organizational stress moderator*

Rita E. Numerof

Organizational life is replete with demands for change and adaptation. In Selye's (1974) terms, such demands constitute stress. Up to a point and taking into account individual differences and coping capacities, these demands are perceived positively—as challenge, variety, and so on. Beyond this point, demands or conditions in the workplace may be perceived as negative and have corresponding negative effects, such as tension, anxiety, frustration, illness, and such. Continuous and unremitting stress in the workplace, particularly where rewards and satisfactions are less than one expected, may lead to a condition that has been defined as burnout, a state characterized by emotional exhaustion, depersonalization, and impaired personal accomplishment (Maslach and Jackson, 1981). Thus burnout can be understood as a segment on the continuum of the much broader concept of stress. While stress includes both positive and negative experiences and extends beyond the work environment, burnout falls on the negative side of the continuum and is confined to the workplace (Numerof and Gillespie, 1984).

Recent research into organizational factors in stress and burnout has identified a cluster of factors associated with work stress. The most prominent of these include supervisory style and support, level of administrative support, the balance between authority and responsibility, degree of discretion over the work being performed, person-job fit, and the conflict resolution process in the work group. These factors can be regarded as stressors, conditions, or events that have the potential for triggering a stress response in individuals. Each of these factors can be managed through team-building interventions to enhance productivity and reduce the negative effects of work-related stress. The focus of this chapter is to identify what organizations can do to promote team development.

DEFINING TEAMS

Before one can talk realistically about team development, one needs to understand what a team is and how it differs from other groups.

Teams are work groups characterized by high levels of energy directed toward accomplishing organizational goals. They are exceptional groups that combine high loyalty, morale, commitment, and effective task performance, often in the face of what appear to be insurmountable obstacles. Their accomplishments have clear relevance to both the team and the organization.

Teams are necessary when the tasks to be performed cannot be achieved by individuals working in isolation. Team effort results in a product or process that is beyond the capacities of any individual team member. Teams are characterized by a shared purpose that is clearly understood by all members. Yet each member has an identified role in accomplishing that purpose, working in concert with other team members. As is true for any work group, a team must confront such difficult issues as leadership style, control, procedures, organization, structure, and the roles of individual members. Successful handling of these issues results in responsive, goal-directed, flexible teams that are able to handle conflict creatively. The open spirit so characteristic of teams encourages intermember support and constructive challenge.

These qualities, in addition to enhancing productivity, can be seen as providing a buffer against organizational stress. Their presence suggests the absence of such stressors as poorly managed conflict, lack of recognition, lack of cohesion, role ambiguity, and lack of identification, all of which have been indicted as harmful in the stress equation (Matteson and Ivancevich, 1979; McLean, 1979; Kahn et al., 1964).

SPECIAL CHARACTERISTICS OF TEAMS

Numerous authors have presented descriptions of effective work groups and outlined their characteristics (Francis and Young, 1977; Dyer, 1977; Patten, 1981). The model presented in Figure 13.1 offers a somewhat different perspective that builds on these earlier efforts. It also extends other (French and Bell, 1978; Quick and Quick, 1984) explorations of team building as primarily a method for identifying, working through, and resolving interpersonal conflicts that evolve in the life of work groups. The model combines elements from role analysis (French and Bell, 1978), effective goal setting procedures (Quick, 1979), research on social support (House, 1981) as well as more traditional concepts of team building as a communications tool for conflict resolution. The model identifies 12 components or characteristics of effective teams. Each component is seen as playing a critical and definitive role in determining the degree to which a particular team can be called effective at any stage of its development. While there are no empirical data that indicate the differential or relative contribution of each component, it seems logically consistent to assume that if each component is optimized a team will be optimally effective. Conversely, any team may be only as strong as its weakest component.

Figure 13.1.   Characteristics of effective teams

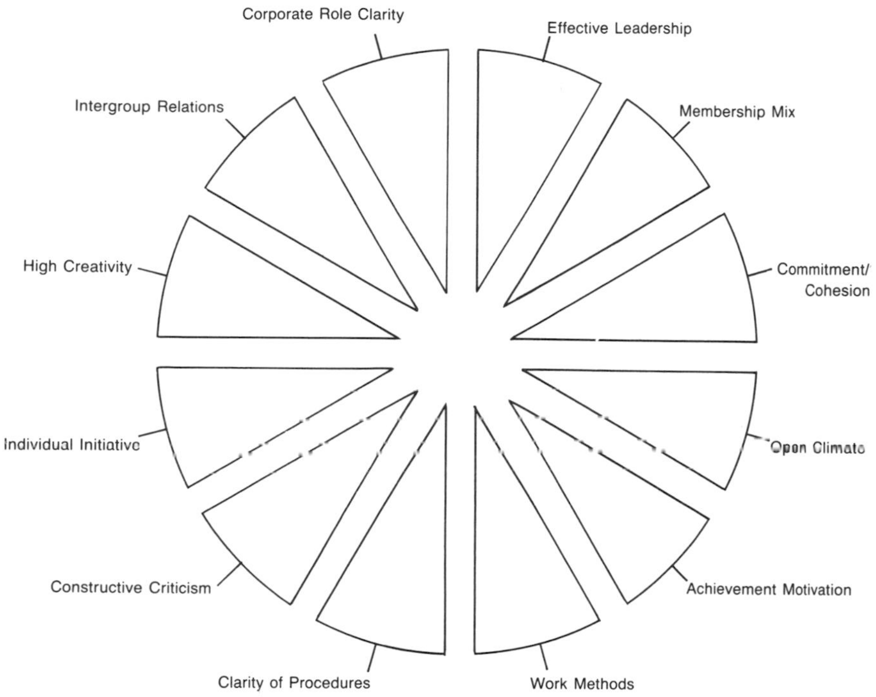

Source: Compiled by the author.

Effective Leadership

Probably the single most important factor in determining the quality of teamwork is the way in which the group is led. Not surprisingly, experience shows that the manager's behavior is, in many ways, more important than what the manager says. The most essential ingredients for success in leading the team are nondefensive and supportive behaviors (Gibb, 1961) that pave the way for an open climate in which willingness to deal with uncomfortable issues prevails. This requires a degree of comfort with personal exposure and openness to feedback (Luft, 1969).

Effective team leadership insures that time is allocated to team-building activities, that leadership roles are shared depending on members' expertise and the nature of the task, that all team members spend time clarifying what they expect and need from each other. In this process it is the leaders' responsibility to see to it that members receive regular feedback about how members see their performance and that they are clear about their individual roles in relation to the team. Decisions are made only after the team has thoroughly discussed available options. As is true for all work groups, the manager performs boundary-spanning functions, representing the team at higher levels of the organization and to other teams. Inherent in these responsibilities is the need for the leader to be sensitive to the needs of each team member and to modify the leadership style according to the demands of the situation. Thus a contingency approach that fosters creativity, autonomy, and full participation becomes essential in leading a team. The manager, although accountable for what occurs within the team, must be able to delegate responsibility across the team so that leadership functions are shared.

Membership Mix

Identifying who should be on the team in terms of individual qualifications and the complement of expertise across members is essential as teams are being formed. This factor is typically not given sufficient attention when hiring decisions are made to fill vacancies that arise in ongoing work groups. Nonetheless, failure to assess appropriate membership mix accurately throughout the life of the group will impede group functioning and may augment the stress experienced by individual members.

As Harrison and Matteson each discuss in their contributions in this volume (see Chapters 7 and 12, respectively), the degree of fit between people and their work is an important factor in job stress. Perhaps most essential is the recognition that attempts at improving fit must be individual. For the person who values latitude in decision making, for example, increasing the amount inherent in the job might increase fit, satisfaction, and reduce stress. The same change would have the opposite effect, however, for the person who prefers little decision-making latitude.

Commitment/Cohesion

Teams require time and attention from their members. Membership in such a work group or committee involves an element of sacrifice because each member gives up some autonomy and self-interest. Often this becomes a serious obstacle, particularly for professionals (such as physicians) whose socialization has emphasized individual decision making (Numerof, 1983). Inevitably, even under the best circumstances, conflicts arise between the interests of the team and the individuals who comprise it. The growth of commitment, often more a matter of feeling than logic, is an important and necessary phase in the development of the team, for it is commitment that assures the team's success in reaching goals. Commitment is more likely when the members believe that the aims of the team are worthwhile and personally satisfying, when they expect that members will be willing to put themselves out for each other. Where there is commitment members continue to value individual goals, but not at the expense of the team. There is a sense of belonging, identification with the group, and a sense of mutual enjoyment. Such mutual support, while providing an important base for team growth and development, can also be potentially detrimental when norms allow or tolerate inadequate performances. If this tendency is managed with ongoing procedures to critically and constructively evaluate performance, commitment will result in increased available energy to build and maintain the team.

Open Climate

The team atmosphere, characterized by open and direct communication and trust, provides the support necessary for members to feel comfortable in taking appropriate risks, thus enhancing opportunities for innovation and creativity. Three interconnecting features of an open climate characteristic of a team include the following:

- Members have skills in interpersonal relations; they possess and employ good communications skills.
- Members convey respect and warmth in their interaction with others.
- Members are supported in their openness by those with power and influence.

Such a climate requires that team members frequently engage in sessions designed to "clear the air." The success of these sessions depends on the group's ability to handle all issues directly, regardless of how difficult and without hidden agendas and political manuevering. In this setting individual viewpoints are strongly encouraged, differences are expressed; conformity, within the limits of deviance the group has defined as acceptable, is not valued. Not surprisingly, the leader's active role and behavioral modeling in establishing and maintaining norms that foster the open climate is critical.

There are obvious advantages to an open climate. These include closer personal relationships, constructive confrontation, high energy levels, minimum inner frustration, greater efficiency, and better morale. What is not as obvious are the disadvantages of an open climate, particularly in the short run. These include individual vulnerability, discomfort owing to increasing awareness of real problems, pressure on the leader, and the risk of honest conflict getting out of hand.

Achievement Motivation

Teams are characterized by high achievement motivation: There is a sense of stretching oneself and devoting energy to achieve specific results.

Performance goals are high but realistic; quality or excellence is a norm to which members subscribe. Group pressure is present to maintain high standards of performance. Perhaps most striking is the group's commitment to regular performance review to assess strengths and weaknesses to determine where improvement may be made. Groups characterized by high achievement motivation are more likely to reach their objectives. Their energies are channeled into productive routes to achieve tangible results. Team members reflect on the return on their own investment— examining if their efforts are producing results and how efficiently and effectively resources are used.

Effective Work Methods

Teams are characterized by task-oriented, structured meetings that follow agreed-upon procedures systematically. Attentive listening occurs to viewpoints expressed; decisions are made after thorough discussion. There is a notable absence of passive/aggressive (for example, withdrawal, sarcasm, manipulation) or aggressive (disruption or criticism) behavior. Meetings are used to resolve issues the team must face. Decisions reached are recorded, implementation is decided, and follow through occurs consistently. Perhaps most striking to team functioning is that members take responsibility for planning meetings and prepare for them. Such activity is not merely the responsibility of the leader.

Clarity of Procedures

Procedural clarity requires that team members are clear about their individual roles relative to the team as a whole. Structural and administrative procedures are in place of support team efforts. These are reviewed and evaluated periodically with regard to their efficacy. While clear procedures are available to the team and are followed, they are not rigidly applied when situations require flexibility. In order for this process to work smoothly, objectives and priorities are reviewed regularly. Integration among individual objectives is sought. Inherent in evaluating clarity of procedures is an evaluation of the team's decision-making process. While no single decision-making style is universally applicable, processes that facilitate broad-based team participation appear to be most useful.

Constructive Criticism

Teams have already been characterized as possessing an open climate. One aspect of that climate is the ability to engage in the process of constructive criticism for the purpose of learning from one's mistakes. The fallacy of perfectionism is not part of team functioning. As a corollary to this, regular reviews of team activities are seen as positive learning opportunities. Impartial assessment of one's work is encouraged. Critical in this is the avoidance of personal attacks and an emphasis on performance improvement. Team members avoid the tendency to store, put off, or bury difficulties. Rather, an exploratory approach to problems is adopted, one that investigates what can be done to understand and resolve them. Thus, team members have the ability to analyze each others' performance strengths and weaknesses and give feedback without rancor. Individual members are thus in a position to use this feedback constructively, growing from error.

Individual Initiative

With a commitment to performance excellence and performance improvement, it is easy to see that teams would encourage members to develop and extend their individual interests. The team that encourages strong individuals enhances its own development through individual contributions. In addition to an emphasis on initiative through individual development, team members are encouraged to constructively question established team procedures and to question each other. Individuals, when they change their minds, do so through a reasoning process, not through pressure or from threat. Team members are also encouraged to move outside the team to broaden their personal knowledge and skills. While the team has clear boundaries, the boundaries are not rigid and do not discourage interaction with nonteam members. The result is that individuals are prepared to take risks for the betterment of the team and are able to be open about their positions. This risk-taking ability ties in directly to the team's ability to be creative.

High Creativity

Some organizations and work groups are characterized by excitement, others by repetition and boredom. Teams are recognized by outside observers by their unusually high degree of creativity. They are often characterized by vision; they have a reputation for innovation. Within the team new ideas are regularly generated, expanded upon, evaluated, prioritized, and selected ones implemented. Critical to this process is the ability to identify a need or perceive missing links, generate new ideas and workable plans for carrying them out, test the plans and implement them.

In order for these steps to occur innovation must be rewarded—new approaches need to be welcomed and openness to difference and disagreement encouraged. This last point is critical from two perspectives.

In addition to setting the stage for creativity, it builds in protection for the team against "groupthink," the tendency for highly cohesive groups to take action that no individual alone would be likely to endorse (Janis, 1968).

While reward for innovation is essential, it mut be accompanied by tolerance for risk. Risk can never be eliminated completely from creativity. Even the most highly trained and experienced people continue to make errors.

Support for creativity comes from many sources in the team including the following:

- Individuals know that their work is valued.
- Ideas, as opposed to people, receive criticism.
- Difficulties are expressed and shared among trusted colleagues, thus breaking down isolation.
- Resources for testing ideas are available.
- Individuals are not punished if things go wrong.

Positive Intergroup Relations

Teams and team-building activities are often criticized as divisive, atomistic units in the organization—a prime example of suboptimization at work. Unfortunately, where the team becomes an isolated and closed entity, the team-building process has broken down. In the model described here, the team is characterized as one integrated unit functioning collaboratively within a larger whole—the organization. In this context the team is seen as having solid working relationships with other groups; it is interested in and responsive to the needs of other groups within the organization. Unresolved conflicts between the team and other groups are rare. Instead, the team is seen as having solid working relationships with other groups. Members have personal relationships with members from other teams. They are, as Likert (1961) suggests, "linked." Teams such as these recognize that effective communications with other groups keep the team from costly errors. Effectiveness is enhanced through collaboration— not only within the team but with other groups.

Corporate Role Clarity

What makes positive intergroup relations possible is the ability of the team to see its existence and its contributions deeply embedded in the organization as a whole. Its work is related directly to organizational objectives and carried out within strategic guidelines. The team sees its own distinctive role contributing to organizational productivity, but it sees itself as offering one part to the whole. Just as team members are clear about the team's contribution to the organization, the team's contributions are clearly understood by the rest of the organization. In light of the team's importance, the organization would feel its loss if the team were to leave. The organization makes use of the vision and skills the team possesses; the team's work is complementary to what other groups do in the organization.

Inherent in this discussion is the notion of a team as a special kind of group. The qualities described present an ideal situation. Teams in organizations will differ in the degree to which they embody these characteristics. To the extent that they do one is likely to see increased productivity, increased commitment, and reduced stress. As can be seen from the descriptions, such groups can reduce stress because they minimize such known stressors as role conflict and ambiguity, lack of administrative support, poor integration and coordination, lack of subordinate participation, inadequate feedback, and poor interpersonal relations.

BUILDING EFFECTIVE TEAMS

The Developmental Process*

The evolution of a group into a team is a developmental process. The fact that a number of people are engaged in a common enterprise does not ensure that a team will emerge. Groups get stuck at various points in their growth for a variety of reasons. They may have poorly defined structures for decision making, members may lack commitment, the group may be plagued with lack of clarity regarding goals, inappropriate leadership, and unrecognized and unresolved conflict.

The relative scarcity of well-functioning teams points to the complexity of the developmental process. Good teams rarely happen by themselves. They must be created deliberately. The essence of team building is to create the conditions supporting and to remove the blockages preventing the development of highly effective groups. There are five stages in the development of teams, each of which is outlined next.

Stage 1: Ambivalence. Stage 1 involves the testing or approach-avoidance that is characteristic of any newly formed group. Despite eagerness for membership, there are doubts about the group's suitability, interpersonal compatibility, and personal anxiety about belonging and acceptance. During this phase people seek to learn about each other, gradually exchanging information concerning their values, attitudes, task-related abilities, communications styles, and expectations for the group. The leader plays an important role in encouraging exploration and

---

*This section has been adapted from R. E. Numerof, *Managing Stress*. Reprinted with permission of Aspen Publishers Inc. © 1983.

ensuring that a noncritical, nonjudgmental stance is maintained. Issues are handled at a primarily superficial level but a degree of comfort is achieved when members are relatively satisfied as others evidence initial interest and commitment to the group. The group has not yet begun to work. However, even at this stage, norms are set with regard to how the group should proceed: for example, if and how one should be considered. As Schein (1985) notes, the process of responding (or, for that matter, failing to respond) helps to develop alliances where there has been agreement, or encourages potential factions where there has been disagreement.

Stage 2: Power and Control. This stage entails the testing of individuals' influence and the limits of the group regarding its tolerance of disagreement and conflict. While the team leader has authority by virtue of that position, this authority is challenged overtly and covertly by team members. It is at this stage that the group is struggling with how it will go about its business. The norms are set with regard to issues of control (that is, who controls the team and how that control is exercised) and deviance (how much and what kind is tolerated, how it is managed).

While there are no prescriptions for groups to follow in resolving these issues, certain typical problems set the stage for team blockage. For example, where the leader does not facilitate the open and constructive exploration of disagreement and conflict among all members, conflict is avoided but is expressed destructively through passive means (for example, resistance to group discussion, sabotage of group effect, failure to contribute to group projects). Because personal views are not freely expressed and encouraged, the development of trust is impeded. The team is likely to become stalemated, characterized by low energy, low morale, and less than optimal performance. Control difficulties must be worked through in order to move on to Stage 3.

Stage 3: Affiliation and Work. This stage is characterized by positive intermember relations, increased degrees of coordination, commitment, and energy toward the group's task and its completion. Individual differences are set aside as members improve their ability to listen receptively to one another. The team becomes concerned about efficiency and reviews performance, looking for alternative and better ways of accomplishing projects. A communications shorthand develops among members as the group strives to improve its methods of operation, becoming more flexible and creative in the process. This stage requires genuine understanding of various perspectives and that the members remain open to reevaluating team operating procedures, searching for improvement while keeping the goal in mind continuously. Without these latter elements, the group is likely to settle for performance adequacy as opposed to excellence. The leader's behavior is critical in developing norms to achieve such excellence.

Stage 4: Differentiation/Integration. This evolves from Stage 3. The emphasis is on the development of individual team members, supporting each to excel to the fullest capacity. This development occurs in the context of cooperation among team members and the integration of different talents for the benefit of the group that, in turn, gives support for individual growth. While the formal leader is likely to remain in that position, members all have become skilled at leader and member roles. The result is a fluidity of leadership, depending on the requirements of a particular task or subtask and the abilities of particular members. Outside observers readily identify the tight-knit aspect of the team and its ability to accomplish work. However, the team is not an isolated unit within a system. Rather, it sees its role and function as intricately tied to the broader goals and objectives of the organization of which it is a part. At this stage, in particular, links to other teams and units in the organization need to be strengthened in the efforts to enhance interteam integration.

Stage 5: Dissolution. This entails the process of terminating the team. No group is forever. Many teams are formed to accomplish time-limited specific projects. Once the need is met and the team has no other mandate, it prepares for its ending. Because of the bonds that have developed and the immense satisfaction of working well with colleagues, resistance to the termination occurs at this stage. The effective team, however, will recognize the roots of such resistance and not create projects of small significance merely to keep itself alive. The team also experiences a form of dissolution with the loss of one or more of its members, even if it continues as an entity. This occurs because the identity and interactions of the team are modified with the loss of any member or the addition of a new one.

The Importance of Cohesion

One of the most striking characteristics of the effective work group is its high degree of internal cohesion. This "stick-togetherness" results from forces that act on group members, causing them to remain in the group. These forces involve the attractiveness of the group itself and the lesser attractiveness of alternatives. There are a number of determinants of group cohesion: the incentive properties of the group, the motive base of its members, the expectation of outcomes, and how the group compares to others (Cartwright and Zander, 1968).

If group cohesion is high, it is accompanied by the following desirable consequences:

• Team membership will be maintained over time, thus increasing opportunities for the development of interpersonal relations characterized by trust.

- Long-term maintenance of membership also produces short-term benefits, such as lowering absenteeism.

- The group will demonstrate high levels of loyalty and participation and will be able to exercise power and influence over its members.

- A degree of personal security will be experienced by each individual member, whose self-evaluation also will be high because of identification with the group.

SETTING A CLIMATE TO REDUCE ORGANIZATIONAL STRESS: OVERCOMING RESISTANCE

Aside from specific stressors related to the work itself and to the match between people and their jobs, the interpersonal environment of an organization, particularly from the standpoint of management-subordinate and interprofessional relations, plays a critical role in determining the level of stress in the organization. The challenge facing organizations is how to set a climate to reduce organizational stress. Trust and three other critical factors are most important: (1) participation in decision making relevant to the work being performed, (2) excellent communications, and (3) a commitment to collaboration. While these three factors, forming the cornerstone of team-building interventions, seem intuitively appealing and straightforward, their integration into the culture of an organization is often a difficult undertaking. The difficulty stems from two major obstacles: threat and resistance to change.

We can begin our exploration of these obstacles with participation. From the standpoint of management practices, managerial behavior directly affects subordinates' participation or perceived level of input in decision making and goal setting. Specifically these practices include but are not limited to: (1) the extent to which employees involved are asked for their ideas when problems occur in the work flow, (2) the extent to which employees are asked for their ideas and opinions on matters that affect them, (3) the extent to which employee input is considered in setting goals for specific jobs and the tasks of the work group, and (4) the extent to which supervisors make changes based on employees' ideas (Numerof and Associates, 1984).

To bring about high levels of participation as defined above takes absolute power out of the hands of the manager and places it squarely in the arena of interdependence: shared between manager and subordinate. Team building, if it is to be successful, requires a redistribution of power. The threat for the insecure manager is obvious. The manager must recognize, nurture, and be able to use the ability of subordinates. That ability for creative problem-solving may exceed the manager's in certain situations. To give recognition requires a sense of personal competence and security, the knowledge that managers do not hold a monopoly on good decision making, and the understanding that the manager's survival

Table 13.1.   Sources of resistance to team building

Lack of awareness that problems exist
Denial of the existence of problems
Fear of uncovering hidden problems and issues
Fear of exposure
Fear of conflict
Fear of loss of control
Fear of failure
Lack of trust

Source: Compiled by the author.

depends ultimately on the work group's performance. Some managers approach these realities with the feeling that they have lost control. Afraid of exposure, not trusting their subordinates' decision-making abilities, afraid of uncovering hidden problems or issues and the ensuing conflict, they hide from awareness of the fact that problems do, indeed, exist.

Threats, however, do not lie solely within the domain of the manager. Employees, unaccustomed to being involved in decision making, are understandably afraid to take risks. Leaving it to someone else, while stifling creativity and undermining identification and involvement, may afford refuge from responsibility, particularly where failure may be a possibility. These threats, combined with the real pressure of daily demands, serve to strengthen general resistance to change and thus maintain the status quo. Unless managers are expected and committed to coach employees in participation, it is unlikely that change will occur.

In the area of communications, similar threats exist. Access to communication and privileged information constitutes power for the manager. To share such communication with subordinates may be perceived by some managers who withhold information as diminishing power. With the constant pressures of time, information is often not communicated, communicated inadequately, or communicated in such a way that critical feedback does not occur. Risk–taking apprehension in communicating reactions and ideas among subordinates also exists for the reasons noted above. Together, these threats undermine team–building efforts. Table 13.1 summarizes related sources of resistance to team building.

Commitment to collaboration exists to differing degrees in organizations, primarily as a function of unit suboptimization. Suboptimization refers to the tendency of individuals and groups to regard their own efforts as significantly more valuable than those of other groups, and to fail to take into account the degree to which their own success is linked to the successful performance of others. This type of situation is manifested where there is low commitment to the organization but high loyalty to the work unit or department. It is also seen in situations where strong professional identification exists, such as in laboratory research, nursing, or medicine. It is seen in situations where strong functional identification exists, such as in manufacturing, sales/marketing, and research and development. When suboptimization occurs here, little or no identification with corporate goals is seen. Problems are blamed on other divisions of the organization, or on other professional groups.

Administration often colludes with this phenomenon. For example, it may orient personnel in an atomistic manner. Little, if any, time may be spent on integration—orienting people as to how their particular unit connects with others or what the impact of an employee's job and department is. Communication between departments may be discouraged. This may occur very subtly, even when the intended outcome is enhanced communication. For instance one organization, trying to overcome problems of suboptimization, convened monthly mandatory management meetings to encourage an exchange between senior and middle management. Typically, 90 people were in attendance. Not surprisingly, few interactions took place and the meetings were disbanded after six months. Senior-level managers perceived middle managers as resistive and unwilling to deal openly; middle managers perceived those in senior levels to be closed to their genuine participation. The intervention was recognized by both sides as a dismal failure in collaboration. At one level the meetings were doomed from the beginning. As a forum for open exchange the sheer magnitude of the group and its structure precluded the kind of dialogue required to enhance communication. At best it reflected a costly naivete on the part of senior managers. It also reflected an underlying resistance to the open dialogue these managers at least verbally desired.

Suboptimization also occurs where organizational objectives may not be communicated. Worse yet, these objectives may not be defined or may change often, increasing uncertainty and stress in the environment. Suboptimization becomes most serious in the case of the work group. It occurs when the group consists of atomized players, each with a specific role without clear integration with the roles of other players. Each player may have obtained that position by a different route and has made no commitment to other group members or to the organization itself. Under these conditions, cohesion is essentially absent; stress is high.

Reward structures in a large number of organizations pose a serious obstacle to team–building interventions. Typically, rewards in organizations are directed at individual performance, not the performance of groups. In organizations that emphasize the identification of "HIPOS" (high potential individuals), there also tends to be an emphasis on mobility, which in turn tends to destabilize well-performing groups. Even where there are productive groups, typically only senior management is rewarded contingent on performance. Thus, existing reward structures in most organizations mitigate against team performance. Under these conditions, rethinking the present reward system and finding opportunities for alternative rewards based on group performance is a precondition for team building. Organizations tend to get what they reward.

Team productivity and the quality of overall team performance can be undermined in yet another way. Where individuals working in a group perceive that their efforts are inadequately rewarded (that is, they believe their rewards are less than their individual performance warrants), they may be likely to shirk their responsibility (Jones, 1983). There may even be an incentive to shirking, if individuals are allowed to coast along on the group's performance, and if individual performance is difficult to measure. With many group members subscribing to this orientation, overall group performance can decline. Thus the failure to reward individual as well as group performance can diminish overall group effort.

The informal structure of the group and factions within the organization may also pose an obstacle to team-building efforts. Take, for example, the not uncommon divisiveness that exists between sales and marketing divisions or between manufacturing and research and development. Where the incumbent leader has power because of the status quo, a redistribution of power will be seen as threatening and thus will be resisted. Similarly, where coalitions exist within a division or work group, changes in the status quo may be seen as undermining the present power basis. If team-building efforts are to be successful under these conditions one must neutralize the resistance of these power forces by carefully identifying what they have to gain under the new arrangement. Without this, the power of the informal mechanisms will subvert team efforts.

Despite the distinct advantages of teams in improving organizational performance and reducing stress brought about by poor integration, lack of goal clarity, low levels of participation, trust, and the like, team building creates stress in the short run for members. If they are to be effective, teams require a degree of openness and self-disclosure that many individuals, regardless of their positions, find threatening. Because conflict is dealt with openly, those uncomfortable with its expression are likely to experience temporary stress and may try to block team development. These factors demand that the team leader be a strong, confident individual with the ability to facilitate discussion and development even when support seems minimal or lacking altogether. Often this requires specialized training.

Team building has particular relevance in organizations in which the work is characterized by high levels of interdependence, frequent problem-solving efforts, and high demands for accuracy and/or timeliness. Given the nature of health care environments, for example, the utility of teams and team building should not be underestimated, whether in the case of committees needing to work together, physician-nursing-administration collaboration, administration-board interaction, patient care teams, support service groups, and the like.

Despite strong resistance to teams, the need for team-building interventions exists in organizations. One of the most promising ways to overcome resistance and introduce team-building efforts involves the identification of a "felt need" (Dyer, 1977) among key members of the organization or work group.

IMPLEMENTING TEAM-BUILDING INTERVENTIONS

Team-building activity, whether it occurs at the level of the work group or permeates the organization as a whole, involves a change in the culture of the group. Interest in corporate cultures has been in evidence for the last several years and has taken a position of respect in the scientific as well as popular literature. All cultures, including organizations, seek to inculcate their members with relevant values. They do this more or less effectively through the selective use of jargon, rituals, symbols, and rites of passage into the culture. In an organizaton the most obvious initial rite involves the entry into permanent, as opposed to probationary, status. Organizations also attempt to strip away, to varying degrees, old identifications as they socialize new members. Striking examples are the military and IBM. The first requires the giving up of civilian clothes, the taking of a uniform; the use of a new terminology and manner of addressing superiors, in particular; the gaining of a number for identification, the loss of more personal forms of address. For IBM the ritual and symbol use is less severe but nonetheless powerful. There is an accepted corporate dress. The process of socialization is enhanced by fairly frequent corporate relocations every couple of years for those selected for and interested in moving ahead. The process of moving tends to strip away other social attachments, neutralizing the effect of competing value systems and identification groups, strengthening the identification with the current group.

Unlike the military, organizations cannot forcefully strip away prior or competing identifications. Organizations cannot control the lives of their employees to that extent. Much more free choice is involved. The challenge is to offer people viable, desirable alternatives to the competing identifications and values they might have.

People choose to join organizations for a reason; typically it is more than for a paycheck. Most people respond positively to the knowledge that their activity makes a difference. They tend to respond negatively when they perceive that their contribution is not meaningful to the whole. Organizations lose a great deal in human productivity and create unnecessary stress when they fail to understand that people need to perceive that they are making an important contribution, and that the organization perceives it as well. The tendency to overlook the importance of these needs is most striking in the area of support services in hospitals. While housekeeping performs a critical role in terms of infection control and the overall impressions patients and visitors have of the hospital, it is unusual for members of the department to get recognition for their role. Similarly, employees who transport patients and attendants in the parking garage all have an important and generally overlooked role as marketers of the hospital and employees in support of patient needs. It is a fairly simple matter to institute programs that spotlight the contributions of all components of the health delivery team, yet most organizations fail to do so.

Team building moves beyond merely strengthening the relation between the worker and the organization, however—a relation suggested by social exchange theory (Blau, 1964). It strengthens the bond between employees relative to organizational activities. To accomplish this there must be explicit rewards for team players that are both visible and valued. To base integration merely on the relation between the organization and the individual or to fail to integrate the strong group with the organization leads to problems.

The former fosters isolation and impedes cohesion, creativity, and productivity. The latter, however, is a problem also associated with great cost. Take, for example, the strong research team that finds its interest best served by leaving the organization en masse and forming a separate corporation. The rate at which this has occurred in the computer industry speaks to the problem when teams and organizations miss some of the critical elements—in this case corporate role clarity and positive intergroup relations. Table 13.2 identifies some of the most common reasons team-building efforts fail. Some of the reasons reflect limited knowledge

Table 13.2.   Why team-building efforts fail

Lack of commitment from senior management
Lack of preparation from senior management
Lack of clarity in team objectives and procedures
Lack of time devoted to team-building efforts
Lack of appropriate sequencing of activities
Failure to manage group process effectively
Inappropriate leadership style
Avoidance of conflict
Inadequate team-building tools
Failure to reward team-building efforts
Implicit rewards for suboptimization
Failure to hold people accountable for team building
Failure to monitor team-building efforts

Source: Compiled by the author.

and skill (such as lack of preparation of team members, lack of appropriate sequencing of activities, inappropriate leadership style). Others reflect critical problems in reward structures and accountability (such as failure to reward team-building efforts, implicit rewards for suboptimization, failure to monitor team-building efforts). Attention must be paid to each of these factors to insure success of any team-building efforts.

Change in any organization or group never comes from complacency and comfort. Effective change begins with the realization that the status quo is less than satisfactory and can benefit from improvement. At this point feelings are important: the need for change must be experienced (that is, felt) by those with power in the organization. The need may be the identification of specific problems, the presence of poorly handled stress, the desire to increase productivity, or the wish to be proactive in improving overall functioning. Without some felt need by those who carry weight, no change will occur. The need must be followed by a technical analysis of what is wrong. One must identify the problem(s) and prioritize the needs. Inherent in the assessment is a vision of where one wants to go. As Dyer (1977) has so aptly noted, managing organizational and group change is similar to taking a trip. It's important to know where one wants to go. The questions of what one wants to see a year hence and where the group members want to be at that time must be asked and answered. Once the vision has been articulated specific goals and strategies must be devised for getting there. Moreover, they need to be monitored on a regular basis so that progress can be assessed continuously.

While there are many different approaches to the implementation of team-building efforts, several factors cut across them. First, there needs to be a commitment from the manager that team building is a good idea. Second, there must be recognition of interdependence as a critical aspect of organizational functioning. Third, where team building is a recognized value, people need to be held accountable for insuring that it happens. One way of accomplishing this is through the systematic measurement of management practices throughout the organization. The implication is that employee participation and feedback and subordinates' perceptions of the behavior of their managers are important aspects of organizational life. In this way the team-building foundation—participation, collaboration, communication—can be woven into the fabric of the organization's culture.

Collaboration structures such as task forces can be established within the organization to facilitate the solving of interdepartmental problems on an ad hoc basis or to ensure the implementation of strategic planning efforts on an ongoing basis. In order for these task forces to succeed they must be under the management of a strong team leader who can teach by example the techniques of team building. In addition, they must be backed up with high-level attention, held accountable and rewarded for results achieved.

Team-building efforts are often initiated by off-site retreats of two to three days with administration and middle managers assessing the need for and viability of a more systematic effort. During these sessions, generally led by an outside consultant, the language of team building is explored and participants are engaged in sessions to identify forces encouraging and impeding the development of a more teamlike organization. In this process it is important to understand existing and potential reinforcers as well as prices for team efforts.

The process is similar to a force field analysis (Lewin, 1951) in which the organization is "unfrozen," new behaviors are introduced, and the new behaviors then reinforced and "refrozen." The following discussion presents a model that is helpful in structuring the change process.

MANAGING THE CHANGE PROCESS

Introducing team-building interventions involves change. Whenever change is anticipated resistance must also be anticipated as it entails a deviation from how things are done now, shifts in power, and some degree of uncertainty. The most effective change efforts seem to reduce uncertainty to manageable proportion and build on the status quo. Thus the linkages between where we are and where we are going are made explicit. Change seen as a reframing or reconceptualization of what is happening in the organization now (Kantor, 1985) can provide the necessary linkages to minimize threat and uncertainty. However, even here there are specific barriers to be overcome.

Kantor (1985) outlines three stages of the change process: reframing or vision phase, coalition-formation phase, and mobilization or implementation phase. The vision phase entails the provision of "discrepant information," which challenges the way things are currently done. This information may be negative (for example, there are symptoms of problems) or positive (for example, we can be even better) and offers new explanations and challenges old assumptions. The leader who envisions more team-like performance as a means for reducing stress and enhancing commitment and productivity serves as a catalyst for change. This vision will be challenged by organizational problems of homogeneity ("I talk only to people who think like me"), insularity (decentralization ensures that each unit gets only a limited view of the enterprise; no one takes responsibility for putting it together), and professional bias (training and specialization decrease one's ability to see the need to do things differently). History (that is, precedent) may also serve to reinforce the way things are done as will the fear of being wrong and thus running the risk of loss of face.

Where segmentation, professional bias, and history exert minor influence, vision can be held back by structural barriers. These barriers include biases toward consensus, conformity, and correctness. Under these conditions, being able to predict correctly is more important than being innovative; discrepant information is shunned.

Table 13.3.   Ten guidelines for successful change

---

1. Clearly understand the real strategy behind the change
2. Connect the change effort to the status quo
3. Identify structural barriers to change
4. Ensure that discrepant frameworks are introduced
5. Identify and work with power sources
6. Establish support for the vision
7. Act quickly or premises and priorities may change
8. Ensure persistence
9. Plan for stability and reassessment
10. Focus on short-term visible results

Source: Compiled by the author.

Stage 2, coalition formation, entails the acquisition of organizational capital (that is, power), which adds legitimacy to the vision and ensures the support necessary to realize it. This process requires more than getting the commitment of those people who will be involved directly in the change effort. It necessitates a systematic approach to change—one that recognizes that putting things together differently (that is, change) sets other forces in motion. If one department changes it has reverberating effects in the system. To be effective, questions asking how and to what extent others will be affected must be asked. Others' ideas must also be solicited. Budget and time must be allocated. Effort must be channeled specifically to the team project and not siphoned off in many directions or nothing will happen.

Assuming the effort advances through Stage 2, roadblocks must be overcome in Stage 3, mobilization or implementation. Most noteworthy are problems in maintaining commitment and ensuring sufficient long-term support (for 18 to 24 months) for the effort to occur. Table 13.3 summarizes the guidelines for a successful change effort.

A structural process for implementing team-building interventions in the organization may be mobilized easily for interventions occurring at the divisional or work group levels (see Numerof and Associates, 1984). Inherent in this approach is the need to establish an initial level of interest on the part of managers of the group in question. A commitment to explore the applicability of team building is the only necessary condition to move into the retreat.

The process identifies the need for a retreat facilitator. Whether this person should be in-house or selected from outside the organization depends on two critical factors: expertise available and degree of resistance in the organization. The facilitator must be expert in group dynamics and group process, thoroughly conversant in team-building and conflict management, and, perhaps most importantly, be recognized by the participants as an expert. With regard to the second factor, where resistance is high experience suggests that outside facilitation can be more effective in identifying and breaking through barriers. Regardless of whether the facilitator is internal or external to the organization, the senior manager is still responsible for the development of team activity. The consultant/facilitator serves an important catalytic and unfreezing function in the introduction of "discrepant information" but is not responsible for the actual accomplishments of the team.

Where the team-building effort centers on a work unit as opposed to an initial organizational introduction, other factors guide the decision to use a facilitator external to the work group. If group members typically feel free speaking up honestly, generally work together without undue conflict or apathetic withdrawal, and are committed to the group, the manager can be an effective facilitator as long as the following conditions apply: (1) the manager feels comfortable trying out something new, (2) the manager's style is compatible with the leadership aspects of team building, (3) the manager is knowledgeable about team building, and (4) the manager is not the source of the problem.

The retreat phase of the structural approach serves as an unfreezing mechanism. Held off-site it provides an opportunity for members of the organization to interact in different surroundings away from the day-to-day pressures of the work and usual roles that are occupied. Retreat objectives can be structured to include:

- an introduction to team-building concepts
- an exploration of forces driving and restraining team behavior in the organization
- an initial assessment of level of commitment to team-building activity.

Follow-through is critically important if the initial effort is to have any lasting impact beyond the retreat site. Structured small group discussion can generate a rich source of interventions that, if implemented have the potential to change the culture of the entire organization over several years, (Numerof and Associates, 1984). These questions and programs utilizing them were developed by the author and used very successfully in a wide variety of organizations interested in exploring or implementing team development programs. The questions are triple-tiered—they investigate rewards and liabilities regarding team behavior within the work group (such as a department), across departments, within senior management. In addition, time frames are established that ask participants to think strategically about the changes that could be made and the expected times for accomplishing them. Such involvement at this stage paves the way for commitment at later stages to those things that are actionable. Establishment of a task force with visibility provides continuity for follow-up activities. Without this the initial enthusiasm generated at the retreat is likely to dissipate. Assuming a commitment to move ahead is made, a demonstration site must be selected and broad structural supports must be in place. Many of the latter supports will have been identified at the retreat. Finally, the systematic implementation, the real work of the effort, must be done.

Several approaches can be employed during implementation. One structure combines the retreat format and ongoing meetings and thus has the advantage of being integrated into the regular operations of the group. More specifically, a one- or two-day retreat is scheduled. If the group members did not attend the prior retreat, the objectives are similar to those outlined before. The discussion focus is on the internal rewards and liabilities in team behavior and the organization in general. Assessment of current team functioning on the 12 dimensions described in the team model (Figure 13.1) occurs through paper-and-pencil questionnaires designed for that purpose. Once individuals assess the group, scores are combined to reflect average ratings and are entered on charts that show relative strength across all dimensions. Discussion centers on each area separately, with the goal being a thorough understanding of what the scores reflect. Minority opinion must be carefully explored. Group discussion is then structured to arrive at a consensus on what dimensions are top priorities for team intervention. Brainstorming activity centers on specific interventions within the dimension with careful attention paid as to how that intervention will affect other parts of the larger system. Force field analysis can be successfully applied to the intervention and time frames and responsibility for accomplishing parts of the intervention assigned.

Weekly, bimonthly, or monthly meetings can be established to monitor goal accomplishment, depending on the needs of the group. Reporting progress via newsletters and other communications to senior management helps to insure continuity and accountability for results. Once goals have been reached successfully, evaluation has occurred, and new scores charted on the dimensional comparison sheets, new areas are selected from the priority list generated earlier and the process continues. The successes and failures of the demonstration site guide the actions of subsequent efforts.

IN CONCLUSION

From one perspective the advantages of teamlike work groups in organizations are patently obvious and the process of getting there common sense. The question that follows is, If it is so obvious, why doesn't it happen? The answer may lie in the failure of people in organizations to recognize the interdependent nature of their roles and in the misuse of power. For the manager who wants to be the sole source of power ("I've got it, you don't"), it is easier to treat people as individual units as opposed to integral parts of a whole. This mechanistic view of people's functioning in the organization increases stress and is the antithesis of team building. If one were to take several machines and put them together in one room they wouldn't perform any better than if they were working in isolation. The same is not true for people.

If the manager saw him- or herself as a consultant to the work group whose job was to create a self-sustaining entity capable of managing the day-to-day operations, the manager would be able to take on the longer range tasks of thinking about and planning for the future. If managers were held accountable for creating work units that could function independently, they might be forced to look for and develop the potentials of their subordinates to contribute to the team. These subordinates might then be able to provide some of the many dimensions of leadership that are too often hoarded by the manager who refuses to relinquish absolute control.

Team-building efforts, while not a panacea for whatever ails an organization, can provide a framework for work groups and organizations that can diminish the frequency and intensity of work-related stressors and pave the way for increased productivity. Team building, as it is presented here, involves change in the distribution of work and of organizational power, change in the allocation of rewards, and change in the nature of what is to be rewarded. Integrating people into highly effective work groups—teams—will become increasingly important, particularly as organizations are being forced to do more with less. The model presented here implicitly assumes that members of work groups have the keys to improving performance and reducing stress—they need the structure for recognizing and realizing it.

REFERENCES

Blau, P. 1964. *Exchange and Power in Social Life.* New York: John Wiley.

Cartwright, D. and Zander, A. 1968. *Group Dynamics: Theory and Research,* 3rd ed. New York: Harper & Row.

Dyer, W. G. 1977. *Team Building: Issues and Alternatives.* Reading, Mass.: Addison-Wesley.

Francis, D. and Young, D. 1977. *Improving Work Groups.* San Diego: University Associates.

French, W. L. and Bell, C. H. 1978. *Organization Development.* Englewood Cliffs, N.J.: Prentice-Hall.

Gibb, J. R. 1961. Defensive communication. *The Journal of Communications,* 9(3): 141–148.

House, J. S. 1981. *Work Stress and Social Support.* Reading, Mass.: Addison-Wesley.

Janis, I. R. 1968. Group identification under conditions of external danger. In Cartwright, D. and Zander, A. (Eds.). *Group Dynamics: Research and Theory*, 3rd ed. New York: Harper & Row.

Jones, G. H. 1983. Transaction costs, property rights, and organizational culture: An exchange perspective. *Administrative Science Quarterly*, 28: 454–467.

Kahn, R. L., Wolfe, D. M., Quinn, R. P., and Snoek, J. D. 1964. *Organizational Stress: Studies in Role Conflict and Ambiguity*. New York: John Wiley.

Kantor, R. M. 1985. Micro Changes and Macro Effects. Paper presented to 45th Annual Academy of Management Meeting, San Diego.

Lewin, K. 1951. *Field Theory in Social Science*. New York: Harper & Row.

Likert, R. 1961. *New Patterns of Management*. New York: McGraw-Hill.

Luft, J. 1969. *Of Human Interaction*. Palo Alto, Calif.: National Press Books.

Maslach, C. and Jackson, S. E. 1981. The measurement of experienced burnout. *Journal of Occupational Behavior*, 2: 99–113.

Matteson, M. T. and Ivancevich, J. M. 1979. Organizational stressors and heart disease: A research model. *Academy of Management Review*, 4(3): 347–358.

McLean, A. A. 1979. *Work Stress*. Reading, Mass.: Addison-Wesley.

Numerof, R. E. 1983. *Managing Stress: A Guide for Health Professionals*. Rockville, Md.: Aspen Systems Corporation.

Numerof and Associates. 1984. "Measuring Managerial Practices." St. Louis: Numerof and Associates, Inc.

Numerof, R. E. and Gillespie, D. F. 1984. Predicting burnout among health service providers. Paper presented at the 44th Annual Academy of Management Meeting, Boston.

Patten, T. H., Jr. 1981. *Organizational Development Through Team Building*. New York: John Wiley.

Quick, J. C. 1979. Dyadic goal setting and role stress: A field study. *Academy of Management Journal*, 22(2): 241–252.

Quick, J. C. and Quick, J. D. 1984. *Organizational Stress and Preventive Management*. New York: McGraw-Hill.

Schein, E. H. 1985. *Organizational Culture and Leadership: A Dynamic View*. San Francisco: Jossey-Bass.

Selye, H. 1974. *Stress Without Distress*. New York: J. B. Lippincott.

14 Job security, job loss, and outplacement: implications for stress and stress management

Richard S. DeFrank and Judith E. Pliner

Employment has a multitude of meanings for people around the world. It provides a wage so that one may live more or less well. It provides structure to one's daily, weekly, and yearly existence. It often provides opportunities for interaction with a variety of people in a variety of settings and situations. It may also provide intense physical and psychological stress, unremitting boredom, and continual reminders that one is not achieving at the level one could, or should. Even so, the issue of job security is extremely important to workers, especially in times of slow economic growth or retrenchment. Keeping one's position and control over the decision to leave it are central concerns to employees everywhere. These concerns often manifest themselves in contract negotiations.

For example, the Kansas City Star newspaper and the International Typographical Union argued for five and a half years over job security contract provisions and finally agreed to limited security through 1990 for those employed when the previous contract expired. The 1984 agreements between General Motors, Ford, and the United Auto Workers established a Job Opportunity Bank-Security Program that would avoid layoffs of workers because of improved technology, obtaining parts from other sources, and so on. The program would provide such options as job training, transfers to openings in other plants, and increased unemployment benefits. A third example is the strike by 6,000 nurses in Minneapolis-St. Paul in 1984, in which job security played a major role. Provisions of the contract that was eventually agreed upon included the spreading of cuts in work time among all nurses in a unit before the elimination of jobs, and the freedom to use half of each individual's tuition reimbursement allotment for job retraining programs. All of these settlements reflect the central importance of job security to many workers. Investigators in the area of job satisfaction have noted this trend as well, since many measures of this construct including the Job Diagnostic Survey (Hackman and Oldham, 1975) and the Minnesota Satisfaction Questionnaire (Weiss et al., 1967) contain items or subscales relating to the perception of security as an element of job satisfaction.

JOB LOSS

Present Situation

The other side of the coin is also true, however: the threat and the reality of job loss are constantly present in our society. The perception of this threat is made clear by the following quote from a recent issue of the *AFL-CIO News*:

Suppose you take the population of New York City, Chicago, and Los Angeles. That's about 13 million people. Then add in the population of Atlanta, New Orleans, Pittsburgh and Boston. That's another 2 million, raising the grand total to 15 million. Now imagine those 15 million people—who might include you—without jobs or working part-time because there are no full-time jobs. This gives you some idea of the real size of America's big, forgotten, ignored economic problem—persistent, high unemployment in the midst of relative affluence (Roberts, 1985: 5).

Although these population figures may be underestimated, the sense of threat and the magnitude of the problem are not. Of the 15 million people mentioned, about 8.5 million are the "officially unemployed" as of April 1985, totaling 7.3 percent of the work force. An additional 5.7 million workers are involuntary part-time employees, and 1.3 million are discouraged workers who have dropped out of the labor market. While official levels of unemployment are down from a high of 9.7 percent in 1982, it is important to realize that loss of work is still occurring at a significant rate. For instance, in 1983 24 million workers—20 percent of all persons who worked or looked for work during the year—underwent a period of joblessness, and the figures are likely to be comparable for 1984. The most recent figures from 1985 suggest that the average length of unemployment is 16 weeks, with 1.3 million or 16 percent of the unemployed having been so for 27 weeks or more. This is *twice* the rate experienced in 1979. In 1984, when a monthly average of 8.4 million were unemployed, only 2.9 million of these were receiving any kind of unemployment benefits. It is also clear that few sectors of the economy are immune to layoffs. A pertinent example here is the health care industry. In 1984, as observed in a recent article in the *Monthly Labor Review*,

health services exhibited a lower rate of employment growth than in previous years. An actual decline in hospital employment in 1984 explains the slower pace, as hospitals streamlined management and staff in response to lower demands and pressure for more cost-effective health services (Devens, Leon, and Sprinkle, 1985: 7).

This example additionally notes some of the reasons behind terminations, specifically in response to marketplace issues. Large-scale layoffs can occur as a function of divisional cutbacks, plant closings, or relocations and mergers. The recent spate of mergers in the United States, especially in the oil business, has produced significant instances of job loss, as in the purchase of Gulf Oil by Chevron. There are many other reasons for termination, however, as suggested by Donald Monaco (1983). These include "Peter principled" employees or those promoted beyond their capabilities, "plateaued out" individuals who are bored and frustrated and ultimately become subpar performers, employees poorly matched to their jobs, employees having interpersonal differences with their supervisor, and workers exhibiting maladaptive behavioral characteristics. Few of these reasons, it should be noted, are related to pure incompetence, which is especially true for white-collar positions (Morin and Yorks, 1982).

Job loss not only has many causes but it also may have significant impacts on the people who experience it. That losing a job is a major stressor for most individuals is observed in the formulation of the widely used Holmes and Rahe (1967) life change scale. Various sample groups were asked to rate a number of life events as to the degree of adjustment required to cope with those situations, marriage given an arbitrary value of 50. The event "fired at work" consistently ranked eighth or ninth out of 43 events with a mean value of 47. Clearly there may be great individual differences in the perception of job loss as negative, with some people devastated by such an occurrence and others welcoming it as a chance to explore various desirable options. There is a growing body of literature, however, that suggests the impact job loss has on the individual may go beyond emotional reactions and adjustment problems.

Health Effects of Job Loss

Indexes of physical health and physiological functioning have been examined in a number of studies of the unemployed. Some of these reports have focused on general, self-reported health status and have found a tendency for poorer health ratings to accompany longer durations of unemployment (Cook et al., 1982; Warr and Jackson, 1984). In one of the most comprehensive studies of job loss effects, Kasl, Gore and Cobb (1975) observed that laid-off men who did not have a job after two years had high levels of illness complaints. However, for the rest of the unemployed sample (who were able to locate jobs), the highest illness reporting occurred just prior to the expected plant closings. There is some evidence indicating higher rates of particular physical disorders such as bronchitis, ischemic heart disease, and psychosomatic complaints among the unemployed than the employed (Cook et al., 1982; O'Brien and Kabanoff, 1979), and higher hospitalization rates in general (Lajer, 1982).

The possibility that job loss may affect health-related behaviors and physiological factors that put people at risk for future health problems has also been explored. There is some evidence that cigarette smoking (Cook et al., 1982), alcohol abuse (Buss and Redburn, 1983), and tranquilizer/ sleeping pill use (Jennings, Mazaik, and McKinlay, 1984) are more prevalent among the unemployed than among those still on the job. A number of biochemical indexes related to stress such as serum cholesterol, glucose, and uric acid were found to be elevated in the unemployed sample studied by Kasl and Cobb (1982). These and other more commonly used stress measures such as cortisol, epinephrine, and norepinephrine have been observed to be especially high among those individuals *anticipating* job loss (Cobb, 1974; Fleming et al., 1984; Levi et al., 1984). It appears that the time surrounding a layoff or termination is particularly stressful and that interventions might profitably be targeted for that period.

Similar findings can be cited for the mental health area, as the prevalence of psychiatric symptoms is higher among the unemployed (both young people and older workers) and that greater length of unemployment is associated with greater symptomatology (Banks and Jackson, 1982; Finlay-Jones and Eckhardt, 1981; Jackson et al., 1983; Hepworth, 1980; Jennings et al., 1984; Bebbington et al., 1981). Some work has been done on specific disorders, with depression showing a modest relationship to job loss (Kasl and Cobb, 1082; Pearlin et al., 1981; Buss and Redburn, 1983; Figueira-McDonough, 1978; Donovan and Oddy, 1982). Suicide has been noted to occur more frequently in unemployed groups (Sainsbury, 1955; Tuckman and Lavell, 1958; Humphrey, 1977; Shepherd and Barraclough, 1980), along with higher levels of anxiety/tension (Kasl and Cobb, 1982; Schlozman and Verba, 1978; Coates, Moyer, and Wellman, 1969), and use of psychiatric services (Lajer, 1982; O'Brien and Kabanoff, 1979).

A word of caution when considering these results: Some studies have not found the effects cited above, many studies are less methodologically sound than is desirable, and an unfortunately small proportion of this work has been done in the United States. Given the limitations, however, the available data suggest that job loss can produce significant physical and psychological difficulties for many people. By extension, there are important impacts on the fabric of our society as well. Family structures are often severely disrupted by the breadwinner's loss of employment, necessitating many changes in life-styles, role structures, and interpersonal relationships. If job-loss stress translates into physical or mental difficulties, it is impacting people who typically have grave problems dealing with the cost of treatment, placing the burden of care on society. Job loss also impacts the community by decreasing the tax base, overloading social services, and decreasing the desirability of life in that locale. Thus the impacts of job loss extend from the sphere of the individual employee to communitywide concerns.

MANAGING JOB LOSS STRESS

Motives for Organizational Involvement

Given that most negative effects of job loss impact on the individual and the community, and that a company or employer may have both self-serving and humanitarian interests, what then are the factors that influence the decision by the employer to provide services directed at reducing the stress associated with job loss? These factors can be roughly divided into three areas: those related to the company, those related to the terminating manager, and those related to the terminated individual.

With respect to factors related to the company, its public image is in some measure a function of the manner in which it treats its departing employees in addition to how it treats those who are retained. Sophisticated job seekers may investigate a prospective employer's policy regarding outplacement, severance pay, and "golden parachute" agreements. Companies that get the reputation of "throwing people out in the street" have a more difficult time recruiting than those with a more humane approach to termination. In addition to the impact a company's policy has on individuals outside the organization, the intraorganizational effect of separating employees needs to be examined. Demoralization, resentment, and anxiety about the future and a feeling of "the stayers got a worse deal than the leavers" are typical reactions of the varied employees who are left behind after a company reorganization or termination of a group of employees. Anxiety about the future possibility of job loss seems to be prevalent whether economic conditions are good or bad, as suggested earlier, and the catalyst of witnessing a colleague from one's own organization lose his or her job makes the threat of job loss more imminent. Given the curvilinear relationship between anxiety and performance, it is logical to conclude that the job performance of those who react too strongly to this threat may deteriorate and thus increase the likelihood that they, too, will lose their jobs.

Another source of influence affecting a company's decision regarding the provision of assistance to displaced employees is the threat of litigation based upon wrongful discharge. In the past few years the number of wrongful discharge lawsuits has risen dramatically. In California, an estimated 80 percent of cases that go to a jury trial result in a judgment against the employer, with awards averaging $500,000 to the plaintiff (Bakaly and Grossman, 1985). Until recently, employment-at-will, or the rule that enables both employee and employer to terminate their relationship in the absence of a contract at any time for any reason, was operative. However, exceptions to the employment-at-will concept have emerged, at both the legislative and judicial levels. It is becoming clear that the employment-at-will doctrine can no longer be relied upon as protection against wrongful discharge liability. While outplacement and related services for the separated employee should never be seen as a way to prevent wrongful discharge litigation, they might be appropriately viewed as a deterrent to nuisance activity. In the minds of many fired executives, the thought of suing the employer is present, and it can either be fueled or defused through interaction with an outplacement counselor. The posture taken by many counselors is to acknowledge the client's anger and need for regaining a sense of control, while at the same time asking the client to reflect upon the consequences of taking legal action. This is often sufficient to channel the client's energies into job-search activity.

A discussion of the impact of terminations on the retained employees would be incomplete without mentioning the effect on the terminating manager. In instances of reorganization or downsizing that involve a significant number of employees, or even in discharging an individual employee, the distress experienced by the terminator may be significant. In fact, the symptoms of stress experienced by individuals who are fearful of job loss are often quite similar to those experienced by the individuals who take responsibility for a termination decision or who are charged with executing someone else's decision. Knowing that the terminated employee is going to receive assistance generally serves to reduce the guilt and anxiety that the terminator experiences. Some firms provide a terminator training service as part of the group of services included in the outplacement package. The training may consist of giving information about typical reactions to a termination and how to handle each as well as straightforward advice about when the termination should take place, Equal Employment Opportunity Commission considerations, and what to include in a severance package. This training reduces the trauma associated with carrying out a termination.

A final motivation for companies to take an interest in reducing the negative effect of job loss on an individual is strictly humanitarian. How much of a particular company's concern about terminating employees stems from humanitarianism is probably impossible to measure. It will be a function of the individual decision makers, including their concern for their employees and their ability to shape company policy.

Notification

Assuming a company is motivated to reduce stress associated with job loss, what are the steps that may be taken once the decision has been made to close a facility, reduce the work force, or terminate an individual? One variable that appears to have a relationship to the amount of distress experienced by the displaced worker is the timing of the announcement. George Shultz and Arnold Weber (1976) in *Strategies for the Displaced Worker* concluded that a minimum of six months is needed by a company to organize services and programs, and for employees to evaluate their options and make plans for their future. Often companies initiate their planning activities six months in advance without notifying affected employees until weeks, days, or even hours before their termination. The lack of advance notice is likely to magnify the trauma involved for displaced workers. Not only does it prevent them from planning for the job change and making necessary financial adjustments and arrangements, there is another important psychological effect—that of feeling "ambushed." Workers who are notified of termination and are "taken out" of their work areas immediately report feeling humiliated, like "criminals." In situations in which employees are simultaneously terminated and escorted out of a plant or office, the usual rationale given is that it is a security measure. In some cases, access to highly sensitive information contained in a data system might be an irresistible temptation to an upset employee seeking revenge. At a high tech company located in the Southwest, upon notice of termination a design engineer "dumped" several of the designs he had been working on, thus obliterating months of effort. Obviously the psychological needs of employees and the need for information that affects their future often conflicts with the security/productivity needs of a company. In some European countries, Sweden and Germany for instance, companies are required to provide advance notice of a plant closing or layoff. Recently, several unions in the United States have succeeded in getting advance notice provisions in their contracts, but white-collar employees in the United States at this point appear to have little assurance of advance warning when a layoff is planned.

Severance Pay

The provision of severance pay or a supplement to unemployment insurance is a major factor in reducing stress associated with job loss. For professional employees the length of severance may be as short as one week for every year of service or as long as one month for every year of service. For nonexempt or hourly paid workers, some companies provide pay that supplements unemployment benefits. Generally, the limit for both is 26 weeks with duration of the supplemental pay based upon length of service. A number of options for disbursing severance pay are available, each with advantages and disadvantages for the company and the terminated employee. Severance pay may be paid in either a lump sum at the time of termination or in payments based on the employee's pay schedule. In the latter case, benefits are likely to continue as well. Some companies that provide severance in the form of regular payments have a policy of terminating payments when the individual secures employment, while others pay out the entire amount specified in the severance agreement regardless of the individual's employment status. If payments are made on a scheduled basis, the worker is considered to be employed and therefore ineligible for unemployment benefits. On the other hand, if the worker receives severance in the form of a lump-sum payment, then that individual will be considered unemployed and, therefore, eligible for benefits. Several hypotheses might be drawn regarding the relationship between type of severance (lump sum or payments) and duration of severance and the motivation to search for work that might be expected of an individual who has a lengthy severance period to be paid out incrementally regardless of employment status. Higher stress could be expected of an individual with a lump-sum payment that provided the equivalent of salary only for a brief time.

Outplacement

In addition to the advance notice an employee may or may not receive about termination, and the type of severance package awarded, the provision of outplacement services represents a third major variable influencing the amount of stress associated with job loss. Outplacement counseling is defined by Morin and Yorks (1982) as a systematic process by which a terminated person is trained and counseled in the techniques of self-appraisal and securing new employment appropriate to his needs and talents. They quickly add the disclaimer that outplacement counseling does not assume the responsibility for placing the person in a new job. A complete outplacement program is more broadly focused than on training and counseling solely, however, and involves a number of adjunct services. Some of these services are addressed to the company and some to the individual being terminated. *Pretermination consultation* is designed to help management think through their options, objectively choose a solution that is consistent with corporate policy, review the package of support services for those being terminated, and prepare the manager to conduct the termination interview. If this phase of the process is handled well, the trauma to the individual being terminated should be reduced. Assistance in setting up a *career center* is another consultative service that readily can be provided by an outplacement consultant. A career center on or near a company location provides more ongoing service to individuals after seminars or workshops have been completed. Typing services, job postings, use of telephones for long-distance calling, informal supportive self-help meetings, and resource materials are generally made available.

The outplacement counseling process per se is the heart of any outplacement program. It may be done individually (usually at a midmanagement level or above) or in groups. It begins at the time when the client(s) meets the outplacement counselor, which is generally moments after the termination. For all practical purposes, this phase of the process is crisis intervention. The counselor's role is to encourage ventilation of negative feelings, process events leading up to the termination, facilitate an adoption of the attitude of positive anticipation about the outplacement process, and give information. If the client is part of a group, a seminar will be held either at company facilities or outside facilities shortly after termination. These clients receive an intensive several-day program that includes most of the information and training offered to executives over a larger time period. If the client is an executive who will receive individual services, the process then resumes at the consultant's office as soon as possible. Together they review the individual's career history, define job accomplishments and skills, and clarify interests. Generally, a fairly extensive battery of psychological tests designed to assess interests, abilities, and personality is given to the client with feedback of the results done by a licensed psychologist.

Once the assessment phase of the process has been completed, the next important task is the development of a career objective. When the client has determined the specific direction she or he will take, the consultant assists in the formulation of a marketing/search plan. This comprehensive plan involves developing and using a contact network, interfacing with executive recruiters, writing a marketing letter and sending it to targeted companies, and carefully making use of advertised position announcements in the professional journals and daily newspapers. A client also receives training in the techniques of interviewing and salary negotiation, and approaches job interviews armed with knowledge about interpersonal communication styles and how to adapt one's own style to enhance rapport. Regular debriefings are held after job interviews to evaluate performance, and the consultant and client continue to meet periodically until new employment has been secured.

Outplacement Benefits. Insofar as the majority of clients seen by a firm providing outplacement services tend to be talented individuals who have demonstrated initiative and direction in their career activities, what benefits accrue to the individual who may be likely to locate employment without assistance? Though not documented empirically, there seem to be three major areas of benefit to the individual: (1) faster reemployment into a position of better "fit," (2) positive cognitive changes, and (3) positive affective changes.

The length of time that it takes an individual who has recently lost a job to find a new one is dependent on a number of factors. The most obvious ones are the individual's profession or trade and the demand for it in the marketplace, the health of the industry in which the individual seeks to work (such as energy, high tech, financial institutions, or whatever), the individual's geographic flexibility, the level of the position being sought, and the manner in which the job-seeker conducts his or her search. The last factor, job search strategy and techniques, is one that may be directly affected by the provision of outplacement services, and logically it should help to reduce the time necessary to secure new employment. The mechanism through which this occurs is primarily by helping the client adopt a "marketing" attitude. In order to "market" a product successfully, the seller must know the product well, be able to articulate its features and benefits, package the product artfully (resume, marketing letter), strategically plan the product's introduction to potential "buyers," and present the product well in a demonstration (or interview). Most jobseekers lack marketing skills required to do an efficient and successful job search. Additionally, outside of an outplacement situation, most jobseekers do not have a consultant available to them on a regular basis to help review materials, offer strategic advice, serve as a sounding board, and debrief meetings and interviews. In short, outplacement counseling is a service that can assist the jobseeker by helping him or her to do it "smarter."

Other benefits that would be expected to be enjoyed by pesons receiving outplacement services are positive cognitive and affective changes. Because these are related, with the cognitive often influencing the affective, they will be discussed together. At the simplest level, the acquisition of self-knowledge and job-search technology provides an advantage for any job seeker. For many clients who have been separated from their jobs, this is the first time they have ever looked for a job. It is not uncommon for outplacement clients to be persons who took positions with companies right out of high school or college and have worked for the same firm for 20 or even 30 years. Even the basics of how to look for a job elude them. One of the authors recalls meeting a refinery manager in Louisiana who went to work for a major oil company the day after he received his degree in chemical engineering. Almost 30 years later he was terminated, asked to clean out his office, and be off the premises, all on the same day.

The fact that a person has been in the same type of job or has worked for the same company for a long time does not necessarily insure that the person was happy and satisfied there. An estimated 80 percent of American workers are ill-suited to do the kind of work in which they are engaged, but because of circumstances and inertia fail to make a needed change. The opportunity for a thorough assessment of one's interests, abilities, motivation, and personality both from one's own perspective and from an objective point of view provides an individual with invaluable data upon which good decisions about future career moves can be based.

Armed with self-knowledge, job-search technology, and a strategic plan for redirecting a derailed career, a very important cognitive change usually takes place. That is, the individual gives up a reactive orientation to job seeking and adopts a proactive stance. In other words, some perceived control of the situation is gained that helps to reduce the anxiety and depression often associated with job loss and subsequent job seeking.

When the job seeker views interviewing as a mutual selection process rather than another opportunity for rejection, the outcome is likely to be more positive. In addition, when the individual has secured new employment, expectations about future employee-employer relationships are likely to be more realistic. Prior to their termination, many workers lived under the impression that as long as they were loyal employees and worked reasonably hard, they would always have a job and the company would take care of them through their retirement. Finding out that this was an illusion runs a close second to financial insecurity in causing the psychological devastation associated with losing one's job. Giving up the illusion that jobs are secure and companies offer family-like loyalty is an important developmental step for outplacement clients. In one sense it protects workers from being hurt in the future by their unrealistic expectations, but more importantly it serves as a catalyst for avoiding complacency and keeping one's job options open continually.

The pain of losing a job can be intense. When a person simultaneously loses financial security, opportunities to be productive, important social/work relationships, chances to compete in a way that is condoned, and a critical part of one's identity, there is a great sense of loss. Having psychological support from outside of as well as from within one's family can be as important as all the content learning that takes place in outplacement counseling. When there are other clients with whom one may share common experiences and derive support, the group therapeutic factors that Yalom (1975) discussed also are present (particularly installation of hope, universality, imparting of information, and altruism).

Outplacement Evaluation. The potential benefits of providing outplacement services, both to the company and to the terminated individual, have been outlined above and are substantiated by anecdotal reports. However, there are few or no empirical data to support these hypothesized benefits. Outplacement is generally not systematically evaluated; and when it is, the provider of the service is most often also the evaluator. In some cases, the clients themselves are asked to assess the quality of services they received.

There are several questions of concern from the client's perspective that need to be addressed. Does outplacement, in fact, lead to faster reemployment? Does it reduce stress-related outcomes of job loss? Is it effective across professional groups and levels of employment (hourly, nonexempt, exempt)? What techniques are most effective for the various types of clients? If outplacement is effective, what factor(s) is (are) operative (for example, confidence building, support group characteristics, learned skills, or simply attention given to the client)? From the company's perspective, how do the costs and benefits of outplacement impact the bottom line; that is, are the direct costs of providing services to an employee regained through ease of recruiting new talent, increased efficiency of company operation, and reduction of unnecessary manpower?

Also, what impact does a single termination or a force reduction have on those who retain their jobs? For example, after a layoff, what are the impacts of concern for one's own job security and the stability of the company, loss of friends and colleagues, increased work load, and accompanying stress? Will these adjustment issues cause productivity problems after a layoff? How can some attention be given to the "survivors" to prevent productivity declines? Some investigators have begun to address these concerns (for example, Greenhaigh, 1985; Krackhardt and Porter, 1985), but generally this area is wide open for research.

Another issue that needs to be addressed is any possible difference in the outcome of outplacement when it is provided by an outside firm or by the company's own staff. When services are provided by an outside firm, the client may feel more free to express negative emotions regarding the company and the termination. The consultant generally has little or no preconceived notion about the client, so their relationship begins with fresh impressions. Also, the client's view that an outsider is an "expert" may create heightened receptivity to the help being offered. On the other hand, companies who have staff capable of providing outplacement services may provide it more consistently owing to the probable lower costs. The providers themselves may also have more in-depth knowledge of their industry, and therefore be better equipped to counsel individuals regarding potential job opportunities. In-house programs could conceivably be better attended if companies tied other benefits to the outplacement services (for example, having a representative from the Employment Security Commission present to sign up people for unemployment benefits).

All of these issues represent fertile areas for discussion and future research. Because of the potential high profit margin, the provision of outplacement services is being offered by many individual practitioners and firms. In order to assure high quality, these questions need to be explored so that consumers of outplacement services can make educated decisions about vendors and what services are needed in different situations.

THE ROLE OF HEALTH CARE PROVIDERS

Finally, where do health care providers fit into this picture? One way relates to the delivery of health care. Given the ongoing levels of unemployment and the resulting potential physical and psychological effects, professionals in the health field need to be sensitive to the employment difficulties of their clients beyond their ability to pay for treatment. This will be especially true of those who deal with lower socioeconomic status and indigent patients. It also could be suggested that the provision of preventive health services would be especially valuable for those undergoing or about to experience job loss. While this is undoubtedly true, it is not clear who would pay a health provider for carrying out these activities. An employer would have considerably less motivation for supporting such measures than for an outplacement program (as discussed above), and indeed sponsoring preventive programs might be construed as an admission by a company that layoffs lead to adverse health consequences. Since employers are unlikely to pay, other sources of funding would be needed to carry out health-promotive activities for such an at-risk population.

Finally, health care providers, especially large-scale ones such as hospitals, might become consumers of outplacement services. In view of the emphasis on cost containment and the consequent downturn in health-sector employment levels being experienced, outplacement for terminated employees would have the same benefits for the organization and the individual as outlined earlier for companies in general. Additionally, the typical high-stress experiences of many health care workers (such as nurses) that might be exacerbated by staff cutbacks would suggest the value of outplacement in reducing some of the nonwork tension undergone by retained employees. In sum, health care providers will be impacted in a number of ways by job security and job loss issues, and they will need to consider creative ways to deal with these problems for their own benefit and for the well-being of their organizations and their communities.

REFERENCES

Bakaly, C. and Grossman, J. M. 1985. *How to Avoid Wrongful Discharge Suits*. American Management Association Publication #0025–1895/85/0006–0044.

Danks, M. H. and Jackson, P. R. 1982. Unemployment and risk of minor psychiatric disorder in young people: Cross-cultural and longitudinal evidence. *Psychological Medicine*, 12: 789–798.

Bebbington, P., Harry, J., Tennant, C., Sturt, E., and Wing, J. K. 1981. Epidemiology of mental disorders in Camberwell. *Psychological Medicine*, 11: 561–579.

Buss, T. F. and Redburn, F. S. 1983. *Shutdown at Youngstown: Public Policy for Mass Unemployment*. Albany: State University of New York Press.

Coates, D. Moyer, S., and Wellman, B. 1969. The Yorklea study of urban mental health: Symptoms, problems, and life events. *Canadian Journal of Public Health*, 60: 471–481.

Cobb, S. 1974. Physiological changes in men whose jobs were abolished. *Journal of Psychosomatic Research*, 18: 245–258.

Cook, D. G., Cummins, R. O., Bartley, M. J., and Schaper, A. G. 1982. Health of unemployed middle-aged men in Great Britain. *Lancet*, 5: 1290–1294.

Devens, R. M., Leon, C. B., and Sprinkle, D. L. 1985. Employment and unemployment in 1984: A second year of strong growth of jobs. *Monthly Labor Review*, 108: 3–15.

Donovan, A. and Oddy, M. 1982. Psychological aspects of unemployment: An investigation into the emotional and social adjustment of school leavers. *Journal of Adolescence*, 5: 15–30.

Figueira-McDonough, J. 1978. Mental health among unemployed Detroiters. *Social Service Review*, 52: 383–399.

Finlay-Jones, R. A. and Eckhardt, B. 1981. Psychiatric disorder among the young unemployed. *Australian and New Zealand Journal of Psychiatry*, 15: 265–270.

Fleming, R., Baum, A., Reddy, D., and Gatchel, R. J. 1984. Behavioral and biochemical effects of job loss and unemployment stress. *Journal of Human Stress*, 10: 12–17.

Greenhaigh, L. 1985. Job security and disinvolvement: Field research on the survivors of layoffs. Presented at the annual meeting of the Academy of Management, San Diego.

Hackman, J. R. and Oldham, G. R. 1975. Development of the job diagnostic survey. *Journal of Applied Psychology*, 60: 159–170.

Hepworth, S. J. 1980. Moderating factors of the psychological impact of unemployment. *Journal of Occupational Psychology*, 53: 139–145.

Holmes, T. H. and Rahe, R. H. 1967. The social readjustment rating scale. *Journal of Psychosomatic Research*, 11: 213–218.

Humphrey, J. A. 1977. Social loss: A comparison of suicide victims, homicide offenders and non-violent individuals. *Diseases of the Nervous System*, 38: 157–160.

Jackson, P. R., Stafford, E. M., Banks, M. H., and Warr, P. B. 1983. Unemployment and psychological distress in young people: The moderating role of employment commitment. *Journal of Applied Psychology*, 68: 525–535.

Jennings, S., Mazaik, C., and McKinlay, S. 1984. Women and work: An investigation of the association between health and employment status in middle-aged women. *Social Science and Medicine*, 19: 423–431.

Kasl, S. V. and Cobb, S. 1982. Variability of stress effects among men experiencing job loss. In Goldberger, L. and Breznitz, S. (Eds.). *Handbook of Stress: Theoretical and Clinical Aspects*. New York: The Free Press.

Kasl, S. V., Gore, S., and Cobb, S. 1975. The experience of losing a job: Reported changes in health, symptoms, and illness behavior. *Psychosomatic Medicine*, 37: 106–122.

Krackhardt, D. and Porter, L. W. 1985. When friends leave: A structural analysis of the relationship between turnover and stayer's attitudes. *Administrative Science Quarterly*, 30: 242–261.

Lajer, M. 1982. Unemployment and hospitalization among bricklayers. *Scandinavian Journal of Social Medicine*, 10: 3–10.

Levi, L., Brenner, S., Hall, E. M. Hjelm, R., Salovaara, H., Arnetz, B., and Petterson, I. 1984. The psychological, social, and biochemical aspects of unemployment in Sweden. *International Journal of Mental Health*, 13: 18–34.

Monaco, D. A. 1983. Outplacement counseling: Business and profession. In J. S. J. Manuso (Ed.). *Occupational Clinical Psychology*. New York: Praeger.

Morin, W. J. and Yorks, L. 1982. *Outplacement Techniques: A Positive Approach to Terminating Employees*. New York: AMACOM.

O'Brien, G. E. and Kabanoff, B. 1979. Comparison of unemployed and employed workers on work values, locus of control, and health variables. *Australian Psychologist*, 14: 143–154.

Pearlin, L. I., Menaghan, E. G., Lieberman, M. A., and Mullan, J. T. 1981. The stress process. *Journal of Health and Social Behavior*, 22: 337–356.

Roberts, M. 1985. Workers without jobs. *AFL-CIO News* 30: 5–10.

Sainsbury, P. 1955. *Suicide in London: An Ecological Study*. London: Chapman & Hall, Mandsley Monograph No. 1.

Schlozman, K. L. and Verba, S. 1978. The new unemployment: Does it hurt? *Public Policy*, 26: 333–358.

Shepherd, D. M. and Barraclough, B. M. 1980. Work and suicide: An empirical investigation. *British Journal of Psychiatry*, 136: 469–478.

Shultz, G. and Weber, A. R. 1976. *Strategies for the Displaced Worker*. Westport, Conn.: Greenwood Press.

Tuckman, J. and Lavell, M. 1958. Study of suicide in Philadelphia. *Public Health Reports*, 73: 547–553.

Warr, P. and Jackson, P. 1984. Men without jobs: Some correlates of age and length of unemployment. *Journal of Occupational Psychology*, 57: 77–85.

Weiss, D. S., Davis, R. V., England, G. W., and Lofquist, L. H. 1967. *Manual for the Minnesota Satisfaction Questionnaire*. Minneapolis: University of Minnesota Industrial Relations Center.

Yalom, I. D. 1975. *The Theory and Practice of Group Psychotherapy*. New York: Basic Books.

15   *A labor view of stress management*

William W. Winpisinger

THE INTERNATIONAL ASSOCIATION OF
MACHINISTS AND WORK STRESS

As an organization the International Association of Machinists (IAM) got into work stress and health care by a rather circuitous route. My experience with the IAM spans the last 40 years (Winpisinger, 1978). Some years ago—after 50 years of trying—we finally achieved the Occupational Safety and Health Act. The passage of "OSHA," as we call it these days, caused a flurry of activity among many of the unions. These unions, including the IAM, established a corollary department within the organization to deal with shop floor worker problems. Of course, when dealing with such problems one always has the outreach that leads well beyond the workplace.

For example, one of the early things we realized was that we seemed to have an inordinately high number of cancer deaths among our railroad membership. Because of this consistently high level of cancer deaths we commissioned a study through our Occupational Safety and Health Department. We are one of the few unions—perhaps the only one—that has maintained complete records of anyone who has ever been a member. Bear in mind that our union is approaching 100 years of age and was founded in a locomotive pit by 19 machinists in Atlanta, Georgia, in 1888. Since we have always had a death benefit program, we are the recipients of a copy of the death certificate in each case involving a death claims benefit. We started a systematic review of these death certificates and found that the incidence of cancer was very, very high. This, we think, is traceable to the fact that steam-age locomotives, with which most of our deceased members worked, were full of asbestos-coated lagging that was used to hold in the boiler heat and to produce steam. It was the inhaling of the asbestos dust that we believe accounted for the very high rate of cancer.

In spite of the high cancer rate (Anonymous, 1978), we found that the average age at death of these locomotive machinists was 74 years. When we looked at their modern counterpart (the airplane mechanics in the air transport industry), the average age of their deaths was 64—a full ten years less without the high incidence of cancer. This, of course, piqued our curiosity and we moved promptly to attempt an explanation of the difference. Hence our first exposure to what can properly be identified as job stress. It is our experience that it is virtually impossible to make a firm distinction between job stress and stress outside the workplace. It is also

210

very difficult to define specifically the kind of stress in modern job categories.

When we began looking at the air transport industry and contrasting it to the older railroad industry, what did we find? We found that the typical railroad worker lived in country towns spaced roughly 50 miles apart along the railroad. He had a typical family life of that vintage with a wife who stayed home and was the cook, the housekeeper, and the child raiser. He walked to work with a lunch pail and ate every day in very dirty circumstances. Even though he worked daily in dirty, noisy, and frequently very cold or brutally warm places, he and his co-workers seemed to have that camaraderie that is so important as a work stress reducer. Nothwithstanding all of those conditions and notwithstanding a hearing loss level that was very, very high compared to the general population, he still managed to live to the average age of 74 years.

Then we looked at his modern counterpart. He works in an environment that is equally noisy, perhaps more so. Protective hearing devices are readily available and mandatory on most airline ramps and in most airline environments. He lives in the suburbs because he is relatively affluent, drives long distances over crowded freeways to work, and probably arrives at the job in a very stressed condition. (I experience this every day and some day will invent a way to have American drivers move when you want them to move—a technique that has not yet been mastered.) He has a far, far cleaner environment within which to work. But the 365-day-a-year, 7-day-a-week emphasis on doing the job well, doing it right, doing it to protect the lives of the traveling public, being on time even though there is oftentimes not enough time to get the job done according to the book—all this seems to take its inevitable toll, which is high stress and shorter life span.

REENGINEERING THE WORK ENVIRONMENT

The situation of high stress concerns us very much and we are actively trying to pursue ways to address the problem (Shostak, 1980). In general manufacturing, for well over half a century, we have existed in an environment encouraged by the writings of Frederick Taylor. Taylor (1911) described the original model for U.S. industry as being mass production with repetitive tasks. Industry then interpreted this model as requiring every move all day long to be monitored religiously by a stopwatch, up to and including personal time used for biological necessities. Trade unions have railed for decades against the continued employment of the stopwatch in industry. We have tried instead to loosen up the work environment and to initiate numerous experiments in quality of work life. In addition, notwithstanding popular rumor, we have experimented very substantially with improvements in the work environment.

One of the problems we find with improvements in the work environment is that when things are made a bit more hospitable, and therefore less stress-producing for an employee, it simply is a stress transfer mechanism; the stress moves from the employee group on to the supervision group, which begins to show all of the signs of job stress. Our first loyalty, of course, is to our member—he or she who performs the work. But we do not see that transferring stress to supervisors is a very decent bargain; certainly it is not a very strategic bargain when stress is simply transferred from one group to another. Over time we have talked with management and we have been able to address the problem, to reengineer the performance of work and to reengineer the environment of work, including the physical plant. Most of the unions have developed some degree of expertise in this type of workplace reengineering.

THE STRESS OF JOB INSECURITY

Employment security remains at the very top of the list of stress producers and I want to point out that there are both micro and macro treatments to the problem. On the micro basis we bargain for specific relief in the workplace or in a group of workplaces. However, this is often not a solution to the problem because it is local in its effect; it does not proliferate and as soon as you solve one problem you breed another stress-producing problem. There are a lot of macro activities that are called for and that is why you see the trade union movement today embarking on some of the courses that it pursues. We can say that people's job security is simply a function of their own talent and their own drive. I guess in the largest measure perhaps that is true, but in general we say "hogwash." Essential to job security is opportunity and without opportunity you do not get rid of the stress of job insecurity.

Take myself. I think I've got all kinds of drive, initiative, and a certain degree of knowledge—notwithstanding my high school drop-out status. But there is not much of a market for "used" union presidents; you know if you get turned out to pasture by the membership for lack of doing what they perceive to be a decent job you are going to have a time landing a job that has anywhere near the kind of rewards that mine has at the moment. Fortunately I'm over sixty now and I'm on the home stretch, so I don't have to worry about that. It's not a source of stress for me, but it surely is for a great many people in this country.

We stand today on the very threshold of the most pervasive revolution in the performance of work: the technological revolution. I see many learned journals and seminars that are coming to grips with various aspects of what I think is an overall problem.

How much confidence can a young worker today have that he or she will even get a job? Many Americans are disadvantaged in terms of employment today. We see the invasion of robotics into America's workplaces and it transcends all collars—pink, white, blue, new, you name it. It invades and every time that invasion goes forward another notch there is a very, very high level of stress created both in and out of the workplace. A lot of human beings become the jetsam and the flotsam of that maddening rush by which we like to say we meet the world market's competition.

Well, without commenting on the validity of this situation, let me just point out that in the macro sense we have a long way to go, but there are many things we can do as a nation to get at these lingering causes of stress and markedly reduce them. First, we can pursue a full-employment economy. Everyone says that that is pie in the sky: "Can't be done." I submit to you that it can be done and that all it takes is the political will of voter support to get it done. Second, taxpayers should support stress-reducing activities in this country today. To a degree unprecedented in our history taxpayers support the efforts of the Pentagon, a significant chunk of which are devoted to the creation of labor-saving machinery on the altar of cheapening the cost of defending the nation. Companies implement the research that creates the hardware and get it into the nation's workplaces. Because of the contracting power of the Pentagon, it can say to a Lockheed or a McDonnell-Douglas or a Boeing airplane company, "Thou shalt put this machinery in place or thou shalt not get the contract." It is worth billions of dollars in many cases. Obviously labor-saving machinery is put into place.

We then have a high segment of displaced machinists right at that point. The stress level for those who remain is up markedly because those people know it is only a question of time until their turn comes. They look at how those who are displaced are shunted aside as a result of the current political thought that it is too expensive to train or retrain people. When we as a nation cannot afford to spend money to retrain people because we have to spend it all on implements to blow up the world, then I suggest that there is a lot of stress being created.

Let me give you another example. Elsewhere in this volume it is suggested that plant closings are a stress producer of a very high order; I know this first hand. I was at a session recently on Capitol Hill hosted by our union and some other unions for congressmen and their aides. The National Association of Manufacturers was there in force as was the National Chamber of Commerce. At the meeting we unveiled a plant-closing piece of legislation that is already endorsed by over 140 U.S. congressmen and for which we wanted to get more cosigners. This is a piece of legislation that requires only one thing; it does not cost a penny, but requires only that an employer who knows that he is going to shut down an operation of 50 or more people give 90 days' notice to the affected employees. That's all. Those two organizations indicated that they would fight to the death and have made it their number-one legislative priority to defeat this legislation. To this I say, "case closed." If 90 days' notice is too humane a treatment of America's workers when one is aware of a closing—and the bill exempts anyone who faces an emergency—if this is too much on the altar of humanity in this nation, then I say to you that stress levels are going to go clear out of sight.

THE COLLISION OF PROFITS AND PEOPLE

This story could be repeated on and on in terms of the political dereliction of the country. As you can see, the union is involved in efforts to create a climate in which human beings finally get at least a chance at equality between themselves and the profit-making mechanism. Up to now, because we have been a progressive, rapidly expanding nation in terms of our economy and our population, we have been able to handle these revolutions in the workplace in a great many ways and the "profit before people" motive did not impede progress too much. It did not cause enough discomfort, it did not create enough notoriety for anyone to do anything meaningful about it. Now we must have the equal sign in the equation and this results in the collision of profits and people. People at least have to get a fair shake or stress levels are going to arc at an unprecedented degree. I suggest to all of those in management that somehow we must balance this equation. Profits cannot always win in the here and now. What we see today is merely a glimpse of what we think we expect to encounter for the balance of this century and well into the next. What lies ahead of us in terms of displacing human beings in the performance of work is challenging indeed.

Now who knows? I certainly lack the expertise to assess all of this in a very meaningful or very professional way. I do know that displacing workers creates social havoc and I do know that social havoc is a stress producer of a very high sort. I also know that, carried to its logical extreme, the result is social unrest, but I do not think that this is the kind of division that we want in our country. I do not think that this is the kind of America that the young workers coming in today want to see on the horizon.

What do we witness with these young workers? Again, through union involvement, we looked around a little bit and found that new workers are graduates from an educational system that has suddenly become abominable. Managers tell us that a very high percentage of those entering the workforce are functionally illiterate. It seems to me a national effort must be directed at the educational system if we are going to reduce stress after these workers get into the workplace.

INTERVENTIONS IN THE WORKPLACE

In addition to increasing illiteracy, we see increasing drug addiction. It is running so rampant in our ranks that, quite frankly, we do not even know the degree of drug addiction. We know something about alcoholism—far more than we do about drug addiction—and it is running rampant, too. I am not trained to assess whether these increases are produced by stress, whether they are a cultural aberration, or what. But they are there and the only way we can deal with them is to drag them out of the closet. Yet it took us years to get to the point where we could sit down with management in this country and create an awareness that a serious problem with drugs and alcohol existed in the workplace. This was a problem difficult to admit: that companies employed alcoholics, mentally disabled people that needed psychological help and care, and substance abusers. We know these problems are there and now we are beginning to build programs that systematically try to treat these problems. To the extent that these programs are successful, it becomes apparent that a reduction of the kinds of tensions and stress that create problems among the entire workforce has occurred. But we have a long, long way to go.

Another very "at home" experience in terms of stress awareness came one day a few years ago when one of our members became so incensed at his supervisor that he got a gun, walked into the supervisor's office, and shot him dead sitting in his chair. The worker got away, jumped in his car, drove down to the union hall, shot the business agent right between the eyes sitting at his desk, calmly walked over and put down the gun, climbed in a police car and went to jail—very blasé about the whole experience, but he got it off his chest. He killed them both. I guess he did not know which one was responsible for the kind of stress he was experiencing. This kind of malignant aggression is not only destructive of others, but it is also self-destructive (Fromm, 1973).

Mishandled stress is a very real challenge as far as we are concerned and we fight to find appropriate responses. We are fighting primarily in a political arena. Maybe the kind of opportunity and the kind of vision that Walter Mondale attempted to create in the political arena in the 1984 election is more valid than the one we have now. I thought so but obviously the majority of Americans did not. I think any measure of awareness is important if we really are serious about tackling stress on the job. The political climate of the country and the priorities that we set as a nation for dealing with problems are inexplicable to me. Are we going to spend all our money doing everything else except attacking these kinds of problems? If we do, I'll submit to you that they will not be solved. Any institution that attempts to solve these problems is going to be very seriously handicapped and debilitated. We in the union movement know something about institutional handicaps these days.

REFERENCES

Anonymous. 1978. 20% of cancer work-related. *Newsday*, September 12, p. 12.

Fromm, E. 1973. *The Anatomy of Human Destructiveness*. New York: Holt, Rinehart & Winston.

Shostak, A. B. 1980. *Blue-Collar Stress*. Reading, Mass.: Addison-Wesley.

Taylor, Frederick. 1911. *The Principles of Scientific Management*. New York: Harper & Row.

Winpisinger, W. W. 1978. Uphill all the way. *Challenge,* March-April.

16   *Corporate health and fitness programs and the prevention of work stress*

W. B. Baun, E. J. Bernacki,
and J. Alan Herd

That exercise is important for good health is believed to be true by most North American adults (President's Council on Physical Fitness and Sports, 1973; Harris and Associates, 1978; Canada Fitness Survey, 1982). Moreover, responses to a popular opinion poll (Harris, 1978) indicated that those who exercised also believed that regular physical activity resulted in feeling, looking, and doing better. Approximately 15 percent of U.S. adults reported that they participated regularly in exercise equivalent to an hour of walking daily at 3–3.5 mph, a daily 20–30 minute run at 6.0 mph, or one hour's swim at 1 mph on five days a week. Apparently, many adults believe that exercise and physical fitness programs are important for good health, and a few actually act out their beliefs.

Several investigators have reported the effects of corporate health and fitness programs on physiological and psychological parameters (Pauly, Palmer, and Wright, 1982; Folkins, 1976; Folkins, Lynch, and Gardner, 1972). In most studies, significant improvements were found in psychological parameters such as self-concept, trait anxiety, and job satisfaction, as well as improvement in physiological parameters such as resting heart rate and blood pressure, concentrations of triglycerides and total concentrations of cholesterol in blood. In most studies, significant improvements occurred in direct relation to frequency of exercise.

The psychological benefits of exercise are apparent in the mentally well, as well as in those with psychological and psychiatric disorders. Moreover, the growing numbers of habitual exercisers report beneficial cognitive and emotional responses to exercise, and psychological studies validate their reports. For some, habitual exercise fills some strong need that compels their regular exercise. However, it also is apparent that individuals who might benefit the most from psychological, cardiovascular, or weight control benefits frequently are the least likely to begin or maintain a program of regular exercise. Fortunately, the psychological benefits associated with exercise are most likely to be the reason individuals continue to participate. The relationship between perceived benefits or self-efficacy and participation has been studied most thoroughly in corporate health and fitness programs.

PSYCHOLOGICAL BENEFITS OF VIGOROUS EXERCISE

Fitness Acceptability

The promotion of personal fitness by medical and fitness professionals and the health and fitness media blitz of the 1980s have made participation in exercise not only socially acceptable but desirable. More importantly, the majority of adults believe that regular exercise is important for good health and that their own health would benefit from more exercise (President's Council on Physical Fitness and Sports, 1974). However, survey information (Canada Fitness Survey, 1982) has shown that those individuals actively seeking better health through exercise are, for the most part, young, highly educated, affluent, and engaged as a professional or white-collar worker.

An early study by Brunner (1969) interviewed two groups of adult males. One group participated in vigorous activity and the other group was made up of nonparticipants. The participants stated that the primary reason for regular participation was a desire to keep physically fit with an associated feeling of well-being. Nonparticipants indicated "perceived benefits" of exercise were to keep physically fit and feel better physically and mentally. The most common exercise barrier cited by the nonpartici-pants was lack of time. However, what is interesting is that both participants and nonparticipants stated that "feeling better" was a primary reason for exercising on a regular basis.

Levenson, Thornby, and Levenson (1985) in a recent study of the perception of benefits to jogging found the three most common reasons stated were emotional and physical benefits, support of others, and attractiveness/appearance. This analysis replicates Brunner's work and supports his findings that many individuals exercise for mental health reasons. It has been estimated that 85 percent of the individuals who exercise experience a generalized sensation of "feeling better" (Morgan, 1979a). Thus, many individuals exercise on a regular basis to reduce the effects of emotional stress and relieve tension.

Although many individuals believe that exercise makes people "feel better," there are few controlled studies that have been performed to support these claims. The studies that have been completed are plagued by the inability to quantify psychological effects and when they are measur-able they cannot be solely attributed to exercise. The expectation that exercise will yield psychological benefits is oten imparted by a zealous fitness instructor or exercise partner who converts the sedentary person into an exercise enthusiast. Sorting out which psychological effects are specific to the exercise and independent of other social, psychological, or characterological factors is almost impossible.

Effect of Stress and Exercise on the Individual

Selye (1975) believes that an organism that is subjected to chronic bouts of moderate stress in the form of exercise will be conditioned to deal more effectively with confrontations with other stressors. A recent line of research that supports Selye's theories is the impact of stressful life events on physical and psychological health. Roth and Holmes (1985) have shown that subjects reporting more negative life stress and who had lower fitness levels reported more overall difficulty with physical health. Those individuals who were in better physical shape dealt more effectively with stress and saw less deleterious effects on their physical and psychological health.

The direct relationship between emotional tension and neuromuscular tension was first recognized by Jacobson (1979). His extensive research and simple exercises have shown that relief of muscle tension can reduce stress. DeVries (1974) has shown that exercise can reduce the electrical activity in resting muscles more than mild tranquilizers. This supports the theory of Morgan et al. (1970), which postulates that the main psychological benefit of exercise is the maintaining of a low tension state. After exercise, the tension slowly increases again within a 24-hour period.

Exercise and recreational activities have been referred to as a palliative coping technique (Mobily, 1982). This process allows an individual in a situation of anticipated threat to divert his attention and momentarily receive emotional relief through the simple act of exercise. Palliative techniques deal with stress indirectly because they provide a diversion or relaxation. Use of this coping technique (Gal and Lazarus, 1975) suggests that it is best used in advance of the stressor and not in conjunction with a stressor's actual occurrence. This implies that exercise and recreation would be most effective in dealing with the anticipatory stress emotions that are felt prior to a stressful confrontation. Schafer (1981) believes that exercise creates a feeling of competence and control, which he refers to as a "personal stability zone." Within the personal stability zone, individuals have opportunity for creative problem solving. This experience of relaxation and discovery of solutions to problems is similar to that which is experienced during meditation or relaxation exercises.

Both behavioral and psychological processes appear to mediate the psychological benefits of exercise for individuals. Not only does exercise provide a means to deal directly with stress, but it also offers coping strategies. All of these processes help the individual "feel better" about himself, which improves his self-concept. Self-concept or self-esteem has been defined as "that aspect of an individual's concept of self that provides a feeling of value or worth" (Terjung, 1982). A feeling of value or worth impacts positively upon an individual's level of job satisfaction. This has been one of the main arguments for the establishment of corporate health and fitness programs.

Corporate Health and Fitness Programs

The four reasons given for the establishment of health and fitness programs by the Washington Business Group for Health (Small businesses show big interest in health promotion, *Employee Health and Fitness*, 1985) are (1) improve human relations through improving morale, engendering greater commitment to the organization, and enhancing employees' sense of belonging; (2) improve productivity; (3) lower health care costs; and (4) improve the company image with the community.

The idea that a physical fitness program could improve the relationship that management has with its employees, thus improving productivity, has been around since the nineteenth century. John H. Patterson initiated the first recorded corporate fitness program in the United States at National Cash Register. Naisbitt (1982), in his book *Megatrends*, indicated there are over 500 companies with health and fitness programs managed by full-time directors, and that in 1980 the Association for Fitness Leaders in Business and Industry had 1,800 members or a 7,000 percent increase in membership since 1974. Corporate fitness programs are generally found in larger organizations, and the current general trend is to provide services to all employees, emphasizing preventive health practices other than just exercise.

Figure 16.1 reflects a modified model presented by Driver and Ratliff's (1982) perceptions of management's rationale used to justify employee health and fitness programs. Exercise leads to physical fitness, which enhances the wellness process. This, in turn, decreases employee health care claims because of fewer occupational injuries and lower annual medical costs. Exercise programs also result in a strong attachment to the organization. This manifests itself as cohesiveness. Cohesive groups are characterized by friendliness, cooperation, and interpersonal attraction. Cohesiveness will positively affect an employee's level of satisfaction, which management feels will increase employee productivity and decrease turnover and absenteeism.

Is this model realistic in its expectations? The initial step of exercise leading to physical fitness, followed by an improved wellness state, is strongly supported in the current exercise science literature (Serfass and Gergerich, 1984). Until recently, only anecdotal case studies have supported the idea that fitness programs could lead to reduction in health care claim costs. A prospective longitudinal study (Bowne et al., 1984) over a four-year period showed an average reduction in medical costs of

Figure 16.1.   Organizational benefits of a corporate health and fitness program

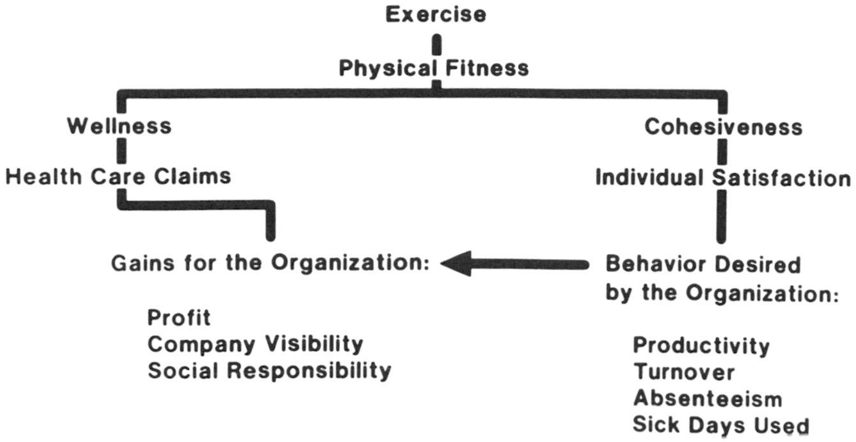

Source: Adapted from Driver and Ratliff (1982).

$262.14 per participant, and a 45.7 percent reduction in the average major medical costs for the postentry year. A recent study (Baun, Bernacki, and Tsai, 1986) showed a difference in health care costs during the start-up year of a health and fitness program for exercisers and nonexercisers. When nonhospitalization costs were separated from total health costs, exercise status significantly affected the average costs reimbursed. The average exerciser cost was only $339 ($p < 0.05$). These studies represent initial research documenting the effects of health and fitness programs on health care costs. Future studies will bring larger populations studied for longer periods of time, which will help provide conclusive evidence that the fitness/wellness link can reduce health care costs.

Can a health and fitness program affect employee cohesiveness? There are many elements to which an employee could feel allegiance within an organization. The diversity of these elements (job, place of work, and work group) offers employees several reasons to make strong attachments to the organization. However, the physical fitness/cohesiveness relationship has not been addressed within the current literature. Cohesiveness infers decreased turnover but, unfortunately, there are no studies of the relationship between fitness programs and turnover rates. Preliminary Tenneco data (Bernacki and Baun, 1984) suggest that the turnover rate of exercisers is 20 percent less than that of their nonexercising counterparts. If this is supported by some in-depth studies, it provides an indication of a possible trend.

If physical fitness leads to stronger cohesiveness, does employee satisfaction follow? Currently, there is no experimental research showing that improvements in mood and self-concept can be generalized into job satisfaction. Thus the linkage between fitness, cohesiveness, and the other behaviors desired by the organization have yet to be supported in the scientific literature.

Research has been completed on some of the other desirable variables that suggests there is a natural tie between cohesiveness and individual satisfaction. Early absenteeism research from Europe supports the contention that fit employees are absent less (Linden, 1969). This author's recent analysis of the Tenneco database (Baun et al., 1986) found there was approximately a one-day difference between exercisers and nonexercisers. The difference between males was insignificant, but a three-day difference was found between the female exerciser (47 hours) and nonexerciser (69) ($p < 0.05$). Shephard, Cox, and Corey (1981) have shown that over a six-month period, individuals who participated in a fitness program developed a 22 percent advantage relative to employees who were not exercising. The combination of the early European studies and recent finding by Shephard and the Tenneco group suggests that exercise can positively affect absenteeism.

The second most important reason for initiating a fitness program given by the Washington Business Group for Health was worker productivity. This implies that employees are not only satisfied with their work group but are supportive of the goals of the organization. Shephard et al. (1981) tried to measure the effects of fitness programming on worker productivity, but small and relatively similar gains in both the experimental and control companies suggested a nonspecific response to experimental intervention, or the Hawthorne effect. A study by the Tenneco research group (Bernacki and Baun, 1984) found a significant ($p < 0.01$) positive relationship between exercise adherence and above-average job performance. There was also an inverse relationship demonstrated between poor job performance and increasing adherence levels ($p < 0.0001$). This has been one of the only studies to find a positive, although probably noncausal, relationship between exercise participation and above-average job performance. Therefore, the need for further studies in this area to confirm these relationships is necessary in order to better understand the linkage between employee satisfaction and increased productivity.

Obviously, there is a great need for more evidence supporting the Driver and Ratliff model. The research investigating within this area should use more rigorous research, applying experimental and quasi-experimental designs. The need for cost-benefit analysis is critical, but should be divided into different time frames to allow for the realization of expected benefits. During the first year of the program, it is the individual participant who benefits most by improved physiology and reduction of coronary heart disease risk factors. Over the next few years, it would be expected that some benefits would occur for the company in terms of reduced absenteeism and improved employee morale. Long-term benefits cannot be expected until around the fifth year, and it is at this time that the first complete cost-benefit study should be completed.

THERAPEUTIC EFFECTS OF VIGOROUS EXERCISE

In addition to psychological benefits reported for healthy individuals with normal psychological characteristics, evidence suggests that vigorous exercise may improve mental health in individuals with psychological abnormalities such as anxiety and depression. However, there have been many problems in demonstrating the therapeutic effects of vigorous exercise. Difficulties include suitable measurements of anxiety and depression as well as problems in providing experimental controls for exercise studies. Self-reports provide information about subjects' perceptions of their psychological abnormalities, and most subjects enter into exercise programs expecting they will benefit. Thus, any experimental study is dominated by perceptions of the subjects and their expectations for benefit. Consequently, data available from numerous studies provide strong support for an associative relationship between vigorous exercise and improvements in psychological status. A controlled clinical trial will be essential to develop evidence for a causative relationship, but the impracticality of administering a placebo control intervention makes the ideal experimental design difficult to achieve.

Anxiety

Anxiety results from heightened autonomic and cognitive responses to real or imagined threats. Complaints such as nervousness, fatigue, headache, and muscular pain frequently accompany physiological states of high heart rate, increased sweating, gastrointestinal distress, and tremulousness. In some individuals, anxiety occurs as an immediate response to some perceived threat and some individuals experience anxiety over long periods of time. The immediate responses to threats are influenced more favorably than the prolonged effects of anxiety. Spielberger, Gorsuch, and Lushene (1970) have developed test instruments that differentiate the immediate from the prolonged effects of anxiety.

The immediate effects of anxiety, called state anxiety, are most favorably influenced by vigorous exercise (Morgan, 1979a; Bahrke and Morgan, 1978; Blumenthal et al., 1982; Folkins, 1976; Lichtman and Poser, 1983; Lobitz et al., 1983). The effects of cardiovascular conditioning on anxiety have been more difficult to demonstrate. However, Kowal, Patton, and Vogel (1978) reported that subjects had a significant decrease in self-reported state anxiety following six weeks of physical conditioning in men. Results from other investigators have shown similar psychological responses to exercise among both men and women (Wilson, Morley, and Bird, 1981; Young, 1979).

Berger and Owen (1982) studied the relationship between swimming and mood. They enrolled 100 college students and assigned them either to swimming classes or lecture-control classes. All subjects completed a self-report inventory of mood states before and after each swimming or lecture class. Results indicated that swimmers reported significantly less tension, depression, anger, confusion, and more vigor after exercising than before. All swimmers changed significantly more than did controls on all scales except fatigue. Although there were no gender differences in the amount of mood change associated with swimming, the women reported significantly less tension-anxiety, depression, anger, and confusion than the men. Figure 16.2 illustrates the pre- and postclass mood change for swimmers in comparison with control subjects. Differences between these groups were statistically significant ($p < 0.05$).

The intensity of physiological and cognitive components of anxiety also influence response to vigorous exercise. Subjects in exercise programs

Figure 16.2.   Relationship between swimming and mood

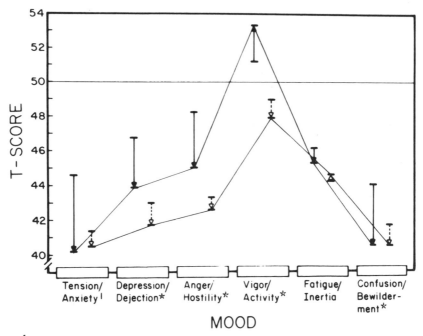

[1]Statistical significance here is $p < 0.06$.

*The pre- and postclass mood changes for swimmers were significantly greater than that for the controls at the 0.05 level.

Source: Reprinted by permission of Elsevier Science Publishing Company, Inc., from "Mood Alteration with Swimming—Swimmers Really Do Feel Better," by B. Berger and D. Owen, *Psychosomatic Medicine* 45, no. 5 (1983): 425–433. Copyright 1983 by The American Psychosomatic Society, (Inc.)

reported less physiological and more cognitive anxiety than subjects involved in a program of relaxation training (Davidson and Schwartz, 1976; Schwartz, Davidson, and Goleman, 1978). In support of this relation, deVries and Adams (1972) showed a reduction in electrical activity of skeletal muscles following vigorous exercise. Electromyographic measurements of forearm muscle tension were made in ten elderly anxious subjects before and after exercise. Results indicated that exercise producing a heart rate of 100 bpm lowered electrical activity in skeletal muscle by approximately 20 percent. Neither meprobamate nor placebo treatments were significantly different from controls. Results of these studies indicated that exercise of relatively light intensity reduced muscle tension.

Although a cause and effect relation between vigorous exercise and reduction in anxiety is difficult to prove, evidence supports the concept that exercise of sufficient intensity, duration, and frequency to produce cardiovascular conditioning can reduce anxiety. Reductions in state anxiety following acute physical activity and physical conditioning also is effective. However, the benefits of vigorous physical exercise in reducing anxiety associated with work stress has not been demonstrated.

Depression

The effects of vigorous exercise in reducing depression have received a great deal of attention. Symptoms of depression include fatigue, irritability, insomnia, lethargy, difficulty in concentrating, and feelings of despair and hopelessness. The antidepressant effects of exercise apparently overcome the clinical manifestations of depression.

Morgan et al., (1970) studied the interrelationships of depression, age, and physical activity in 101 adult males who participated in an exercise program. In these subjects, six weeks of exercise did not produce a significant reduction in depression for all subjects in any kind of exercise program. However, a significant reduction in depression was observed in 11 subjects who were depressed initially. It was concluded that depressed adult males experienced a significant reduction in depression following six weeks of exercise training.

Brown, Ramirez, and Taub (1978) studied the psychological correlates of exercise in normal and depressed subjects. Their studies were designed to demonstrate the antidepressant effect of exercise in relation to intensity, duration, and frequency of physical activity. The objective was to develop a technique for prescribing exercise as treatment for depression.

In the first set of experiments, Brown et al (1978) studied 167 subjects, of which 96 were women (average age 19 years) and 71 were men (average age 24 years). All were given psychological tests including the Zung Depression Scale (Zung, 1965). All subjects kept a journal of their activities in a physical fitness program and recorded pulse rates before and after exercise. Psychological tests were repeated after ten weeks, during which all subjects had been exercising for an average of 30 minutes a day three days a week. Subjects in exercise programs involving wrestling, mixed exercises, jogging, and tennis had reductions in depression scores. However, subjects who played softball or had no exercise routine had no significant change in depression scores.

In the second phase of the study, 561 university students were enrolled in a study program. Students who were clinically depressed according to the Zung Self-rating Inventory were divided into two groups in which 91 undertook an exercise program and 10 served as controls. An additional group of 406 normal controls entered an exercise program while 54 normal students served as no-exercise controls. Subjects chose whether to jog three or five times each week or to refrain from exercise altogether. An Activation-Deactivation Adjective Checklist (Thayer, 1970) and a Multifactor Adjective Checklist (Lorr, Daston, and Smith, 1967) were added to the psychological test battery. Following a ten-week period of exercise, those subjects who jogged five days a week for ten weeks had the greatest reduction in depression. Significant reductions were observed in the depression scores of both the depressed subjects and the nondepressed control group. Similar patterns were exhibited by those who jogged only three days a week for the same period. The subjects who did not exercise

Table 16.1. Depression scores for subjects jogging three or five times per week for ten weeks (Phase 2)

	Before Exercise		After Exercise	
	Mean	*SD*	*Mean*	*SD*
Jogging Five Times Per Week				
Group 1 (N = 54)	42.0	4.42	41.4	6.25
normal controls, no exercise				
Group 2 (N = 23)	35.3	4.27	32.5*	5.17
normal controls, exercise				
Group 3 (N = 10)	54.1	5.90	51.4	13.42
depressed, no exercise				
Group 4 (N = 26)	58.0	7.84	43.4*	8.82
depressed, exercise				
Jogging Three Times Per Week				
Normal controls (N = 383)	40.6	5.29	38.4*	6.51
Depressed (N = 65)	54.5	5.06	46.2*	8.10

Source: Compiled by the author from data presented by Brown, Ramirez, and Taub (1978).

*p < .001

Figure 16.3.   Level of depression as related to aerobic exercise

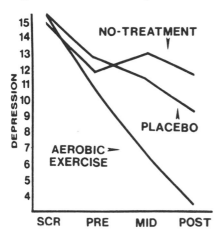

Source: McCann and Holmes, 1984. Reprinted with permission of the authors.

during the same time interval had no change in depression scores. Responses to the adjective checklists indicated that negative affective states of anger/hostility, fatigue/inertia, and tense/anxious were significantly decreased among the depressed subjects who jogged. Positive affective states of cheerfulness, energy, and general activation were significantly increased among the depressed subjects who jogged. When depressed subjects could select their exercises, the most depressed chose the most vigorous. Depression scores for subjects jogging three or five times per week for ten weeks are listed in Table 16.1.

Although the association between exercise and reduction in depression has been shown in several studies, only two randomized controlled clinical studies have been reported: by McCann and Holmes (1984) and by Martinsen, Medhus, and Sandvik (1985). These studies provide controlled evidence concerning the effects of strenuous exercise on depression.

A study of the influence of aerobic exercise on depression was reported by McCann and Holmes (1984). In their study, 43 depressed women were randomly assigned to an aerobic exercise treatment program, a placebo relaxation program, or a no-treatment condition. Subjects were selected from a group of 250 undergraduate women enrolled in a general psychology course who completed the Beck Depression Inventory (Beck et al., 1961). Self-reported depression was assessed before, during, and after the treatment period. As shown in Figure 16.3 subjects in the aerobic exercise condition had significantly greater decreases in depression than did subjects in the placebo condition or in the no treatment condition. Reductions in depression also occurred in subjects who did not exercise, but the extent of improvement was substantially less.

The antidepressive effects of aerobic exercise in hospitalized psychiatric patients was reported by Martinsen et al. (1985). They studied 43 patients with depression, ages 17–60 years (average age 40 years). The diagnosis of depression was made according to the criteria of the Diagnostic and Statistical Manual of Mental Disorders for Major Depression. Patients were randomly allocated to a training group and a control group. For nine weeks, the training group underwent a program of aerobic exercise for one hour three times each week at an intensity between 50–70 percent of maximum aerobic capacity. The control group attended occupational therapy while the training group exercised. Depression was assessed with the Beck Depression Inventory (Beck et al., 1961) and physical working capacity was assessed by submaximal exercise tolerance testing on a bicycle ergometer (Astrand and Rodal, 1977). Mean reductions in the Beck Depression Inventory were significantly larger and physical working capacity was significantly increased in the training group (Figure 16.4). Those patients in the training group who had a small increase in physical working capacity had small reductions in depression scores, whereas those with large increases in physical working capacity experienced larger antidepressive effects. Results of this study suggested that a moderate increase in physical working capacity was sufficient to obtain an antidepressive effect in hospitalized psychiatric patients.

Figure 16.4. Depression as measured by the Beck Depression Inventory and physical working capacity as measured by oxygen uptake.

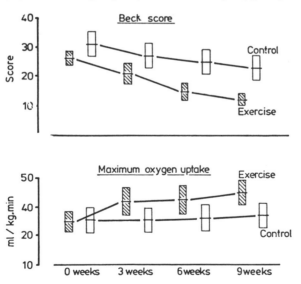

Source: Martinsen, Medhus, and Sandvik, 1985. Reprinted with permission.

The observation that strenuous aerobic exercise reduces depression has led to studies of physiological mechanisms. Since studies of depression have indicated altered biochemical function in the central nervous system of patients with depression, attention has been focused on neurochemical transmitters that might be altered by vigorous aerobic exercise.

The possibility that norepinephrine, dopamine, or serotonin function in the central nervous system might be influenced by vigorous aerobic exercise arises from the observation that these amines may be linked to depression (Coppen, 1972; Goodwin and Bunney, 1973; Schildkraut and Kety, 1967). In general, the major urinary metabolites of serotonin, dopamine, and norepinephrine have been reported to be reduced in depressed patients. Other investigators have reported that exercise increases the secretion of amine metabolites in depressed patients. Ebert, Post, and Goodwin (1972) studied six depressed patients who increased their physical activity for eight hours on one day. This exercise increased the urinary excretion of amine metabolites. However, the majority of catecholamines released into the blood and metabolized arise from sympathetic nerve terminals in relation to exercise and a relatively small amount arises from aminergic synaptic transmission in the brain. Further experiments will be necessary to clarify the relationship between autonomic nervous system activity and amine function in the brain.

Another hypothesis to explain effects of vigorous aerobic exercise on depression is the endorphin hypothesis. This hypothesis is supported by studies showing release of beta-endorphin into the peripheral blood of human subjects during exercise.

Fraioli et al., (1980) reported results of studies with eight professional male athletes who were able to reach their maximum aerobic capacity on a treadmill. Results from athletes who were not able to reach maximum aerobic capacity were discarded. The blood concentrations of adrenocorticotropic hormone rose from 80 pg/ml during basal conditions to 850 pg/ml during maximal aerobic effort. Concentrations of beta-endorphins rose from 320 pg/ml during basal conditions to 1,620 pg/ml during 100 percent maximal aerobic effort. Although increases in concentration of the substances in peripheral blood were demonstrated, there was no information available concerning concentration of the substances in the central nervous system.

Carr et al. (1981) studied hormonal responses to chronic exercise training in seven women (18 to 30 years of age). Blood samples were taken during control sessions at rest, while exercising on a stationary bicycle ergometer, and during recovery from exercise. Results showed that exercise increased plasma levels of beta-endorphin and its precursor beta-lipotropin. Significant rises in beta-lipotropin and beta-endorphin levels were observed during exercise testing at 80 percent of maximal heart rate in four successive months. The average power outputs observed were 70, 90, and 100 watts, indicating increases in physical working capacity. Levels of beta-endorphin and beta-lipotropin in plasma increased in proportion to the increase in work load. Although the higher work loads were associated with increased levels of beta-endorphin and beta-lipotropin, it is difficult to conclude what effects physical conditioning might have had on the exercise-induced secretion of the substances.

Farrell et al., (1982) studied six endurance athletes during submaximal treadmill exercise. Plasma levels of beta-endorphin and beta-lipotropin were measured using immunoreactivity radioassay techniques. Blood samples were drawn before and after 30-minute treadmill runs at a self-selected pace, 60 percent and 80 percent of maximal work load, and during rest. Results indicated that values for beta-endorphin and beta-lipotropin increased two- to fivefold after each run. Although immunoreactivity increased under all three conditions, only the increase for the 60 percent of the maximal work load was statistically significant. However, no measurements were made of rates of secretion, degredation, or excretion. Furthermore, concentrations of beta-endorphin and beta-lipotropin immunoreactivity in the central nervous system could not be determined.

Although the physiological mechanisms whereby vigorous aerobic exercise decreases depression have not been conclusively demonstrated, plausible physiological mechanisms have been proposed. Further research will be necessary to indicate whether either the amine hypothesis or the endorphin hypothesis might be correct.

CONCLUSION

Exercise has been shown to reduce physiological responses to stress (Sinyor et al., 1983; Sime, 1977). However, little is known of the prevalence or incidence of negative psychological effects of exercise. Morgan (1979b) has described "running addiction" in individuals whose commitment to exercise is higher than work, family, or interpersonal relationships. It is not clear if running causes the negative behavior or if certain personalities are predisposed to abuse running to escape coping with other problems.

Exercise appears to improve the accuracy with which an individual perceives bodily states (Hughes, 1984). The potential for stress relief through exercise is largely determined by the individual's physical condition. The poorly conditioned show the greatest psychological improvements in regular exercise programs (Goff and Dimsdale, 1985). It is also the most self-motivated individuals who maximize results (Dishman, Ickes, and Morgan, 1980). Contemporary sport psychology is referred to as the last frontier in exercise science and sport sciences (Straub, 1978). The studies that have been used in this review should indicate that a variety of psychophysiological changes can occur with physical activity.

Normal individuals appear to benefit substantially with exercise in promoting physical and mental health. However, the need for more rigorous research is critical in order to expand the knowledge of the long-term effect of exercise on anxiety, depression, and other abnormal mental states.

REFERENCES

Astrand, P. O. and Rodal, K. 1977. *Textbook of Work Physiology*. New York: McGraw-Hill.

Bahrke, M. S. and Morgan, W. P. 1978. Anxiety reduction following exercise and mediation. *Cognitive Therapy and Research*, 2: 323–334.

Baun, W.B., Bernacki, E. J., and Tsai, S. P. 1986. A preliminary investigation: Effect of a corporate fitness program on absenteeism and health care cost. *Journal of Occupational Medicine*, 26: 18–19.

Beck, A. T., Ward, C. H., Mendelson, M., Mock, J., and Erbaugh, J. 1961. An inventory for measuring depression. *Archives of General Psychiatry*, 4: 561–571.

Berger, B. and Owen, D. 1982. The positive effects of swimming on mood: Swimmers really do feel better. Paper presented at the Annual Conference of the North American Society for the Psychology of Sport and Physical Activity, University Park, Maryland, May.

Bernacki, E. J. and Baun, W. B. 1984. The relationship of job performance to exercise adherence in a corporate fitness program. *Journal of Occupational Medicine*, 26: 529.

Blumenthal, J. A., Williams, R.S., Needels, T. L., and Wallace, A. G. 1982. Psychological changes accompany aerobic exercise in healthy middle-aged adults. *Psychosomatic Medicine*, 44: 529–536.

Bowne, D. W., Russell, M. L., Morgan, J. L., Optenberg, S. A., and Clarke, A. E. 1984. Reduced disability and health care costs in an industrial fitness program. *Journal of Occupational Medicine*, 26: 809.

Brown, R. S., Ramirez, D. E., and Taub, J. M. 1978. The prescription of exercise for depression. *The Physician and Sportsmedicine*, December: 35–45.

Brunner, B. C. 1969. Personality and motivating factors influencing adult participation in vigorous physical activity. *Research Quarterly*, 40: 464–469.

Canada Fitness Survey, 1982. *Canada's Fitness*. Ottawa: Government Printing.

Carr, D. B., Bullen, B. A., Skrinar, G. S., Arnold, M. A., Rosenblatt, M., Beitins, I. Z., Martin, J. B., and McArthur, J.W. 1981. Physical conditioning facilitates the exercise-induced secretion of beta-endorphin and beta-lipotropin in women. *New England Journal of Medicine*, 305: 560–563.

Coppen, A. 1972. Indoleamines and affective disorders. *Journal of Psychiatric Research*, 9: 163–171.

Davidson, F. J. and Schwartz, G. E. 1976. The psycholbiology of relaxation and related states: A multi-process theory. In Mostofsky, D. I., (Ed.). *Behavior*

Control and Modification of Physiological Activity. Englewood Cliffs, N.J.: Prentice-Hall.

DeVries, H. A. 1974. *Physiology of Exercise,* 2nd ed. Dubuque: Wm. C. Brown Co., p. 280.

DeVries, H.A. and Adams, G. M. 1972. Electromyographic comparison of single doses of exercise and meprobamate as to effects on muscular relaxation. *American Journal of Physical Medicine,* 51: 130–141.

Dishman, R. K., Ickes,W., and Morgan, W. P. 1980. Self-motivation and adherence to habitual physical activity. *Journal of Applied Social Psychology,* 10: 115–132.

Driver, R.W. and Ratliff, R.A. 1982. Employers' perceptions of benefits accrued from physical fitness programs. *Personnel Administrator,* August: 21.

Ebert, M. H., Post, R. M., and Goodwin, F. K. 1972. Effect of physical activity on urinary MHPG excretion in depressed patients. *Lancet,* 2: 766.

Farrell, P. A., Gates, W. K., Maksud, M. G., and Morgan, W. P. 1982. Increases in plasma B-endorphine/B-lipotropin immunoreactivity after treadmill running in humans. *Journal of Applied Physiology,* 52: 1245–1249.

Folkins, C. H. 1976. Effects of physical training on mood. *Journal of Clinical Psychology,* 32: 385–388.

Folkins, C. H., Lynch, S., and Gardner, M. M. 1972. Psychological fitness as a function of physical fitness. *Archives of Physical Medicine and Rehabilitation,* 53: 503–508.

Fraioli, F., Moretti, C., Paolucci, D., Alicicco, E., Crescenzi, F., and Fortunio, G. 1980. Physical exercise stimulates marked concomitant release of B-endorphin and adrenocorticotropic hormone (ACTH) in peripheral blood in man. *Experimentia,* 36: 987–989.

Gal, R. and Lazarus, R. S. 1975. The role of activity in anticipating and confronting stressful situations. *Journal of Human Stress,* 72: 538.

Goff, D. and Dimsdale, J. E. 1985. The psychologic effects of exercise. *Journal of Cardiopulmonary Rehabilitation,* 5: 234–240.

Goodwin, F. and Bunney, W. E. 1973. A psychobiological approach to affective illness. *Psychiatric Annual,* 3: 19–53.

Harris, L. and Associates. 1978. *The Perrier Study: Fitness in America.* Vital and Health Statistics of the National Center on Health Statistics.

Hughes, J. R. 1984. Psychological effects of habitual aerobic exercise: A critical review. *Preventive Medicine,* 13: 66–78.

Jacobson, E. 1979. Physical activity: A tool in promoting mental health. *Journal of Psychiatric Nursing and Mental Health Services,* November: 24–25.

Kowal, D. M., Patton, J., and Vogel, J. 1978. Psychological states and aerobic fitness of male and female recruits before and after basic training. *Aviation, Space and Environmental Medicine,* 49: 603–606.

Levenson, P. M., Thornby, J. I., and Levenson, A. J. 1985. Dimensions, benefits, and barriers to jogging perceived by joggers and nonjoggers. *Health Values,* 9: 20–21.

Lichtman, S. and Poser,E. G. 1983. The effects of exercise on mood and cognitive functioning. *Journal of Psychosomatic Research,* 27: 43–52.

Linden, V. 1969. Absence from work and physical fitness. *British Journal of Industrial Medicine,* 26: 50.

Lobitz, W. C., Brammell, H. L., Stoll,S., and Niccoll, A. 1983. Physical exercise and anxiety management training for cardiac stress management in a nonpatient population. *Journal of Cardiac Rehabilitation*, 3: 683–688.

Lorr, M., Daston, P., and Smith, I. 1967. An analysis of mood states. *Educational and Psychological Measurement*, 27: 89–96.

Martinsen, E. W., Medhus, A., and Sandvik, L. 1985. Effects of aerobic exercise on depression: A controlled study. *British Medical Journal*, 291: 109.

McCann, L. and Holmes, D. S. 1984. Influence of aerobic exercise on depression. *Journal of Personality and Social Psychology*, 46 (5): 1142–1147.

Mobily, K. 1982. Using physical activity and recreation to cope with stress and anxiety: A review. *American Corporation*, May-June: 77.

Morgan, W. P. 1979a. Anxiety reduction following acute physical activity. *Psychiatric Annual*, 9: 141–147.

———. 1979b. Negative addiction in runners. *Physician Sportsmedicine*, 7: 57–70.

Morgan, W. P., Roberts, J. A., Brand, F. R., and Feinerman, A. D. 1970. Psychological effect of chronic physical activity. *Medicine and Science in Sports*, 4: 213–217.

Naisbitt, J. 1982. *Megatrends*: 135. New York: Warner.

Pauly, J. T., Palmer, J. A., and Wright, C. C. 1982. The effect of a 14-week employee fitness program on selected physiological and psychological parameters. *Journal of Occupational Medicine*, 24: 457–463.

President's Council on Physical Fitness and Sports. 1973. *National Adult Physical Fitness Survey*. Washington, D.C.: U.S. Government Printing Service.

———. 1974. *Physical Fitness Research Digest*, Series 4, 2: 1–27.

Roth, D. L. and Holmes, D. S. 1985. Influence of physical fitness in determining the impact of stressful life events on physical and psychologic health. *Psychosomatic Medicine*, 47: 164.

Schafer, W. 1981. Running therapy for the depressed. *Topics in Clinical Nursing*, 32: 77–86.

Schildkraut, J. J. and Kety, S. S. 1967. Biogenic amines and emotion. *Science*, 156: 21–30.

Schwartz, G. E., Davidson, R. J., and Goleman, D. J. 1978. Patterning of cognitive and somatic processes in the self-regulation of anxiety: Effects of meditation versus exercise. *Psychosomatic Medicine*, 40: 321–328.

Selye, H. 1975. *The Stress of Life*. New York: McGraw-Hill.

Serfass, R. C. and Gergerich, S. G. 1984. Exercise for optimal health: Strategies and motivational considerations. *Preventive Medicine*, 13: 79–99.

Shephard, R. J., Cox, M., and Corey, P. 1981. Fitness program participation: Its effect on worker performance. *Journal of Occupational Medicine*, 23: 359–363.

Sime, W. E. 1977. A comparison of exercise and meditation in reducing psychological response to stress (abstract). *Medicine and Science in Sports*, 9: 55.

Sinyor, D. 1983. Aerobic fitness level and reactivity to psychosocial stress: Physiological, biochemical, and subjective measurers. *Psychosomatic Medicine*, 45: 205–217.

Small Businesses show big interest in health promotion. 1985. *Employee Health and Fitness*, 6: 1.

Spielberger, C. D., Gorsuch, R. L., and Luchene, R. 1970. *State Trait Anxiety Inventory Manual*. Palo Alto, Calif.: Consulting Psychologists Press.

Straub,W. E. (Ed.) 1978. *Sport Psychology: An Analysis of Athlete Behavior*. Ithaca, N.Y.: Movement Publications.

Terjung, R. L. 1982. Exercise and sport science reviews. *American College of Sports Medicine*, Series 10: 120.

Thayer, R. E. 1970. Activation states as assessed by verbal report and four psychophysiological variables. *Psychophysiology*, 7: 86–94.

Wilson, V. E., Morley, N. C., and Bird, E. I. 1981. Mood profiles of marathon runners, joggers, and non-exercisers. *Perceptual and Motor Skills*, 53: 472–474.

Young, R. J. 1979. The effect of regular exercise on cognitive functioning and personality. *British Journal of Sports Medicine*, 13: 110–117.

Zung, W.W. 1965. A self-rating depression scale. *Archives of General Psychiatry*, 12: 63–70.

17 Preventive law trends and compensation payments for stress-disabled workers

Gilbert T. Adams, Jr.

PERVASIVENESS OF STRESS-INDUCED DISABILITY

Annual costs for medical care in the United States exceed $200 billion (U.S. Bureau of the Census, 1985). Of the medical problems treated, stress has surpassed the common cold as the most prevalent problem in America. Some 80 to 90 percent of all industrial accidents have been related to emotional problems (Mollick, 1983). Stress-related injuries account for more than 70 percent of all job absenteeism and result in losses equal to nearly 10 percent of the total U.S. GNP. The American Institute of Stress calculates that stress-related illness costs the American economy $100 billion a year, ten times more than all strikes combined (*How business beats stress*, 1985). In 1980 the annual cost of executive stress alone in the United States was estimated at $20 billion (Norris, 1980). That figure covers only measurable items such as work-loss days, hospitalization, outpatient care, and mortality to executives. It does not account for ineffectiveness on the job or effects on other employees. Annual productivity losses in the United States as a result of stress-related mental illnesses are estimated at $17 billion (Yates, 1979). Control Data Corporation, the computer firm, found that total *employee* health care costs increased 119% during the period 1980 to 1985 (Johnson, 1986).

The National Institute of Occupational Safety and Health has ranked the ten most serious occupational risks in order:

1. Occupational lung disease (including lung cancer)
2. Musculoskeletal injuries
3. Occupational cancers other than lung cancer
4. Traumatic deaths, amputations, fractures, and eye losses
5. Cardiovascular diseases
6. Reproductive problems
7. Neurotoxic illnesses
8. Noise-induced hearing loss
9. Dermatologic diseases and injuries
10. Psychological disorders (Center for Disease Control, 1983).

There is no doubt that claims for psychiatric injuries are increasing dramatically each year in this country. California presently receives 4,000 psychiatric claims a year, a threefold increase during the last five years (Lublin, 1980). In 1979, 47 percent of all worker's compensation dollars in California were disbursed for cardiovascular and neurotic conditions. The New York Life Extension Institute reported an epidemic increase in the proportions of psychological signs of stress in 1971 relative to 1958 (Lublin, 1980). Insurance companies are concerned about the growing trend. As an example, Aetna Life & Casualty Company spends over $250 million a year in payments for mental health care (Shorr, 1982).

Mental disability occurring in the work environment is due primarily to job stress. Unlike exposure to chemical or physical agents, which can be considered as being specific to a type(s) of industry, job stress is common in some degree to all occupations. Therefore, it can be considered to have virtually unlimited exposure potential. Statistics indicate an increase in psychological job stress during the last two decades, along with a concomitant rise in worker compensation claims for stress-induced disabilities.

HISTORY OF WORKER'S COMPENSATION

Worker's compensation did not develop in the United States. It started in Germany in about 1860 under Chancellor Bismarck. This was part of the Industrial Revolution long before it came to North America. It was Chancellor Bismarck's thought that employees should have a form of medical care and some form of wage supplement to assist them with regard to an on-the-job type of injury. That was a time in history when workers began to quit working for themselves. For example, the shoemaker, instead of just making shoes on an individual basis, went to a factory and started making shoes in the factory. Initially, workers had a problem when injured on the job because the employer would just essentially tell them, "When you get well, come on back." At construction sites and in other physical activities, there was no interest in worker welfare and no social awareness on the part of the employer that there was a need to give some consideration to safety and the cost of injury to people, even if it resulted from some activity at the work site.

Bismarck's form of worker's compensation quickly spread across Europe and by the turn of the century and the Industrial Revolution in the United States it was like a wave that swept across from state to state. State legislators across the United States began to pass individual worker's compensation statutes. They basically required that the employer purchase a form of insurance that would cover certain types of on-the-job injuries, and that insurance would be paid by the employer. It would cover 100 percent of all medical expenses for injuries that were related to or caused by or connected to or aggravated by activity at the worksite. It also provided for some limited form of wage supplementation for the period of time in which the person was disabled. Then, at the point when they were able to return to some form of employment, if they had a permanent loss or partial loss of working capacity it provided remunerative benefits along that line.

For instance, in Texas if someone is totally disabled, partially disabled, or deceased they have a maximum benefit of 401 weeks. Almost every state has some limited form that they place on the number of weeks for compensation. If you are paralyzed from the neck down, totally disabled, can never work again, or dead, you or your beneficiaries are still only entitled to a maximum of 401 weeks of compensation. In Texas now the limit of compensation is $417 a week. It doesn't matter if you were making $1,000 a week or whatever, you can't get more than $417 a week; you can never get more than two-thirds of your average weekly wage. But those are legislated types of compensation that exist throughout this country.

CONTEMPORARY COMPENSATION PRACTICES

Now the courts take different positions with regard to stress-induced or emotionally induced disability (Ivancevich et al., 1985). (The Appendix at the end of the chapter includes a listing of cases by state related to compensation awards.) A number of courts have taken the position that a disabling mental disorder resulting from a work-related emotional stimulus is generally and probably considered an accidental injury, a disease, within the meaning of the worker compensation statutes. Some courts have reasoned that there is no valid justification for distinguishing between the mental disorders that result in disability and the physical disorders, such as a broken bone or something of that nature, that result in disability. The states that have generally followed that line of equalization between physical and mental or emotional disabilities are California, Hawaii, Kentucky, Illinois, Maine, Michigan, Mississippi, Missouri, New Mexico, Oregon, Pennsylvania, Tennessee, and West Virginia.

Some courts have taken the position that a disabling mental disorder induced by a work-related sudden emotional stimulus may properly be considered as an accidental injury or disease within the meaning of the worker's compensation statutes. In the following states it has been held that a worker's compensation benefit may be awarded for a disabling mental disorder that results from a work-related sudden emotional stimulus: Arizona, Illinois, New Jersey, New York, Texas, Virginia, and West Virginia.

A case example occurred in Texas where the court held a disability based on a sudden emotional stimulus. There were two window washers working on a high building, maybe 30 to 40 stories high. One end of the platform that they were on gave way; one man fell to his death. The man who remained on the scaffold was significantly terrified; in fact, he was terrified to the point at which he was disabled from returning to that kind of employment. He had watched his fellow worker fall; he had grabbed and held on for dear life not knowing whether the scaffold was going to fall with him, if he would be next. He was not next, he did survive, and he didn't have any physical injury. But he had that emotional stress, resulting in his inability to resume his former duties. The medical testimony was such that he was disabled from doing that kind of work. This was a new case, a new question that the courts had never before addressed in Texas. The courts ruled that a sudden emotional stimulus of the nature that produced the disability would be covered by the Texas law.

On the other hand, to distinguish between a sudden emotional stimulus and one that is not, the Texas worker's compensation did not cover, for instance, a newspaperman who for 20 or 30 years was under significant stress to write the stories, get the articles published, get out the edition, and so on. Eventually he had a breakdown. The court held in that situation that he was not covered; under the way the Texas legislature wrote the law it is not an accidental injury. It is not an injury within the coverage of the compensation laws of Texas.

Other courts from different jurisdictions around the country take the stance that a disabling mental disorder induced by a work-related nonsudden emotional stimulus may properly be considered an accidental injury or disease within the meaning of their worker's compensation statutes. In the following states the courts took the position that worker's compensation benefits may be awarded for a disabling mental disorder that is caused by a work-related nonsudden emotional stimulus: Arizona, California, Maine, New Jersey, New Mexico, and Oregon. Other courts fall in line with the general viewpoint set out above.

There is another Texas case that illustrates how a physical injury can be related to an emotional or mental injury. This case involved a man who worked as a blacksmith at the Oil City Grass Company in Beaumont. There was a great deal of noise in the place of business. This worker ended up with some significant hearing loss and some permanent ringing or buzzing in both ears. He testified that this ringing and buzzing was in both ears, that he couldn't hear what people were saying or had great difficulty in hearing, that it had created dizziness he had just about every day. He had throbbing and pain in his left ear at all times. The worker had been treated by doctors in Beaumont and Galveston.

Medical testimony to the effect that the worker's condition had on his nervous system was from a psychiatrist from the University of Texas Medical Branch at Galveston. The psychiatrist stated that the worker was suffering from a depression caused by the buzzing in his ears and dizziness and from an anxiety disorder. As a result the plaintiff was disabled from engaging in gainful employment. The psychiatrist also stated the condition would continue unless a way to eliminate this buzzing and dizziness was found, and if the conditions continued for a prolonged time it would leave psychological scars. The Texas court held that an initial physical injury had evolved into a psychological injury.

Now let me mention a Massachusetts case. The court was faced with a question of whether an employee who suffers an emotional breakdown as a result of a layoff or transfer suffers a compensable injury—an interesting case. The court said:

We recognize that layoffs and job transfers are frequent events and that the emotional injuries are more prone to fabrication and less susceptible to substantiation than are physical injuries. Nevertheless it is within the legislature's prerogative to determine, as a matter of public policy, whether one of the costs of doing business in this commonwealth shall be the compensation of those few employees who do suffer emotional disability as a result of being laid off or transferred, and it is also the legislative prerogative to state whether determination of the existence of such a disability is appropriately left to the expertise of the Industrial Accident Board. We construe [and they cite the Massachusetts law] as providing that an employee who suffers emotional disability as a result of layoff or transfer is entitled to worker's compensation and as vesting in the Industrial Accident Board the responsibility to make the relevant factual determination.

This is a 1985 case from Massachusetts. These are issues that are just now reaching the courts.

Another 1985 case from Rhode Island deals with worker's compensation stress-related disabilities. The court held in this situation that the disability was a compensable one. Here the decedent was defendant's newspaper sports editor. After covering a football game the decedent's behavior was erratic, and he became incoherent and was taken to a hospital where he died five days later from a cerebral hemorrhage. His surviving wife brought a claim for worker's compensation benefits, alleging that the hemorrhaging was caused by the combination of her husband's diabetes and hypertension and his job at the newspaper, which included odd and long hours and deadline pressures. The worker's compensation commission rejected the claim, and the appellate commission reversed the decision and awarded benefits. On appeal by the employer the state supreme court affirmed: "An employer takes its workers as it finds them, and then if an employee aggravates an existing condition and the result is an incapacity for work, the employee is entitled to compensation for such incapacity." The court rejected defendant's denial of causation, claiming that

it is immaterial whether the employee's work involved unusual exertion or whether there was a particular incident which brought on the injury. Rather the crucial issue is whether there is a causal relationship or nexus between the work and the attack. In worker's compensation cases we do not equate the term causal relationship with the term proximate cause as found in negligence actions. Here it is enough if the condition and nature of employment contribute to the injury. The court believes the decedent's stressful employment aggravated both the diabetes and the hypertension and the three combined to cause the vascular disease that killed him. Consequently the court finds that there is sufficient evidence to support the lower court's finding that the decedent's death was causally related to employment (Mulcahey vs. New England Newspapers, Inc., 488 A. 2d 681, Sup. Ct. R.I., 1985).

Now that wouldn't occur in Texas, for instance; it is a Rhode Island decision. These are issues that are just now being addressed for the most part by courts around the country.

CASE LAW AND ITS IMPLICATIONS

The legal system in the United States is based on case law, which operates as much on case precedents as it does on legal codes and statutes. There are several important implications of this system for both employees and companies. First, there are no hard and fast rules as to compensation awards or liability when it comes to stress-related disorders. Because of the way case law unfolds, it is critical for employees and companies to be constantly monitoring precedents around the country. Second, although there is no federal legal system, the states vary substantially in the application of local law. We saw this in several cases discussed earlier. This means that state-level trends are critical to follow. Third, the rules of evidence and determination of causality in the legal arena are often quite different than those in the scientific arena. This, coupled with the adversarial nature of the legal process, means that there are strong conflicting forces operating in the establishment of case law. This means that trends can shift, change, ebb, and flow over a several-year period.

In terms of current national trends there are none, from a legal standpoint, that are denying coverage. On the contrary, there is a new awareness of stress-related illness and a new and further consideration of the impact of on-the-job stress to disease, heart attacks, mental disorders, and the like. This means that companies are likely to be increasingly exposed to liability for stress-related illness, and it is through case law precedents that the limits of this liability will be determined.

APPENDIX: CASES INVOLVING COMPENSATION FOR THE MENTALLY DISABLED WORKERS

Alabama
   Abex Corporation vs. Coleman, 386 So.2d 1160 (Ct.App.Ala., 1980)
   Freuhauf Corporation vs. Prater, 360 So.2d 999 (Ct.App.Ala., 1978)
Alaska
   Providence Washington, Inc. vs. Fish, 581 P.2d 680 (Sup.Ct.Alaska, 1968)

Brown vs. Northwest Airlines, Inc., 444 P.2d 529 (Sup.Ct. Alaska, 1968)

Arizona

Owens vs. Industrial Commission, 628 P.2d 962 (Ct.App.Ariz., 1981)

Archer vs. Industrial Commission, 619 P.2d 27 (Ct.App.Ariz., 1980)

Hooper vs. Industrial Commission, 617 P.2d 538 (Ct.App.Ariz., 1980)

Fireman's Fund Ins. Co. vs. Industrial Commission, 579 P.2d (Sup.Ct.Ariz., in banc, 1978)

Arkansas

Bibler Brothers, Inc. vs. Ingram, 587 S.W.2d 841 (Civ.App.Ark., 1979)

Price Lumber Company vs. Adams, 527 S.W.2d 932 (Sup.Ct.Ark., 1975)

California

Albertson's Inc. vs. Workers' Compensation Appeals Board, 182 Cal.Rptr. 304 (Ct.App.,[3rd Dist.] 1982)

Baker vs. Workers' Compensation Appeals Board, 96 Cal.Rptr. 279 (Ct.App.,[4th Dist.] 1971)

Colorado

Casa Bonita Restaurant vs. Industrial Commission, 624 P.2d 1340 (Colo. Ct.App., 1981)

Connecticut

Donato vs. Pantry Pride (Food Fair), 438 A.2d 1218 (Sup.Ct.Conn., 1981)

Delaware

Ramey vs. Delaware Material, Inc., 329 A.2d 205 (Sup.Ct.Del., 1979)

Sturgill vs. M & M, Inc., 329 A.2d 360 (Sup.Ct.Del., 1974)

Sears Roebuck & Company vs. Farley, 290 A.2d 639 (Sup.Ct.Del., 1972)

Florida

Racz vs. Chennault, Inc., 418 So.2d 413 (Ct.App.Fla.,[1st Dist.] 1982)

Franklin Manor Apartments vs. Jordan, 417 So.2d 1159 (Ct.App.Fla.,[1st Dist.] 1982)

Marci Ann Sportswear vs. Busquet, 393 So.2d 1132 (Ct.App.Fla., [1st Dist.] 1980)

Williams vs. Hillsborough County School Board, 389, So.2d 1218 (Ct.App.Fla., [1st Dist.] 1980)

City of Winter Park vs. Bowen, 388 So.2d 1376 (Ct.App.Fla., [1st Dist.] 1980)

Georgia

Hanson Buick, Inc. vs. Chatham, 299 S.E.2d 428 (Ct.App.Ga., 1982)

Glynn County Board of Commissioners vs. MIMBS., 291 S.E.2d 62 (Ct.App.Ga., 1982)

St. Paul Insurance Company vs. Henley, 234 S.E.2d 159 (Ct.App.Ga., 1977)

Hawaii

Royal State Nat. Ins. Co. vs. Labor & Indus. Rel. App. Bd., 487 P.2d 278 (Sup.Ct.,Hawaii, 1971)

Illinois

Collier vs. Wagner Castings Co., 408 N.E.2d 198 (Sup.Ct.Ill., 1980)

Veritone Co. vs. Industrial Commission, 405 N.E.2d 758 (Sup.Ct.Ill., 1980)

Watts vs. Industrial Commission, 394 N.E.2d 1171 (Sup.Ct.Ill., 1979)

Indiana

Campbell vs. Kaiser Corporation & Diecast, 208 N.E.2d 727 (Ct.App.Ind., 1965)

Kansas
   Reese vs. Gas Engineering & Construction Company, 532 P.2d 1033 (Sup.C-t.Kan., 1975)
   Berger vs. Hahner, Foreman & Cale, Inc., and Employers Fire Ins. Co., 506 P.2d 1175 (Sup.Ct.Kan., 1973)
Kentucky
   Ricky Cole Company vs. Adams, 426 S.W.2d 464 (Ct.App.Ky., 1968)
   Commonwealth, Department of Highways vs. Linden, 380 S.W.2d 247 (Ct.App.Ky., 1964)
Louisiana
   Franklin vs. Complete Auto Transit Co., 397 So.2d 60 (Ct.App.La., 2nd Cir., 1981)
   Eagnelly vs. Liberty Mut. Ins. Co., 355 So.2d 595 (Ct.App.La., 4th Cir., 1978)
   Gibson vs. New Orleans Public Sch. Bd., 352 So.2d 732 (Ct.App.La., 4th Cir., 1977)
   Boucher vs. Orleans Parish Sch. Bd., 346 So.2d 1124 (Ct.App.La., 4th Cir., 1977)
   Miller vs. United States Fidelity & Guaranty Co., 99 So.2d 511 (Ct.App.La., 2nd Cir., 1958)
Maine
   McLaren vs. Webber Hospital Assoc., 386 A.2d 734 (Me. 1978)
   Murray vs. T. W. Dick Co., 398 A.2d 390 (Me. 1979)
Massachusetts
   Kelly Case, 477 N.E. 2d 82 (Sup.Ct. of Mass., 1985)
   Albanese's Case, 389 N.E.2d 83 (Sup.Ct. of Mass., 1979)
   In Re Ralph McEwen's Case, 343 N.E.2d 869 (Sup.Ct. of Mass., 1976)
Michigan
   Lopucki vs. Ford Motor Co., 311 N.W.2d 338 (Ct.App.Mich., 1981)
   Deziel vs. Difco Laboratories, Inc., 268 N.W.2d 1 (Sup.Ct.Mich., 1978)
Minnesota
   Lockwood vs. Independent School Dist. No. 877, 312 N.W.2d 924 (Sup.C-t.Minn., 1981)
   Mitchell vs. White Castle Systems, Inc., 290 N.W.2d 753 (Sup.Ct.Minn., 1980)
Mississippi
   Hemphill Drug Company vs. Mann, 274 So.2d 117 (Sup.Ct.Miss., 1973)
   Miller Transporters, Ltd. vs. Reeves, 195 So.2d 95 (Sup.Ct.Miss., 1967)
Missouri
   Boatwright vs. ACF Industries, 463 S.W.2d 549 (Ct.App.,St. Louis, 1971)
   Todd vs. Goostree, 493 S.W.2d 411 (Ct.App.,Kansas City, 1973)
Montana
   Schumacher vs. Empire Steel Mfg.Co., 574 P.2d 987 (Sup.Ct.Mont., 1977)
   Sykes vs. Republic Coal Co., 22 P.2d 157 (Sup.Ct.Mont., 1930)
Nebraska
   Davis vs. Western Electric, 317 N.W.2d 68 (Sup.Ct.Neb., 1982)
   Cardenas vs. Peterson Bean Company, 144 N.W.2d 154 (Sup.Ct.Neb., 1966)
New Hampshire
   Condiles vs. Waumbec Mills, Inc., 58 A.2d 726 (Sup.Ct.N.H., 1948)

New Jersey
  Williams vs. Western Electric Co., 429 A.2d 1063 (Sup.Ct. of N.J., 1981)
New Mexico
  Schober vs. Mountain Bell Tel., 630 P.2d 1231 (Ct.App.N.M., 1980)
  Martinez vs. University of California, 601 P.2d 425 (Sup.Ct.N.M., 1979)
  Ross vs. Sayers' Well Servicing Company, 414 P.2d 679 (Sup.Ct.N.M., 1966)
New York
  Lohlin vs. Burroughs Corp., 427 N.Y.S.2d 78 (Sup.Ct.,3rd Depart., 1980)
  Nizich vs. Robert F. Barreca, Inc., 448 N.Y.S.2d 529 (Sup.Ct., 3rd Depart.,
    1982)
  Ottomanelli vs. Workers' Compensation Board, 436 N.Y.S.2d 442 (Sup.Ct., 3rd
    Depart., 1981)
North Carolina
  Fayne vs. Fieldcrest Mills, Inc., 282 S.E.2d 539 (Ct.App.N.C., 1981)
North Dakota
  Tyson vs. North Dakota Workmen's Compensation Bur., 129 N.W.2d 351
    (Sup.Ct.N.D., 1964)
Ohio
  Szymanski vs. Halle's Dept. Store, 407 N.E.2d 502 (Sup.Ct.Ohio, 1980)
Oklahoma
  Montgomery Ward & Company vs. Johnson, 645 P.2d 1051 (Ct.Civ.App.,
    Okla., 1982)
  Daugherty vs. ITT Continental Baking Company, 558 P.2d 393 (Sup.Ct.Okla.,
    1976)
Oregon
  Matter of Compensation of Maddox, 651 P.2d 180 (Ct.App.Or., 1982)
  Matter of Compensation of Harris, 6532 P.2d 1299 (Ct.App.Or., 1981)
  Wilson vs. Weyerhaeuser Company, 567 P.2d 567 (Ct.App.Ore., 1977)
Pennsylvania
  Mrs. Smith Pie Co. vs. Workmen's Comp., 426 A.2d 209 (Commonw.Ct. of Pa.,
    1981)
  Thomas vs. Workmen's Comp., 423 A.2d 784 (Commonw.Ct. of Pa., 1980)
Rhode Island
  Seitz vs. L & R Industries, Inc., 437 A.2d 1345 (Sup.Ct.R.I., 1981)
  Mulcahey vs. New England Newspapers, Inc., 488 A.2d 681 (Sup.Ct.R.I., 1985)
South Carolina
  Fleming vs. Appleton Co., 51 S.E.2d 363 (Sup.Ct.S.C., 1949)
Tennessee
  Jose vs. Equifex, Inc., 556 S.W.2d 82 (Sup.Ct.Tenn., 1977)
  Intern. Yarn Corp. vs. Cesson, 541 S.W.2d 150 (Sup.Ct.Tenn., 1976)
Texas
  Hood vs. Texas Indemnity Ins. Co., 209 S.W.2d 345 (Tex., 1948)
  Bailey vs. American General Ins. Co., 279 S.W.2d 315 (Tex., 1955)
  Transportation Ins. Co. vs. Maksyn, 580 S.W.2d 334 (Tex., 1979)
  Brown vs. Texas Employers' Ins. Ass'n., 635 S.W.2d 415 (Tex., 1982)
  Texas Employers' Ins. Ass'n vs. Fisher, 667 S.W.2d 589 (Tex.App. – Beaumont,
    1984, n.w.h.)

Scott vs. Houston Independent School Dist., 641 S.W.2d 255 (Tex.Civ.App. – Houston [14th Dist.] 1982 no writ)

Aetna Casualty & Surety Co. vs. Burris, 600 S.W.2d 402 (Tex.Civ.App. – Tyler 1980, Ref'd n.r.e.)

The University of Texas System vs. Schieffer, 588 S.W.2d 588 (Tex.Civ.App. – Austin 1979, Ref'd n.r.e.)

Colonial Penn Franklin Ins. Co. vs. Mayfield, 508 S.W.2d 449 (Tex.Civ.App. – Amarillo 1974, Ref'd n.r.e.)

Virginia

Burlington Mills Corporation vs. Hagood, 13 S.E.2d 291 (Sup.Ct.,Va., 1941)

Washington

Jacobson vs. Department of Labor & Industries, 224 P.2d 338 (Sup.Ct.Wash., 1950)

Peterson vs. Department of Labor & Industries, 33 P.2d 650 (Sup.Ct.Wash., 1934)

West Virginia

Breeden vs. Workmen's Compensation Com'r., 285 S.E.2d 398 (Sup.Ct.W.Va., 1981)

Harper vs. State Workmen's Compensation Commissioner, 234 S.E.2d 779 (Sup.Ct.W.Va., 1977)

Wisconsin

Valedzic vs. Briggs & Stratton Corp., 286 N.W.2d 540 (Sup.Ct.Wis., 1979)

Wyoming

Carter Oil Co. vs. Gibson, 241 P. 219 (Sup.Ct.Wy., 1925)

Admiralty

Petition of United States, 418 F.2d 264 (1st Cir., 1969)

Longshoreman's & Harbor Workers' Compensation Act

Tampa Ship Repair, etc. vs. Dir., Off. of Wkrs.' Comp. P., 535 F.2d 936 (5th Cir., 1976)

American National Red Cross vs. Hagen, 327 F.2d 559 (7th Cir., 1964)

Voris vs. Texas Employers' Ins. Ass'n., 190 F.2d 929 (5th Cir., 1951)

Federal Employees' Compensation Act

Sullivan vs. United States, 428 F.Supp.79 (U.S.D.C., E.D.Wis., 1977)

REFERENCES

Center for Disease Control. 1983. Leading work-related diseases and injuries— United States. *Morbidity and Mortality Weekly Report,* 32: 24–26.

How business beats stress. 1985. *The Economist* (U.K.), 295(7389), April 13, p. 83.

Ivancevich, J. M., Matteson, M. T., and Richards, E. P. III. 1985. Who's liable for stress on the job? *Harvard Business Review,* 64(2): 60–72.

Johnson, B. 1986. Personal communication, November 13.

Lublin, J. S. 1980. On-the-job stress leads many workers to file—and win— compensation awards. *Wall Street Journal,* September 17 (Section 2), p. 33.

Mollick, L. R. 1983. The corporation needs a psychologist. *Occupational Health and Safety,* 52: 36–40.

Norris, E. 1980. Stress: Employers and insurers feel the gains of spreading occupational ailment. *Business Insurance*, 14: 34.

Shorr, B. 1982. Insurers stopped paying for some treatment by psychiatrist and they had doubt about need. *Wall Street Journal*, May 4 (Section 2), p. 31.

U.S. Bureau of the Census. 1985. *Statistical Abstract of the United States: 1986* (106th edition). Washington, D.C. Figure 4.1, p. 94.

Yates, J. E. 1979. *Managing Stress*. New York: AMACOM Publishers.

IV   *Therapeutic interventions*

18   *Therapeutic stress interventions*

Alan A. McLean

   In a sense, the health care delivery aspect of this volume comes into focus in Part IV on therapeutic activities. This section deals not with activities that *might* prove helpful, but with those practices *already in use*. The following chapters suggest models of occupational health and mental health practice that have been, for the most part, demonstrated in the real world by the authors.

Some therapeutic activities merge without clear distinction into the arena of preventive interventions. Fitness programs, for example, may be therapeutic as well as preventive. For some people fitness programs will be as effective as more focused interventions such as risk counseling in alleviating work stress. Even with the most successful preventive stress management activities, however, individuals will still experience stressful demands and resulting physical and mental signs of distress. Thus it is essential that organizations understand the benefits, the costs, and the means of organizing therapeutic stress interventions.

BENEFITS AND COSTS

   Over the past decade a steadily growing number of organizations have incorporated stress-related therapeutic activities into the range of services they offer to their employees. Several factors underlie this trend. At least part of management's motivation appears to be genuine concern for employees' welfare. Fitness programs have been started after an executive has survived a heart attack or other close encounter with heart disease, finds that he feels better (and works better) when he is in good physical condition, and decides that everyone in the company should share the benefits of fitness.

The initiation of therapeutic activities can also be motivated by the hope that stress management programs will help to control spiraling health care costs and reduce costs associated with alcohol and drug abuse, absenteeism, accidents, and poor job performance. In this respect, stress management is often considered an essential aspect of human resources management—the "preventive maintenance" cost for the company's human capital resource. Finally, as Adams pointed out in Chapter 17, claims of stress-related disability increasingly are being sustained by the courts; organizations are looking for ways to control their liability.

Although many organizations have a sense of responsibility for their employees that in itself is sufficient to justify support for therapeutic stress interventions, others need to be convinced of the relative economic costs and benefits of such programs. Fortunately, data from a variety of studies are generally supportive. Reviews of cost-benefit studies indicate that employee counseling programs, stress management training, short-term psychotherapy, and alcohol treatment programs are variously associated with such benefits as decreased absenteeism, increased productivity, reduced use of inpatient and outpatient health services, and lower accident rates. The savings attributed to these benefits ranged from two to eight times the cost of the intervention program itself. (Manuso, 1982; Quick and Quick, 1984).

ORGANIZING THERAPEUTIC INTERVENTIONS

Individual stress management activities can be undertaken through self-study, the employee's personal physician, local counseling and human service agencies, or one of a growing number of independent stress management programs. Increasingly, however, stress management activities are initiated at the workplace through the medical or health department, through employee assistance programs, through the personnel department, through company fitness centers, or through comprehensive health promotion programs.

The diversity of professional skills that can be invoked to staff and manage stress management programs is well illustrated by the perspectives reflected in this section of the book: occupational social work, occupational medicine, occupational psychiatry, psychoanalysis, and clinical psychology. Occupational nurses, union counselors, industrial chaplains, and pastoral counselors may work separately or through medical departments to provide additional services. Just as substantive research and effective prevention activities require an interdisciplinary approach, so too do therapeutic interventions involve a diversity of professionals.

OVERVIEW OF THERAPEUTIC STRESS INTERVENTION CHAPTERS

The following four chapters in this section illustrate well the range of approaches to individual stress management. In Chapter 19, James Francek provides a practical introduction to the history, the conceptual framework, and the operation of employee assistance programs as a strategy for managing stress. Bonnie Seamonds, in Chapter 20, describes the integration of risk counseling into routine health evaluations. The process is designed to assess work and personal stressors, individual coping skills, and general health status. Her published studies indicate that risk counseling and appropriate referral are associated with significant decreases in absenteeism.

Historically, occupational health has been primarily concerned with physical, chemical, and biological factors in the workplace and their impact on occupational diseases and injury. Raymond Suskind, one of the foremost leaders in occupational medicine, describes the objectives and functions of occupational medicine and the increasing focus on diagnostic and therapeutic strategies to cope with psychosocial and organizational stressors (Chapter 21).

Finally, in Chapter 22, John Wolfe and Thomas Robischon look at the role of private psychiatric hospitals in work stress interventions. Their chapter centers on a survey of seven private psychiatric hospitals and one private general hospital that have programs in occupational psychiatry. They note that psychiatric hospitals have viewed stress management programs as a marketing opportunity for inpatient psychiatric services, but conclude that most stress-related problems are appropriately handled in less-intensive outpatient environments. They suggest a rather limited role for private psychiatric hospitals in the management of work stress.

CONCLUSION

The chapters in Part IV do not reflect the full range of therapeutic interventions and organizational structures that can be brought to bear on individual stress management. They do, however, represent the experiences and views of some of the leading practitioners in this field. As such, they provide a valuable overview of recent accomplishments in the management of work stress—and some insights into the areas in which additional work is needed.

REFERENCES

Manuso, J. S. J. 1982. Stress Management and Behavioral Medicine: A Corporate Model. In O'Donnell, M. and Ainsworth, T. (Eds.). *Health Promotion in the Work Place*. New York: John Wiley.

Quick, J. C. and Quick, J. D. 1984. *Organizational Stress and Preventive Management*. New York: McGraw-Hill.

19   *Employee assistance programs: a strategy for managing stress*

James L. Francek

Insofar as our place of work is the source of our financial and physical survival, it represents a major institution within our lives that has a direct effect on the quality of life that we enjoy. Our place of work is the most regular contact we have outside of our home. The majority of our waking hours are spent in the pursuit of resources that we can use in other areas of our lives.

Today, more than any other time in the history of man's employment, we are living on the crest of waves in a sea of change. We can travel the breadth of our earth in a matter of hours; we can communicate instantaneously by satellite, by phone, by computer linkage; the market-places of the world are linked in such a fashion that the world can now be best described as an economic village. People living today have seen the world move through many evolutions. Family farms have given way to collective farms and factories. Factories, long a place of intensive labor, are now giving way to robotics. Offices today are undergoing a rapid transition. Millions of workers trained in the processing and analysis of information are being replaced by computers that do the same work in far less time and with far less difficulty.

If anything is constant, it is the experience of change. In the midst of this unprecedented level of change, we are asked to chart the maps of our personal and collective journey. Yet the target and path keep moving. In the midst of all this change individuals are struggling to survive and to better their situations. Yet the structure of the family, which is the basis and support of our life, is undergoing radical shifts as well. We now have to deal with dual-career marriages, single parenting, sexual roles in transition, and a flood of substances that magically alter the way we function and feel. Traditional values that served as roots in our families, in our cultures, and in our faith have become confused and thrown to the wind.

Standing in the midst of this changing world, one can quickly lose the sense of one's identity. Work is one of the chief ways that one defines oneself. Work uses a significant amount of our energy and our time. Work serves as an anchor and a resource. When we begin to function poorly at work we risk our very survival. For some, the workplace and their fellow workers have become their family. When we begin to feel the effects of multiple changes, we begin to experience stress. When those charged with the running of the workplace are cognizant of the behavior pattern resulting from stress, they are in an excellent position to prevent its full negative effects.

WORK STRESS

Elements of Stress

The elements of stress are threefold: stressor, context, and person (Figure 19.1). The *stressor* is the external action, person, or event that serves as the critical mass that brings the other elements into play. It can be extensive and prolonged, such as a terminal illness, or it can be extensive and short in nature, such as an earthquake. It can affect one individual, as in a layoff, or it can affect a number of individuals, as in the closing of a plant. Some of the potential stressors facing people at work today include relocation, reduction in force, reorganization of the workforce and restructuring the nature of the work, introduction of new technology, and early retirement.

The second element of stress in the *context* of the event, which is defined by the culture in which it takes place, the nature of social support, the geography, the physical environment, and the organizational structure within the community. The third element of stress is the individual *person*.

Figure 19.1.   Elements of stress

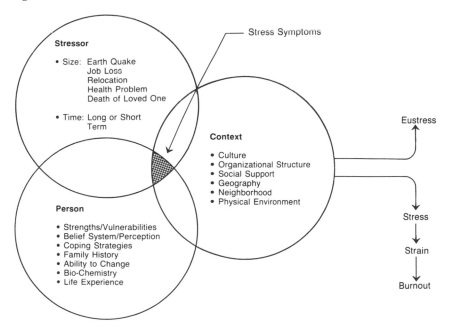

Source: Compiled by the author

Each person comes from a specific family where he or she developed certain coping strategies. Each person has his or her own belief system, strengths, and vulnerabilities. Each person has his or her own life experience that has prepared him or her to deal or not deal with change. It is said that even an individual's biochemistry has a good deal to do with the speed with which he or she responds to situations.

When we combine the concepts of change, work, and stress it is easy to see the similarities between our situation today and that of our predecessors who were hunters of the saber-toothed tiger. Survival skills are as necessary now as they were then. As we live and breathe the air of the twentieth century, we still need to know when to fight and when to flee. We also need to know that the wear and tear of our life-style can be reduced or increased by our perceptions of the world in which we live. While the current economic uncertainty serves as a background of distress for many individuals, if we translate this uncertainty into a life-or-death situation with no certainty of the outcome, then we open ourselves to incredible amounts of stress, strain, and eventual burnout. How we perceive the situation will determine to a great extent how we respond.

Observations about Stress

There are a number of observations about stress in general and stress in the workplace in particular that should be highlighted:

- High demands and low control are often associated with higher levels of strain or distress.
- Stress is cumulative, additive, and interactive.
- The more a period of fear or uncertainty is prolonged, the greater the risk for psychosomatic illness and accidents.
- One's fears are often greater than the eventual reality; planning from a "worst-case scenario" can allow the individual and the organization to capitalize on their creative energy.
- It is not the situation itself but one's perception of the situation that determines one's response.
- The broader the sense of ownership of an organization's problems and responsibility for their resolution, the more likely is a positive outcome.
- Structured group sessions during times of change and crisis can have positive and long-term effects on both the individual participants and the work organization.

Managing stress on a river of change means taking the time to read the river, plan the trip, balance a load, and understand the ebb and flow of the river. It requires taking responsibility for one's own health, one's use of time, the balance that one maintains in various relationships, and one's communication style.

In one important study of people who manage stress well, three key qualities were identified: (1) they perceived change as an opportunity rather than a threat; (2) they had social support systems that allowed them to get the input of other people, help them put corrals around their dragons, and reduce their sense of catastrophe; and (3) they had an internal value system, belief system, philosophy of life, faith—call it what you will—to which they could turn to draw strength (Kobasa, Hilker, and Maddi, 1979). Individuals and work organizations have a tremendous capacity to develop and nurture these qualities. One of the major objectives of employee assistance programs is to contribute to this process.

EMPLOYEE ASSISTANCE PROGRAMS

An employee assistance program (EAP) or employee health advisory program (EHAP) is, in our view, a systematic approach to employees and their dependents, whereby those who are experiencing psychosocial or emotional stress, family or marital difficulties, dependence on alcohol or drugs, or career changes are offered a range of professional and confidential interventions:

- Crisis intervention
- Assessment and differential diagnosis
- Interviewing and counseling
- Motivation for treatment
- Identification and referral to appropriate treatment resources
- Case management
- Orchestration of crises
- Short-term treatment
- Consultation to supervisors, union representatives, medical staff, family members, and others

Of these interventions, the most central one is probably that of case management. EAPs are in the position of being able to assess employees with stress-related problems and orchestrate an appropriate individual intervention plan.

Background

Employee assistance programs started initially in the 1940s as occupational alcoholism programs in response to an increasing awareness of the relationship of absenteeism, health care costs, accidents, and productivity problems related to alcohol consumption. Supervisors were trained to identify employees with alcohol problems and refer them to a relatively few treatment programs or to Alcoholics Anonymous. The formation of the National Council on Alcoholism in the 1940s, the recognition of alcoholism as a disease by the American Medical Association in the late 1950s, and the passage of the Hughes Act in the early 1970s all served to strengthen the occupational alcoholism movement. These programs demonstrated that something could be done, people did get better; there were dramatic improvements. Following the passage of the Hughes Act, occupational alcoholism programs grew rapidly. Today there are nearly 6,000 of them.

One of the critical lessons of this period was that if the work system was oriented to respond to changes in the job performance or behavior of its employees, and made referrals of those cases that did not respond to normal supervisory interventions to a confidential resource for assessment, usually these cases turned out to be early or developing cases of alcohol or drug dependence. Using this same approach, other complex human situations also surfaced.

The shift of occupational alcoholism to broader programs handling a full range of personal problems—now known as employee assistance programs—was gradual. Program counselors found that once they had identified a full range of services for the alcoholic and his dependents, they could adjust to the broader range of psychological, social, emotional, or health problems. As these programs expanded their scope of activities, leaders within management and unions recognized that these programs needed an even more comprehensive set of skills in order to deliver high-quality services. There was also a developing concern about liability questions and the necessity for more comprehensively trained people. This realization set the stage for the involvement of a wider range of professional disciplines, including social work, psychology, nursing, guidance and vocational counseling, and psychiatry. The joining together of these human resource professionals with occupational alcoholism counselors generated a great deal of creativity in EAP development.

Today, EAPs enjoy strong support in many companies from management, from union leadership, and from employees themselves. At Ford Motor Company it is a Health Counseling Program; at Exxon, an Employee Advisory Program; at Metropolitan Life Insurance Company, the Center for Health Help; and at Kimberly Clark EAP is part of the Health Management Program. These programs have changed over time and are constantly adapting to the needs of their environment.

Focus of EAP: The Individual within the System

To be effective, EAPs must consider the individual within the context of his entire family, social, and work systems (Figure 19.2). At the first level,

Figure 19.2. The focus of EHAP—the individual within the system

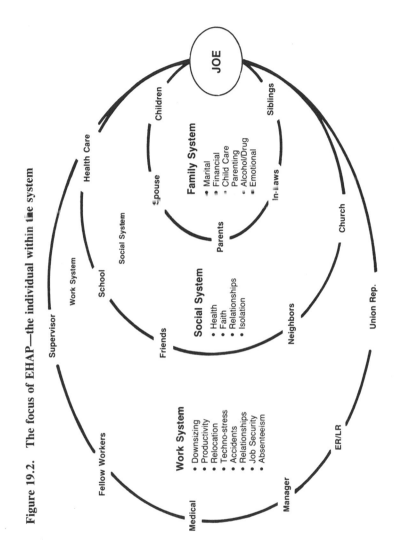

Source: Compiled by the author.

Figure 19.3. Personal inventory of stress and allocation of time

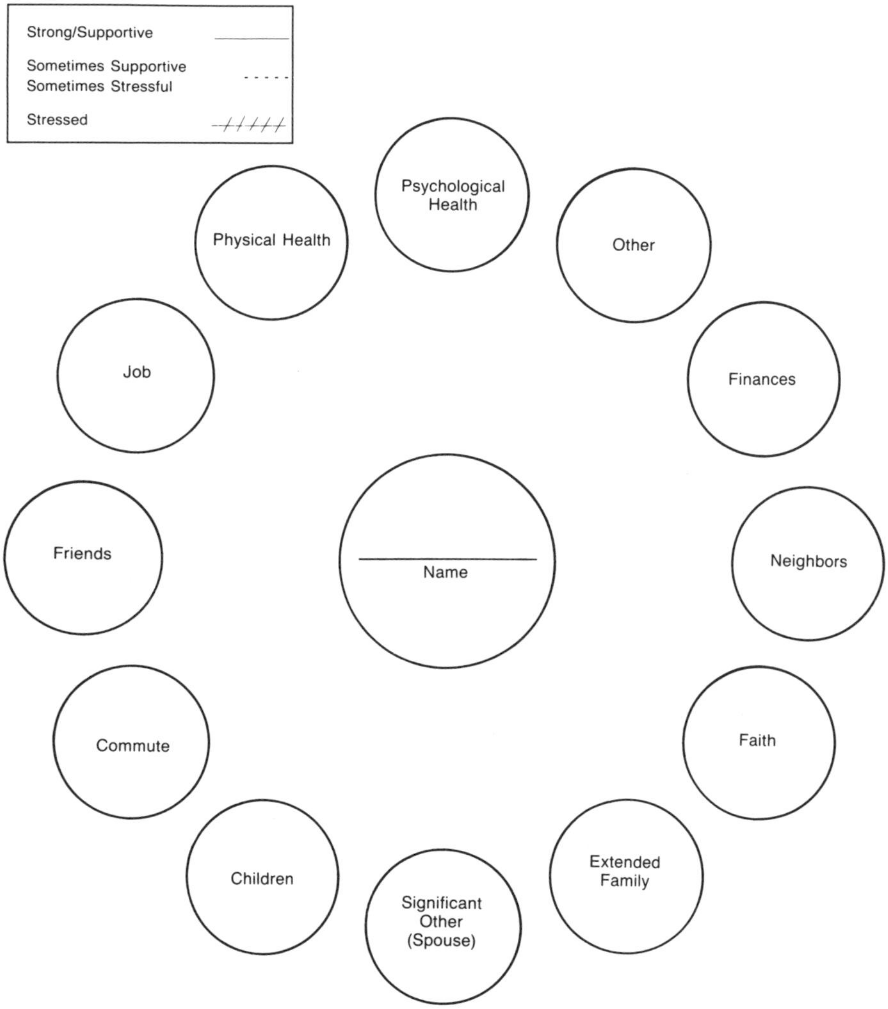

Strong/Supportive _____

Sometimes Supportive
Sometimes Stressful - - - - -

Stressed —/—/—/—/—/

ACTIVITY	HRS/WK	ACTIVITY	HRS/WK
Time with Significant Other		Time for Social Activities	
Time for Self		Time with Family	
Time for Commuting		Time for Work	
Time for Exercise		Other Activities	

Source: Compiled by the author.

an individual is generally part of a family, and there are many things that can be going on in a person's life that relate primarily to the family system. At the second level, an individual is part of a larger social system—his school, his neighbors, the church to which he belongs all affect him in one way or another. There may be problems or there may be positive social supports coming from these areas. Finally, there is the work system, including fellow workers, supervisors, managers, and organizational services such as counseling and health care.

When an individual comes in contact with an EAP we attempt to make a rapid assessment of the individual's relationship to each of the elements in the family, social, and work systems. In our programs we attempt to work quickly. We may see an individual only once and then only for an hour. In that hour we need to bring together the health data, the personal behavioral data, the interview, and other relevant information. Figure 19.3 is the personal inventory we use to help this process. We have used this form both with individuals and with groups.

When we use this form we first tell the person; "Often when you come in to seek advice, you are aware of one area in your life where you are hurting. And yet, if you look, there's more than one thing going on. In order to get a feel for that, would you quickly just put your name in the center here and draw out for me where you are feeling strong support and energy and where you are feeling stress. There may be places where you are getting some energy and feeling some stress." In a quick way we get a feeling for what is on the top of the employee's list of stressors and supports. More often than not in just this simple exchange the employee says, "I didn't know that so much was going on in my life." Or, "I forgot I could get more support from that area in my life."

Next, we have the employee fill out the bottom part of the form. This then provides a very useful comparison or contrast between the way in which the individual uses his or her time and the relationships between the circles on the top of the form. Although the completion of this form is usually only the beginning of the employee's relationship with the EAP, it illustrates the approach we take to assess stress in the life of the individual employee and the importance we place on looking at the individual within his or her system.

EAP Design

EAP programs exist in many styles and structures. An EAP can be described by the answers to three questions: What is to be covered by the program? Who is to accomplish each function? And how is each to be accomplished? An *effective* EAP is generally characterized by the following:

- Confidential services
- Professional EAP staff
- Clear definition of roles for medical, EAP, managerial, supervisory, human resources, staff, and union representatives
- Training for all of the above personnel
- Use of selected, quality treatment resources
- Noninterference with a consistent system of accountability for job performance and behavior

Among the different designs for EAPs are the assessment and referral model, in which troubled or potentially troubled employees are identified and assessed in-house or by an external contractor, and referred to appropriate services; the assessment and treatment model, in which identification, assessment, and basic counseling services are all provided in-house; and the service center model, in which employees are referred to a free-standing, independent service center that provides problem assessment, case consultation, some treatment, referral, and follow-up (Klarreich, Francek, and Moore, 1985). Services can also be provided through external contractors, private individuals, or organizations engaged to provide services ranging from initial assessment to short-term consultation to total coverage. In addition, labor unions have become increasingly involved in working jointly with management or independently in identifying assistance services for union members or in actually providing services.

The range of EAP designs is probably a reflection not only of the diversity of the organizations and individuals that EAPs serve, but also an indication of the creative diversity that various professional groups have brought to the growth of EAPs.

The EAP Environment: A Systems Approach

If there is one conclusion that emerges from the experience of EAPs, it is that their work cannot be done in isolation: there is no single discipline, profession, or organizational structure within a company that can successfully take responsibility for the mental health and well-being of the people in the organization. Thus, a major goal of EAPs becomes one of strengthening the interface between EAPs and allied functions within the organization such as employee relations (ER), medical staff, organizational development (OD), wellness programs, and the variety of activities related to these programs (Figure 19.4). Accomplishing this goal requires a systems approach to EAP.

The American Heritage Dictionary defines a system as "a group of interacting, interrelated, and interdependent elements forming or regarded as forming a collective entity." Before EAPs existed and before any EAP was introduced in a company, management, employees, and

Figure 19.4.   The interface between EHAP, ER/OD, and wellness

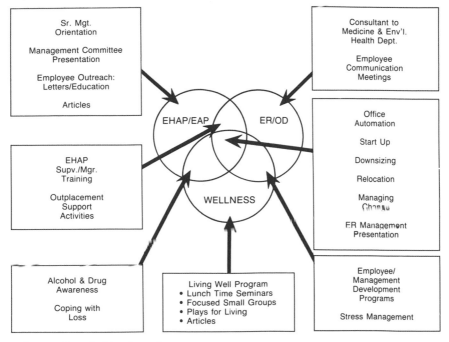

Source: Compiled by the author.

unions existed as systems and systems within systems. To function effectively within these systems, EAPs must take a systems approach; they should understand how power is distributed, how relationships are structured, how roles are defined, and how communication is used to convey messages.

The unprecedented level of change referred to earlier in this chapter is being reflected in redistribution of power, restructuring of work relationships, redefinition of roles, and a virtual revolution in communication patterns. If EAPs are to serve people in this changing environment, they must develop a broad understanding of the environment in which they work.

EAP IMPACT

Although EAPs have not been subjected to the type of research and evaluation on overall effectiveness that have been applied to some areas of work life, case examples and evaluations to date suggest a positive, and in some instances quite cost-effective, impact.

EAP at a Time of Crisis: A Case Example

The potential role of EAPs as a strategy for managing the stress of change in the workplace is illustrated by the following example from one company. A number of years ago employees from a specific division were told that in three months everyone in that part of the company would either be moved to a new position, retired, or transferred to another place. People were told that they would not remain in their present positions, but that they would not know for three months what their status would be. Management was trying to give notice of what was to come in order to allow people to prepare themselves. But three weeks after the announcement the manager of that section came to us and said, "There is nothing happening. There are no phones ringing. Everyone is flat dead in the water. Is there anything you can do to help us?" Obviously we had a huge group of people who were worried about whether they were going to survive; there was a sense of impending catastrophe.

In response to this situation, a group process was designed as a dynamic approach to the problem. Several different approaches were used. First, concepts adapted from Elizabeth Kubler-Ross's (1969) work on the process of death and dying were applied to the experience of major change that involves loss or feared loss. Thus the steps of letting go that she identified in the dying process were applied to marriage breakup, job loss, or any major job change. By the time the workshops were implemented, people had already passed through the phase of denial, so they were asked to do a stress inventory. The Personal Inventory form (Figure 19.3) was used to do this in a quick fashion. Working in groups of 50 people, participants were asked to fill out the form individually for themselves. When asked the simple question, "Are there any surprises? Any observations?" responses included: "I didn't know I had that many strengths"; "I didn't know I had that many stresses"; "now I see where I can get some help." All of these comments came out of the group.

The participants were then asked to take index cards and do two things: On one side, write down what they needed to let go of—maybe their demand for perfection, maybe their demand that the company will always be fair—all the shoulds and the musts. On the other side, they were asked to summarize briefly the emotional effect on themselves and their families during this period of uncertainty. Participants were encouraged to use whatever language suited them best. They then passed the cards to the facilitators who read them aloud and commented on the pain, thoughts, and emotional content. The effect was very powerful; the pain, the hurt, the fear, the anxiety all came out, and it became obvious to each individual that he or she was not alone. They said, "My God, I'm not the only one feeling this way." "Everyone around me is going through the same feelings." Too often in the workplace the emotional and social content is blocked out, and it becomes difficult to deal with the very real impact of this content on the daily life of people at the workplace. In this instance employees were encouraged to express the emotional content and to get support from one another.

The next step was to have each individual look at his or her value system. In groups of six, they were asked to talk about the values they had identified and rated individually. This also can be a very powerful activity. "What is the thing that you do for yourself that gives you power?" "What is the thing that gives you a sense of personal power and control in your life?" After 20 minutes they came back and put the answers on the board, revealing a whole roomful of options people had generated.

In a three-and-a-half-hour session employees came to see that they themselves were resources, that they could be supports to one another, and that the sense of impending catastrophe could be turned around to an opportunity. This is not to say that everyone came away with a positive grip on his or her situation, but that an EAP can have an important impact on mobilizing individual and collective resources.

Evaluation of EAPs

Despite anecdotal evidence of the impact of EAPs, and despite the continued growth of EAPs over the past several years, there has been little substantive research conducted to verify the effectiveness of these programs. Potential measures of EAP effectiveness can be grouped into four major classes (Googins, 1985):

1. Change in behavior—a measure of the degree to which a person has achieved behavioral improvements such as abstinence from alcohol.
2. Change in work performance—a measure of the degree to which the employee has improved job performance.
3. Change in cost reduction—a measure of savings realized through improved work performance.
4. Change in penetration—a measure of the extent to which a program reaches the target population of a given organization.

In the introduction to Part IV on therapeutic interventions (Chapter 18) it was pointed out that some data exist documenting the effectiveness of counseling programs and occupational alcoholism programs in particular. However, Edwards (1975) points out that there are a number of biases that tend to inflate success rates, and that only a subset of programs—possibly the elite, somewhat atypical, well-implemented active programs—have been evaluated. In reviewing EAP program effectiveness, Reidiger (1985) concludes that, despite the lack of numerous or systematic studies of EAP impact, a "few unique programs have demonstrated that the employee assistance concept can work, not only as a rescue mission, but as an integral part of an employing organization's system of human resource management." From these successful programs he identifies the following key concepts associated with effectiveness:

- Comprehensive scope—EAPs should be designed to deal with a comprehensive range of personal problems.

- Integration with the workplace—EAPs should be considered a health plan aimed at the organization and an essential component of good management.

- Support from the employer—This support can be manifested through policy statements, assignment of specific responsibility and accountability for program implementation, development of formal links between the EAP and other parts of the organization, and assurance of adequate funding.

- Professional clinical resource—Either through in-house staff or through outside contracts, clinical services should be provided in a professional and competent manner.

- Positive program definition—The program should be regarded as a fair, positive option, and not associated with coercion or identified with management's disciplinary process.

- Behavior health model—EAPs need to support and cooperate with mental health services and existing community treatment agencies to discover arrangements appropriate for the workplace.

- Program education—Educational programs aimed at individual employees, supervisors, and senior managers are important in developing within each group the knowledge and skills necessary to play their part in the referral, assessment, or treatment process.

- Responsibility for ongoing development—EAPs should see their development as an ongoing process, both in terms of professional skills and in terms of effective integration into the organization.

Thus the lack of systematic evidence documenting the impact of EAPs places the onus on individual EAP directors, coordinators, and counselors to build local support for EAPs and a sense of ownership of the problems to which EAPs address themselves.

FUTURE OF EMPLOYEE ASSISTANCE PROGRAMS

Employee assistance programs have grown and changed remarkably since their origin in occupational alcoholism treatment programs, but the amount of change that organizations are currently undergoing and the diversity of demands that are being placed on people strongly suggest that EAPs must continue to change and develop. EAPs can serve an important function in gathering information on how individuals are functioning within the context of a changing work environment; they can analyze the patterns of change, and provide feedback to management. They need to work closely with other components of the organization, such as organizational development, medical staff, and employee relations professionals, to address systemic problems. EAPs need to continue to develop a proactive approach to alcoholism, drug abuse, and stress-related disorders, bringing these activities into overall wellness efforts.

Finally, practitioners in employee assistance programs can influence the very social conscience and direction of their host organization by appropriately using observations, data, and their credibility to engage the organization's leaders in a full discussion of the changing nature of work and its impact on all of its human resources.

REFERENCES

Edwards, D. W. 1973. The evaluation of internal employee and occupational alcoholism programs. In Williams, R. I.. and Moffat, G. H. (Eds.). *Occupational Alcoholism Programs*. Springfield, Ill: Charles C. Thomas.

Googins, B. 1985. Can change be documented?: Measuring the impact of EAPs. In Klarreich, S. H., Francek, J. L., and Moore, C. E. (Eds.). *The Human Resources Management Handbook: Principles and Practice of Employee Assistance Programs*. New York: Praeger.

Klarreich, S. H., Francek, J. L., and Moore, C. E. (Eds.). 1985. *The Human Resources Management Handbook: Principles and Practice of Employee Assistance Programs*. New York: Praeger.

Kobasa, S. C., Hilker, R. J., and Maddi, S. R. 1979. Who stays healthy under stress? *Journal of Occupational Medicine*, 21(9): 595–598.

Kubler-Ross, E. 1969. *On Death and Dying*. New York: Macmillan.

Riediger, A. J. 1985. EAPs: Barriers to effectiveness. In Klarreich, S. H., Francek, J. L., and Moore, C. E. (Eds.). *The Human Resources Management Handbook: Principles and Practice of Employee Assistance Programs*. New York: Praeger.

20   *Risk counseling as a therapeutic intervention in the workplace*

Bonnie C. Seamonds

Risk counseling interviews are proving to be useful tools in managing the effects of occupational stressors in the workplace. Stressors are defined as changes that occur in one's environment requiring adaptation. Stress reactions are psychological and physiological responses to changes in the work environment that can directly affect motivation and productivity. Risk counseling was developed originally to assist employees in coping with a changing work environment and to help them identify and develop effective coping skills that would decrease their vulnerability to work stressors.

RISK COUNSELING FORMAT

Risk counseling, done as a 20-minute interview between a skilled interviewer and an employee, is designed to do the following: (1) identify job stressors and their effects on the employee; (2) assess other stressors that may impact on the employee, such as family, health, finances, social issues; (3) assess the presence and severity of psychological and/or physical symptoms as reactions to these stressors; (4) assess the level of coping skills the employee has available; (5) determine how well the employee maintains a balance with regard to time for work, for family, for self; (6) develop a plan of action for managing stressors more effectively, adding to the skill levels and making appropriate referrals where necessary; and (7) provide opportunities for organizational change by reducing unproductive stressors.

The interview was limited to approximately 20 minutes as time lost from work was a major consideration. Employees were given a comprehensive medical evaluation that included a computerized medical history, laboratory work, X-ray, electrocardiogram, a risk counseling interview, and finally, an examination by a physician. This entire process was generally completed within two hours.

During the interview referrals were suggested and resources identified where appropriate. Employees were encouraged to report back as additional referrals were needed. During the research phase of the risk counseling effort, follow-up data on employees were gathered by telephone and questionnaire after eight weeks. Table 20.1 and the paragraphs that follow describe the risk counseling format.

Table 20.1.   Risk counseling format

Job stressors	• Type/severity/frequency
Personal stressors	• Family/marital/health/financial/social
Symptoms	• Psychological/physical
Coping skills	• Adaptive/maladaptive
Life style balance	• Work/family/self
Action plan	• Strategies/goals/resources
Executive commitment	• Culture/commitment/planning/change

Source: Compiled by the author.

IDENTIFYING JOB AND PERSONAL STRESSORS: Type, severity, and frequency of occurrence of job and personal stressors have to be identified. It is suggested that a standardized questionnaire be used to ascertain these factors such as Kahn et al.'s (1964) occupation stressor scale or McLean's (1979) self-assessment scheme. A job stressor questionnaire can be administered in conjunction with other interventions such as medical examinations or health risk appraisals, if desired.

The actual effect of these stressors on the individual employee can best be examined as part of the risk counseling effort. It would be ideal to have a copy of any medical examinations at hand in order to learn about physical symptoms that could be part of reactions to various stressors.

ASSESSING THE PRESENCE OF SYMPTOMS: Questions are asked during the risk counseling interview about specific reactions to any work stressors highlighted by the employee on the medical exam, the questionnaire, or by the interviewer. These reactions may manifest as psychological in nature (irritability, absent-mindedness, lack of concentration, hyperactivity, loss of sense of humor, and such) or may be physical in nature, such as muscle tension, headaches, gastric upsets, palpitations.

The task is to look for a change—something that has recently occurred that had not been present before or at least did not occur as frequently as it is occurring now. How does this employee know when he or she is under stress? How does this state show itself?

ASSESSING THE LEVEL OF COPING SKILLS: What coping skills does the employee bring to the stressful situation? Are they adaptive or maladaptive? What behavior and attitudes does the employee have that determine how he or she will cope with these stressors?

Questions such as "How are you able to cope as well as you do?" "What are the strengths you have that enable you to perform so well?" "What gets in your way when you are faced with these problems?" are designed for the interviewer to focus on the level of coping the employee is experiencing at the moment. The interviewer can then assist the employee in planning different responses for the future.

LIFESTYLE BALANCE: THE MANAGEMENT OF TIME FOR WORK, FAMILY AND SELF: Very often job demands supersede other demands, particularly from the family. With long commutes, leaner staff, and higher productivity, employees often find themselves pulled in several directions at once. In many instances, the last person on the list to find time for is the employee. Families can be very supportive if the employee maintains good lines of communication and actively enlists family support.

How satisfied is the employee with the way in which he or she manages the time between work, family, and self? Is the employee examining priorities periodically to make sure that everyone is getting their fair share of time and attention—particularly the employee?

The most common excuse for lack of exercise or relaxation programs from the employee's point of view is: "I don't have the time." This excuse bears closer examination and is often the result of lack of organization or inadequate priority setting on the part of the employee. Of course, in the short term, there may be pressing business goals where all else becomes secondary, but this should be only a short-term problem. With appropriate priority setting, the employee should be able to get back on track after the crisis event is over—unless the employee allows him- or herself to be managed by crises. Taking charge of one's time versus operating in a reactive mode is an important assessment to make during the interview.

Most of us have various stressors that impact on our ability to cope, and many are not job-related. We may have aging parents that are of concern to us, or financial problems, marital problems, or problems with children that contribute to our general stress levels. An inquiry into other stressors the employee is experiencing can help the employee understand the cumulative effect these concerns can have on his or her ability to perform well on the job. The interviewer can be most helpful in this area by encouraging the employee to prioritize these stressors and to make some determinations as to what he or she can and cannot influence directly and in the short term. Taking proactive steps to solve some of the problems can help remove some of the feelings of being overwhelmed that can be experienced when many stressors converge at once.

DEVELOPING AN ACTION PLAN: The goal of the interview is to work with the employee to diagnose his or her stress reactions, identify stressors, and assess coping skills. A plan of action is developed jointly to reduce stressors where possible, develop or acquire new coping skills through skills training, increase one's support system, and to create new opportunities to cope with stress such as exercise or relaxation programs.

EXECUTIVE COMMITMENT: Executive commitment to risk counseling should be obtained prior to putting the program into effect. This can be accomplished through well-designed proposals that include an evaluation of the program's effectiveness. A pilot project of specified duration is more acceptable than an open-ended one. Executive commitment gives needed credibility and helps ensure participation by all levels in the organization. It is important to avoid the problem that many EAPs have where senior management utilization is very low. Risk counseling should be part of the health promotion effort and not be seen as targeted for a specific part of the workplace population.

This commitment may also result in the development of an avenue for real problem solving throughout the organization. In one company, it became apparent through numerous interviews that a major stressor for employees was role ambiguity. On closer examination of that stressor it was learned that unclear job descriptions in several areas had led to competing lines of reporting, duplication of services, and some animosity between departments. Because senior management was cognizant and in full support of risk counseling efforts, this information was fed back and acted upon.

Senior management should be apprised of any trends, observations, or concerns that employees have while maintaining strict confidentiality. This is most easily done through summary reports about major stressors and anonymous input from the interviewed employees as to what might be done to resolve the effects of these major stressors. Periodic evaluations of the risk counseling efforts should be done with senior management as well in order to plan future direction.

KEY ISSUES IN RISK COUNSELING

Who Will Benefit Most from Risk Counseling?

Individuals who are experiencing the effects of job stressors need to be identified. Managers cannot afford to ignore the issues of occupational stress. Stress will always be a part of our daily lives, but excessive stress costs everyone—in terms of health, turnover, motivation, productivity, and job dissatisfaction.

Risk counseling programs can benefit not only the manager but also the employee and the organization. As a preventive program, it helps pinpoint some of the major stressors, identify employees who are not coping well, and also enables everyone to learn from the individuals who are thriving in a highly pressurized environment.

Who Should Do Risk Counseling?

Risk counseling involves working with personal as well as job stress. The interviewer, therefore, must have significant expertise and experience in interpersonal skills. Professional training in psychology, communications, managing people, research, and medical skills should result in an interviewer who has credibility with senior management as well as other employees.

Since information obtained during risk counseling is confidential, it is probably best to have an outside consultant conduct these interviews rather than a fellow employee. It is often true, for example, that senior staff members do not often avail themselves of in-house counseling programs out of concern for their own job security or their corporate image. This experience must be made as safe as possible in order to get the maximum amount of data in the least amount of time to produce a worthwhile experience for the employee.

What Factors Are Most Important in Risk Counseling?

The interview outline in Table 20.2 is an example of the format of a typical interview. An explanation of each section follows:

1. Presenting Problem. The reason for the employee coming to the interview may appear as a part of a general health evaluation, as a score from a job stressor questionnaire, or through eliciting the information at the beginning of the counseling session. It will be necessary to help the employee define his or her stress issues while providing a relaxed and safe environment for this to occur.

2. Relevant History. Has this problem occurred in the past? Is it a problem the employee has carried for some time? Does the employee's current sleep problem, for example, relate to the specific work situation or are irregular sleep patterns the norm? Complaints about an unresponsive boss may not be due to insensitivity but could be a function of the employee being unable to ask directly for recognition, make requests, say no to extra work, or ask for assistance.

3. Health Status. What is the employee's current level of health? Does he or she smoke, drink heavily, overeat? What facts from the latest physical exam would be important when assessing coping skills?

4. Stress Symptoms. The employee may be experiencing easily identifiable symptoms or may not have made any connections, for example, between tension headaches and being bored on the job. The interviewer wants to help the employee explore possibilities but come to his or her own conclusions in the process. Major stressors can be identified throughout the interview. Focusing on both job and personal issues helps the employee to understand the cumulative effect of stressors that may come from both areas of life.

5. Life Balance. Survival issues according to Knippel (1980) are basic attitudes and behaviors related to general health maintenance. Included in this section are major survival issues: diet, exercise, sleep patterns, environment, and recognition. Several questions related to these areas provide both the interviewer and the employee with a checklist. For example:

- Are the hours worked conducive with a healthy life-style?
- How does the employee go about getting what he or she needs or wants from the work environment?
- Is the work environment safe and healthy? Ergonomic factors such as ventilation and work station design should be assessed.

- Are there identified people who are available to provide support and feedback for this employee?
- Is the employee using leisure time to restore his or her energy, reduce stress levels, and provide a balance?

6. Major Life Changes. What is currently going on in the employee's world to contribute to the amount and severity of change he or she is experiencing? Holmes and Rahe's (1967) scale on social readjustment measures effects of cumulative change and some of their parameters are used here.

7. Levels of Satisfaction. This involves professional and personal aspects of the employee's life. It is important to listen to the employee's perception of how stress affects him or her and what they want to do about it. The employee may need skills training, for example, to learn assertive behavior at home or on the job.

Table 20.2. Interview format for risk counseling

1. Presenting problem
2. Relevant history
3. Health status (include habits, behaviors)
4. Stress symptoms/identification of major stressors
5. Life balance
   nutritional status
   exercise program
   sleep pattern
   recognition pattern
   environmental conditions
   support systems (at home, at work)
   leisure time activities
6. Major life changes (number and kind)
   death/spouse, family member, friend
   marriage/separation, divorce
   communication problems/work, spouse, family, friends
   changes in health/family, self
   change in responsibility and/or status at work
   change in financial status
   sexual difficulties
   birth of child/other life-style changes
   problems with children
   relocation
7. Levels of satisfaction
   job: tasks, status, interpersonal, salary
   home: climate, interpersonal, style
8. Professional and personal skill levels
   negotiation, assertiveness, time management, conflict resolution, stress
      management
9. Assessment and referral

Source: Compiled by the author.

8. Skill Levels. This involves assessing the various professional and personal skills that the employee possesses. Strengths and limitations are determined here. Subsequent skill development activities may then be undertaken in specific areas of need, such as time management, assertiveness training, and stress management.

9. Referrals. At this point the interviewer refers the employee to the appropriate resource. These referrals require the interviewer to be familiar with the in-house resources in the organization, as well as external ones in the community.

Inside Resources

Corporate inventories should be taken by the risk counseling interviewer in order to identify and evaluate the resources that exist within the organization for effective stress management. Following are some examples of resources that may already exist in an organization. It is not difficult to see how these programs may enhance risk counseling efforts.

- **Skills Training.** Courses, seminars, and training programs in coaching skills, time management, managing conflict, communication, stress management, and such, can help reduce the effects of job stressors. Executive round tables, strategy meetings, quality circles, participative management meetings, and so on, can become forums for changing unproductive job stress.

- **Counseling Services.** Medical facilities, employee assistance programs, educational and career counseling may be sources for follow-on for the employee after risk counseling.

- **Health Benefits.** Mental health insurance covering private counseling, risk reduction programs, and health promotion efforts can add to more effective stress management.

- **Organizational Tools.** Performance appraisals, preretirement planning, job descriptions, and such, can provide opportunities for stress reduction within the organization.

Outside Resources

Community resources that can be used in stress reduction are numerous. Programs in exercise, smoking cessation, weight reduction, and meditation are available in most areas. Opportunities to gain needed skills in educational facilities, private counseling hospital clinics, and various recreational activities may all lend themselves to the reduction of stress reactions.

Risk counseling efforts should include a brief assessment of the interviewee's level of knowledge about community resources. Expanding this knowledge will provide more options for the employee to manage much of his or her stress levels.

It is ultimately up to the employee to obtain the assistance he or she needs. Diagnosis, assessment, and goal setting are part of risk counseling. Implementation and utilization of resources are up to the employee.

SUPPORTIVE RESEARCH

Risk Counseling and Illness Absenteeism

In a research project in 1982 and a follow-on study in 1983, I measured the effects of risk counseling on illness absenteeism in a group of 1,000 employees of a major financial institution (Seamonds, 1982, 1983). Twenty-minute risk counseling interviews were done in conjunction with a medical examination that included Kahn's (1964) job stress inventory in the computerized medical history. These interviews were designed to assess stress-related symptoms and coping abilities related primarily to work stress. Referrals and education materials were given as part of the interview process. The results showed that the risk counseling process can have a significant impact on the reduction of illness absenteeism.

Subjects whose absentee rates for specific time periods were above established norms were categorized as high absentee employees. These subjects became the experimental group. Experimental subjects were matched to control subjects resulting in 292 pairs for statistical analysis (see Figure 20.1). Control subjects were matched by sex, job classification, job stress score, and had had a medical examination during the same time interval as the experimental subject. Control subjects did not have risk counseling.

Subjects were grouped according to job stress scores (Y axis) with high/low scorers grouped together as a result of Selye's work (1956) demonstrating that deprivation of stimuli as well as excess is accompanied by an increase in stress. Weiman's work (1977) confirmed this hypothesis by showing that disease/risk factors occur more frequently when employees are either deprived of stimulation or are overloaded.

Illness absenteeism for both groups (short-term absences shown on the X axis) was monitored for six months prior to the risk counseling time period (PRE-EXP for the experimental group and PRE-CON for the control group) and for six months after the risk counseling interval (POST-EXP for the experimental group and POST-CON for the control group).

In all three groupings, the experimental groups exhibited a decrease in average rate of absenteeism in the period following the interview. Over that same time period, the control subjects in all three groupings displayed an increase in the average number of days absent. The data were subjected to a regressed change analysis in which the effects of sex, job classification, and job stress score were eliminated prior to correlating the effect of risk counseling and levels of absenteeism. When evaluated by a hierarchical regression analysis, the significance of the relationship between the interview and the absenteeism in the second six-month period becomes apparent ($F = 5.261$, $p \leq .01$).

The data indicate that some illness absenteeism is a result of job stressors. Personal stressors seemed to be a factor with high absentee

Figure 20.1.   Before and after measures of absentee rate. Absentee rates for experimental groups (those who had the health evaluation interview) were measured six months prior to interview (PRE-EXP) and six months after interview (POST-EXP). Absentee rates for control groups (those who did not have the interview) were measured for the same periods, six months prior (PRE-CON) and six months after experimental group had the interview (POST-CON).

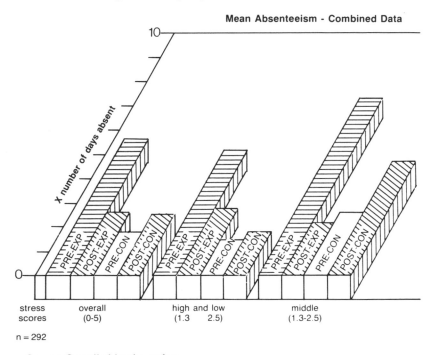

Mean Absenteeism - Combined Data

x number of days absent

stress scores

overall (0-5)

high and low (1.3   2.5)

middle (1.3-2.5)

n = 292

Source: Compiled by the author.

employees who indicated only a moderate level of job stress. It became obvious, however, that preventive steps to enable employees to improve health benefits, behaviors, and attitudes could be taken regardless of the kind of stressors experienced.

It became clear during these studies that employees often did not have the information necessary to manage their own stress reduction, particularly in learning to differentiate between stressors they could and could not control. Employees, with guidance, were able to reassess their health practices, their work habits, their reactions to stressors, and their attitudes about maintaining optimal health in the workplace.

Almost half of the employees interviewed expressed difficulties in coping with work stress. Symptoms related to these coping difficulties presented as mild but persistent psychological and physical symptoms such as fatigue, irritability, sleep disturbance, "nervous" stomachs, and muscle aches, to more severe symptoms such as chronic headaches, marked anxiety, heavy smoking, and weight gain. On follow-up eight weeks later, 73 percent of those with milder and more recent symptoms reported a significant reduction in stress-related symptoms. Of those with more severe symptoms, 55 percent reported a reduction in symptoms through some health management plan established during risk counseling.

Risk counseling efforts are cost–effective and can directly impact on short-term absenteeism that affects productivity and motivation. In addition, organizational stress can be dealt with by senior executives who have been involved in the risk counseling process from its inception and see it as another valuable benchmark for organizational health.

High Tech Stress and Risk Counseling

Risk counseling was also used as part of a recent study by myself and C. Weiman (1985) in which we investigated the effects of video display terminals used by 75 operators on stress levels. These subjects completed a comprehensive medical examination, a job stress inventory, and a risk counseling interview. The interview format in Table 20.2 was followed as well as an additional format outlined in Table 20.3.

The purpose of this investigative study was to offer employees who use VDTs four or more hours per day an opportunity to contribute to a general knowledge base as to what staff and management could do to help with the effective integration of computer technology into the workplace. We also wanted to learn whether stress reactions were different in the high tech environment from the general office workplace previously investigated.

A comparison was made with 75 employees who had undergone a medical examination, completed a job stress inventory, but did not use VDTs at all or for less than two hours per day. Risk counseling efforts uncovered stress-related symptoms and concerns expressed by VDT operators. Employees reported fear of what long-term use of VDTs would be. The lack of information contributed greatly to general stress levels with regard to health and safety.

Table 20.3.   High tech stress interview format

Office environment	● Lighting/air quality/noise/space
Work station	● Equipment/cabling/furniture
Work practices	● supervisory style/job design/training
VDT operator	● Training/attitudes/work habits/coping skills

Source: Compiled by the author.

- **Fatigue:** Employees complained of stationary work conditions, sedentary jobs, and repetitive tasks in the VDT group as well as in the control group.
- **Vision Symptoms:** Symptoms were much greater in VDT user group and were accounted for, to a larger extent, by ergonomic factors. Glare, harsh lighting, poor copy, poor resolution of letters on the screen, and poor work habits such as staring into the screen when thinking were highlighted.
- **High Tension:** Tension levels appeared to be about the same for both groups.
- **Musculoskeletal Symptoms:** Aches and pains of muscles in joints were reported with similar frequency in both groups. Back pain accounted for most complaints in 61 percent of the VDT user group and 64 percent of the control group. Shoulder, wrist, and finger pain was reported in less than 10 percent of employees in both groups.

Several trends became apparent during this study:

- Physical and psychological symptoms associated with VDT use do not seem appreciably different from nonusers with the exception of reported eye strain.
- Job design seems to be a major contributing factor in stress in an automated environment. During interview sessions, VDT users complained of repetitive, boring tasks or stressful customer service interactions.
- The methods currently used in introducing computer technology into the office need improving. Educational materials, ergonomic standards, supervisory and VDT user training in how to reduce stress-related symptoms in this environment are currently being designed to meet the needs uncovered during the risk counseling interview process.

A resistance to change seems to be occurring in this workforce studied and may be a result of job design, training efforts, and ownership problems—that is, a lack of autonomy and control of important aspects of one's job—particularly in a high tech environment. These findings are being studied further with a view to assessing specific high tech work environments with appropriate ergonomic, psychosocial, and organizational development parameters.

SUMMARY

Risk counseling is having a positive effect in the workplace in assisting the employee to gain the information and tools necessary to maintain optimal health in the workplace and in supplying organizations with crucial information about work stressors than can result in organizational change to promote a healthier place in which to work.

Risk counseling efforts allow the interviewer to assist the employees to cope more effectively with job-related and personal stressors; to teach employees to better manage much of their own health care, particularly in the area of stress management; to help lower absentee rates that are, in part, a result of stress-related issues; and to direct employees to appropriate resources. Risk counseling can also highlight major stressors and trends in the area of work stress for management, help generate data on the impact of computer technology in the workplace, and provide information that may help reduce high tech stress. Finally, there is some evidence that risk counseling can promote healthier employees *and* healthier organizations.

REFERENCES

Holmes, T. and Rahe, R. 1967. The social readjustment rating scale. *Journal of Psychosomatic Research*, 1: 213–218.

Kahn, R., Wolfe, D., Quinn, R., Snoek, J., with Rosenthal, R. 1964. *Organizational Stress*. New York: John Wiley.

Knippul, G. 1980. The survivor's checklist. *Journal of Transactional Analysis*, 10: 61–67.

McLean, A. A. 1979. *Work Stress*. Reading, Mass.: Addison-Wesley.

Seamonds, B. 1982. Stress factors and their effect on absenteeism in a corporate employee group. *Journal of Occupational Medicine*, 24(5): 393–397.

————. 1983. Extension of research into stress factors and their effect on illness absenteeism. *Journal of Occupational Medicine*, 25(11): 821–822.

Seamonds, B. and Weiman, C. 1985. *High Tech Stress and the Impact of Video Display Terminals in the Workplace*.

Selye, H. 1956. *The Stress of Life*. New York: McGraw-Hill.

Weiman, C. 1977. A study of occupational stressors and the incidence of disease/risk. *Journal of Occupational Medicine*, 17: 119–122.

21   *Occupational health and stress*

Raymond R. Suskind

Several questions need to be addressed when considering the main issues in the field of occupational health. These questions include: what is the role of occupational medicine in health care delivery systems; what are the primary concerns and activities of the occupational physicians; what do other members of the occupational health team contribute; and, finally, what are the activities and problems that deal with stress reactions? I shall attempt to answer these questions by drawing from my own four decades of experience, first as a participant in and subsequently as a director of a comprehensive university-based occupational health program for 16 years.

For a period of almost three decades there was an active collaborative clinical, teaching, and research program at the University of Cincinnati involving the Department of Psychiatry and the Clinical Section of the Department of Environmental Health. Out of this joint effort Ross (1956) wrote his pioneering textbook, *Practical Psychiatry for Industrial Physicians*.

Within the health care delivery system occupational medicine provides the resources, the clinical and administrative expertise, as well as the research capabilities to identify and quantify the biological, chemical, and physical hazards that result in disease or injury. *The major role of occupational medicine is to prevent and control occupational diseases and injury.* When adverse effects are suspected, the body of scientific, clinical, and therapeutic knowledge and the skills of the trained physician and associated professionals are utilized in a coordinated fashion in the evaluation and management of the problem.

HISTORY OF OCCUPATIONAL HEALTH

The health of workers has been the subject of social concern for several thousands of years. One of the earliest records is the Edwin Smith papyrus dated 3000 B.C. in which the severe injuries sustained in the building of the step pyramids Sakkarah at Memphis in Egypt are described. Of particular interest is the detailed description of head injuries and their prognoses. Hippocrates, who was concerned about the effects of air, water, and workplaces on health, clearly described lead colic in miners. Pliny the Elder and Galen carefully described workplace stresses and how to diagnose and treat such illnesses. In the sixteenth century the Swiss physician George Bauer—known as Agricola—in his treatise *De Re Metallica*, recorded the dreaded lung disease of Carpathian mountain miners before it was recognized as cancer of the lung. At the end of the nineteenth century, the ore was found to contain pitchblende from which radium was extracted by Madame Curie. The pioneer occupational physician, Bernadino Ramazzini, wrote a comprehensive treatise on occupational diseases and insisted that the only way to understand occupational diseases was to study them in the work environment itself.

During the first half of the twentieth century, there were some organized efforts to use existing knowledge and skills for the diagnoses and treatment of occupational disease. Official recognition of occupational medicine as a specialty was established in the early 1950s through the creation of a certifying board. The first degree-granting program in occupational medicine was initiated by Dr. Lyle Hazlitt at the University of Pittsburgh. In 1947 the residency training program was developed at the University of Cincinnati by Dr. Robert A. Kehoe. He pioneered in environmental health research and education. In 1945, just after World War II in Europe was over, he delivered a lecture in the Hall of the Worshipful Society of Apothecaries in London in which he clearly described the essential objectives of occupational medicine, the requirements of an effective training program, and the multidisciplinary nature of the resources in an effective occupational medicine program (Kehoe, 1946). He described the essential character of this new field, including the marriage of the academic occupational health disciplines and clinical practice. By the year 1975 there were more than 100 physicians who had graduated from the residency program at the University of Cincinnati. Currently there are about 12 federally supported residency programs in occupational medicine.

TRAINING IN OCCUPATIONAL HEALTH

Although in occupational medicine there is a body of clinical and scientific knowledge that is utilized in its effective practice, occupational medicine depends on and coordinates its efforts with a number of other related occupational health disciplines. These include: toxicology, industrial hygiene, occupational safety, nursing, biostatistics, epidemiology, and radiologic health. It is also dependent for both diagnostic and therapeutic management on internal medicine, surgery, and their respective specialities. The field of occupational medicine has grown significantly in the past 40 years and there are now a number of subspecialities and specialists within the field of occupational medicine, such as occupational psychiatrists, occupational pulmonary physicians, occupational dermatologists, occupational allergists, occupational ophthalmologists, occupational otolaryngologists, and the list is growing.

The objectives of the graduate training program in occupational medicine are for the trainee to develop proficiency in:

1. The diagnosis and management of illness common to occupational medicine including the management of emotional and social factors.
2. The practice of preventive medicine in an industrial setting.
3. The planning and implementation of health care and surveillance programs.
4. The use of epidemiological and biostatistical methods for the development of critical information about hazards and their adverse effects.
5. The use of industrial hygiene and toxicology as the basis for designing, implementing hazard control programs, and for making policy decisions about such hazards.
6. Training the physician to develop research programs in occupational medicine (Suskind, 1977).

The training curriculum program includes at least one year of academic courses: toxicology, industrial hygiene, epidemiology and biostatistics, industrial safety, public health management, radiologic health—both introductory and advanced courses in these subjects. The academic curriculum also includes courses in applied psychiatry, dermatology, pathology of cellular injury, environment law, environmental quality management, as well as laboratory courses in pulmonary function.

The clinical year includes attendance in the occupational medicine clinic within the university hospital as well as clerkships in the medical departments of regional industries, clerkships in the Emergency Department of the University Hospital and elective clerkships in dermatology, psychiatry, radiology, cardiology, as well as a required clerkship in the Poison Center.

For the physician who may be unable to spend two years in a full-time residency program but who does have occupational medicine responsibility in industry or government agencies, there is available a mini-residency program that includes a two-week intensive short course followed by two weeks of additional short-course work (one week each year over a period of two years). This mini-residency is a most popular continuing education training effort.

Unfortunately, occupational medicine is often practiced by physicians without any special training. In some plants the physician may provide minimal services such as sick call or be available when needed. In many small industries occupational medicine is often practiced by the nurse who sees a problem initially and may offer medication or refer the case to an emergency facility or to a nearby hospital.

Most of the physicians who have been through a full residency program have many career options. They may serve as plant physicians or as plant or corporate medical department administrators. They may serve in a variety of essential capacities in federal and state agencies studying populations at risk, carrying out health hazard evaluations or industrywide studies, or providing occupational medical expertise in regulatory decision making.

OCCUPATIONAL HEALTH AND OCCUPATIONAL STRESS

The primary concern and responsibility of the occupational physician is the prevention of occupational disease and injury. All of the other concerns and responsibilities flow from that objective. The occupational physician should have an in-depth knowledge of the processes and materials used in a plant or industry. He or she is responsible for developing an inventory of these and establishing a surveillance program for those that require monitoring. In this regard the details of processes and use of materials require the professional effort of the industrial hygienist. His or her responsibility is to know and to understand the processes and materials used and their potential hazard. The hygienist's functions are to sample and provide analyses of chemicals used and identify and quantify physical agents, to become familiar with the hazard potential and make recommendations regarding reduction or elimination of the hazardous exposures. The hygienists or safety professionals in a plant should be knowledgeable about the physical factors such as thermal stresses (high and low temperature), nonionizing and ionizing radiation, and vibration to which workers are exposed. They should be knowledgeable about lifting heavy loads, the inappropriate uses or improper design of tools that lead to fatigue and physical injury.

One can classify stress factors into the following groups: (1) The physical, chemical, and possible biologic factors; and (2) psychosocial and socioeconomic factors. The worker may become fatigued, injured, or distressed by the type of physical activity in which he or she is engaged. The chemical agents may induce symptoms of intoxication or the biologic agents may affect workers, as in agricultural pursuits. The worker may become fearful of such potential adverse reactions. The adverse physical reactions often can be enhanced or increased by emotional and social factors. The length of shift, excessive overtime, and nightshift work may all contribute to the worker's weariness and dissatisfaction.

Among the psychosocial stresses are discrepancy between the job demands and its opportunities and the worker's capacities, expectations, and personal needs. The effects of these stresses may be behavioral, leading to abuses of alcohol or drugs or excessive smoking, or may be manifest as medical complaints such as nervousness, irritability, sleep disorders, or disturbed organ functions such as skin complaints (itching and scratching) gastrointestinal, cardiovascular, and pulmonary complaints as well as eating disorders.

There is sufficient information to recognize that long continued stresses may be associated with hypertension, peptic ulcer, colitis, as well as psychiatric disorders. The observant occupational physician should be in a position to assess the ecologic and psychosocial stresses. He or she is in a position to stimulate management to provide more satisfactory physical or social environments or mitigate the effects of stressful tasks. Change of job assignment or the rotation of jobs can be recommended.

Studies have been carried out on the ergonomic factors that lead to a physical distress and injury in specific industries. These have led to a number of modifications of tool design or processes. There have also been a number of studies of groups of employees who have had behavioral manifestations of work stress.

There is a recent report on the excess days lost at a Ford Motor Company plant as an index for identifying jobs with ergonomic stress (Anderson et al., 1985). The report also describes methods of identifying problem jobs based on risk rate measures and excess risk measures.

The occupational physician is keenly aware of the stress factors that lead to medical complaints and in many instances the ascribing of disability.

CONCLUSION

Occupational medicine requires the expertise of and depends upon the resources of psychiatry, clinical psychologists, and professionals in the behavioral sciences and counseling to assist in developing remedies for the psychosocial stresses and their clinical manifestations.

This presentation has provided a broad overview of the objectives and functions of occupational medicine, of the physicians who work in the field, as well as the critical nature of the team effort to determine the nature and level of ecologic stress factors in the workplace. It has described the occupational physician's role in initiating diagnostic and therapeutic strategies to cope with the psychosocial and organizational stressors.

REFERENCES

Anderson, C. K., Fine, L. J. Herrin, G. D., and Sugano, D. S. 1985. Excess days lost as an index for identifying jobs with ergonomic stress. *Journal of Occupational Medicine*, 27(10): 740–744.

Kehoe, R. A. 1946. Medical education, research and practice in relation to industrial health. *The Medical Press and Circular*, 225: 5567.

Ross, W. D. 1956. *Practical Psychiatry for Industrial Physicians*. Springfield, Ill.: Charles Thomas.

Suskind, R. R. 1977. Perspectives in education: Occupational medicine graduate training. *Journal of Occupational Medicine*, 19(3): 211–214.

22 Private psychiatric hospitals and work stress therapeutic interventions

John C. Wolfe and Thomas Robischon

Stress management's successful track record and its promising results for productivity have been recognized by business and industry (Goldbeck, 1982). In fact, the need for such programs is said to be as great as the need for chemical dependency programs (Hurst, 1985). Private psychiatric hospitals (PPHs) have been portrayed as being "in the ideal position to respond with innovative programs" (McDonald, 1982); and services dealing with stress reactions and other mental health issues in work organizations have been called a PPH marketing opportunity (Hurst, 1985).

However, a recent survey conducted by one of the authors found that the number of PPHs with occupational psychiatry programs reflects neither the kind of growth that has occurred in this division of psychiatry nor the "increasingly significant" role of the psychiatrist in the workplace ("Report of the Task Force . . .," 1984 [hereafter "Report," 1984]). The survey was based on interviews with six administrators of hospital-related occupational psychiatric programs, three of them administrator-physicians, and an industrial health care planning expert. The seven PPHs and one private general hospital covered in this survey were the only ones found to be involved in some form of occupational psychiatry after a Medlars II literature search and inquiries with the National Association of Private Psychiatric Hospitals and the American Psychiatric Association's (APA) Task Force on Psychiatry and Industry.

Only one of the PPHs operates a program as part of its regular psychiatric services. Two other programs were originally divisions within PPHs but are now separate corporate entities, and one educational program with a strong occupational psychiatric component is an "educational companion" separate from a PPH. Three additional PPHs are developing programs as part of a series of "special symptom programs," but they are also separate from the PPHs. Only one hospital-related program was found to have an explicit workplace stress orientation, but it is part of the psychiatric department of a private general hospital.

The 1984 report of the APA's Task Force on Psychiatry and Industry called on psychiatrists to become involved in occupational psychiatry and declared that the failure to do so would mean an equal risk to psychiatry and to the business world. There was no mention in the report, however, of the role of PPHs ("Report," 1984).

A special issue of *The Psychiatric Hospital* devoted to psychiatry and industry referred to workplace stress and described three PPH-related occupational psychiatric programs; however, the role of the PPH in providing services for dealing with workplace stress was not addressed (Brody, 1982).

Only one other piece of literature on occupational stress and hospital psychiatry exists. It reported on a study that measured and ranked the potential of 61 sources of stress among psychiatrists in Saint Elizabeth's Hospital in Washington, D.C. (Dawkins, Depp, and Selzer, 1984).

This chapter will examine the seven PPHs and one private general hospital that have programs in occupational psychiatry. It will discuss three issues directly related to PPH involvement in such programs: the mission of the PPH, alternative views of the nature of stress and its connection with the workplace, and the role of the PPH in dealing with it. Finally, the chapter will explore several issues surrounding marketing of therapeutic interventions in this area, with special reference to the PPH.

THE PROGRAMS

St. Joseph Stress Management Center (Wichita, Kansas) is the only hospital-related program found in the survey with an explicit orientation to workplace stress. It is also part of the psychiatric department of a private general hospital.

In addition to a standard day hospital for follow-up and transitional care and an evening hospital for working people, St. Joseph offers services to people who are reluctant to come in as psychiatric patients but want to deal with tension, stress, or other personal problems. The year-and-a-half-old center is staffed by two full-time specially trained RNs and a part-time community liaison RN who works with industrial nurses (Porter, 1985).

St. Joseph found that while they are prepared to go to the workplace to help individuals with stress and other problems, people seem to prefer to come to the center. Many patients discover that St. Joseph's staff are "okay and not monsters." Patients reportedly are amazed to see staff members become sensitive to self-defeating patterns in a person's life, and they decide to do something about it. This has led to the utilization of more corrective services; however, St. Joseph's basic contract is to teach stress reduction and relaxation techniques, both as individual and as group efforts. A stress telephone line is also widely advertised in the community, and the services of a consultative stress team are also available for patients of hospital physicians. Programs on stress are presented at the workplace upon request.

The inpatient component of the St. Joseph center is a ten-bed stress management day unit with two nurses, a clinical director, and a part-time social worker. Although it is not officially called such, it resembles a psychosomatic unit. The staff differs from the rest of the hospital staff and is grafted on to what was an underutilized, standard open psychiatric unit in another section of the building. Only one shift of special services is provided, with the evening and night nurses coming from the regular psychiatric ward.

Thus the inpatient component is "completely different and separate" from the psychiatric unit, with the program running through the waking day, six days a week, and reverting to regular psychiatry in the evening and night. All patients must have diagnoses, attending physicians, charts, and utilization reviews.

Some patients in the inpatient program are referred from the outpatient clinic. Others are referred by family physicians and internists who are encouraged to co-manage their patients. Those who become therapy patients through the clinic may be on inpatient status, or may have a therapist who will start seeing them in the hospital.

The center's outpatient component is a stress management clinic with 25 to 30 openings for active patients. Census is 18 patients in the evening—their busiest time since so many patients are employed—and 7–8 during the day. Patient census has increased greatly since the initial opening.

South Oaks Hospital (Amityville, New York) does not have a program that specifically addresses stress, believing rather that stress finds expression in a variety of other disorders. This PPH became involved with industry in 1971 by hosting a conference on industrial psychiatric medicine devoted to alcoholism in industry (Carone and Krinsky, 1982). They established an inpatient alcoholism program with separate units for patients who did not see themselves as having psychiatric disorders. Free, outpatient alcoholism clinics and group counseling workshops were later established. Today, more than 300 people attend South Oaks's free weekly clinics and some 500 people utilize its charge clinics each week. Recently, South Oaks opened a 56-bed alcoholism unit (Carone, 1985).

Recognizing that many industrial workers were reluctant to enter the hospital for alcoholic rehabilitation, South Oaks established an Alcoholics-Anonymous–oriented detoxification unit with a stay of five to seven days. As a result of their experience in that unit, some patients were willing to remain for a more extended rehabilitation.

More than 500 people have now been trained by South Oaks in alcoholism treatment, many of them union counselors or representatives, as well as medical directors and executives. As an outgrowth, several other free services for the industrial community were created, including a 24-hour alcoholism hot line, a speaker's bureau, and consultant services. In addition, South Oaks now offers an adolescent program, a residential therapeutic community for drug-abusing adolescents, and a unit for acting-out adolescents with substance abuse problems (Carone and Krinsky, 1982).

Since its first industrial psychiatric medicine conference, South Oaks has invited 250 to 300 representatives each year from the professions, academia, management, labor, and government to two-day conferences devoted to such topics as "The Aging Employee," "Drug Abuse in Industry," "Misfits in Industry," and "Women in Industry." Annual psychiatric conferences for clergymen and other religious workers, including individual conferences for school psychologists and teachers, are also offered (Carone, 1985).

After operating an outpatient program in metabolic disorders, South Oaks recently opened an inpatient program for disorders with psychogenic factors, an outgrowth of its relations with industry and with the general public. "If you develop a sufficient number of outpatient departments, you can cut down the inpatient length of stay and transfer them to the OPD, (Outpatient Department)," explained Dr. Pasquale Carone, South Oaks's recently retired CEO (Carone, 1985).

Industrial workers are apt to look upon a PPH as an alien camp, an institution catering to the very rich where employees would be merely tolerated, at best. Realizing this, South Oaks took special steps to train its staff for this new kind of patient who was unaccustomed to the intensity of care to which psychiatric patients were accustomed. The staff learned that these patients were frightened more than anything else, and that they would demonstrate hostility as a protective mechanism. As a result, South Oaks has been successful in encouraging its staff to accept them more readily (Carone and Krinsky, 1982; Carone, 1985).

More recently, a "tremendous change in the socio-economic level" of South Oaks's patients has been reported. The hospital has discovered that unions have declined in their power and influence, and a concomitant decline has occurred in workers' awareness of their mental health benefits and available services. Management is increasingly more "in the driver's seat," increasingly aware of its benefits payments, and is now dictating its needs to insurance companies (Carone, 1985).

An increased need is still predicted for the PPH among blue-collar workers by South Oaks, but it is not as optimistic as it was two or three years ago. In 1982, South Oaks was operating at full capacity with a waiting list for the first time in its history (Carone and Krinsky, 1982). By mid-1986 it was not full but "working at very high capacity." For South Oaks, the outlook is still "very encouraging" (Carone, 1985).

At *Growth Associates* (Newton, Kansas) formerly a division of Prairie View Hospital (a PPH) staff serve as consultants with business and industry, in organizational behavior issues, such as morale, turnover, conflict, organizational structure, and career counseling. Their work also includes stress management and motivation, but their specialty is working with organizational problems (Raber, 1985).

A staff of four at Growth Associates provides continuing education for health professionals with a wide range of seminars for business and industry. Monthly luncheons for business and industry representatives feature a speaker and discussion that allows Growth Associates "to be in the frontline with business and industry around pertinent problems," its director reports. However, Growth Associates does not try to "make everything they do a psychiatric problem" (Raber, 1985).

Prairie View Hospital is involved in a sheltered workshop, through which the Associates places patients with its contacts in industries.

Lakeside Hospital (Memphis) formerly called Organizational Resources, provides services for the "people problem" areas of industry (Ross, 1982). The approach of this PPH is four-pronged:

- training individuals and groups to address communication problems in their organizations,
- providing psychological testing as an assessment for an EAP, or as a tool for specific employees, including pre-employment screening, career assessment, and career planning,
- providing counseling dealing with employee relations and the stress often associated with a transfer, and
- developing and operating EAPs (Ross, 1982).

Another group, *Charter Medical Corporation,* had started Employee Assistance Services (EAS) patterned after Lakeside's Organizational Resources and invited Lakeside to join forces. Lakeside decided it would be advantageous to devote the two FTEs (full-time equivalents) in its program to other projects with industry within the hospital, and in May 1984 Organizational Resources joined Charter's EAS as a separate sister organization of the hospital (Thornton, 1985).

Even though Lakeside's former administrator once singled out psychiatric hospitals as the first places to which industry could turn for assistance on issues in communication, employee relations, and organization fitness (Ross, 1982), the operation of Lakeside's former program has been turned over to EAS. The decision to move the program was as much a result of Lakeside's desire to redirect those two FTEs as it was financial. The nature of the Organizational Resources program did not lead the hospital to make the move. If EAS had not existed, Lakeside would still have its program (Thornton, 1985).

Lakeside Hospital itself has a coordinator working with business and industry who can draw on the resources of any staff member. This may include educational or training programs for a business that already has an

EAP, or for a small business. In the majority of cases, the service is a free community program, unless it is something unusual or a major project. The number of presentations is described as "very large, though not overwhelming," with approximately ten industries and businesses involved (Thornton, 1985).

EAS and Lakeside Hospital are connected "only loosely" in a relationship that enables the hospital to train supervisors or provide employee educational programs. The hospital might provide a free alcoholism seminar or a seminar on stress for a company with its own EAP. If, however, a company wants a comprehensive program involving a long-term commitment, EAS would handle it. EAS would also be called in if a company with which the hospital is working decides to set up an EAP (Thornton, 1985).

This relationship gives EAS the freedom to refer patients to hospitals other than Lakeside. It has been claimed that some hospitals in the business of setting up EAPs are actually creating service contracts. Lakeside's assistant administrator cited instances where a patient from an industry under contract requests Lakeside but is transferred because the patient is part of a service contract. It may be an unwritten agreement, but "it obviously is there" (Thornton, 1985).

Neither Lakeside nor EAS has ever had service contracts that require all patients to be referred to Lakeside. "While we think we have a quality facility and many of the patients do come here, nothing in our contracts say they have to come to Lakeside" (Thornton, 1985).

Lakeside's administration declines to reveal the exact number of patients the hospital receives from EAS, but said it is "not large ... we get our appropriate share of referrals, we have been very ethical about that." Lakeside believes there are "a lot better ways" to receive referrals without establishing an EAP branch—unless you want to go into the EAP business (Thornton, 1985).

The Education Center of Sheppard Pratt (Baltimore) began implementing its "total EAP concept" in 1979, as a separate entity from the Sheppard Pratt Hospital, with 67 programs designed to provide supervisory training, counseling, intervention, treatment, as well as health promotion through preventive education ("Information for Patient Referral," 1983 [hereafter "Information, 1983"]).

Included in its division of professional and public education is health promotion and education about mental health issues; collaboration in evaluating an organization's policies and procedures for health awareness and employee well-being; training for supervisors to carry out a continuing EAP schedule at the company; referral of troubled employees for individual care at Sheppard or another appropriate agency; and implementation of a cost-effective plan for each company client. Sheppard provides some faculty and staff for their program, but the majority are drawn from outside (Mitchell, 1985).

Today, Sheppard Pratt's education center offers over 300 programs to a projected audience of 12,000, most at the hospital center, under the headings of "Organization," "Managers/Supervisors," and "Self-Development." The latter includes workshops on "Managing Stress and Change," "Managing Stress for Success," and "Self-Hypnosis for Stress Management" ("Information," 1983). The center also offers consulting services, invitational breakfast lectures for employee assistance practitioners, a speaker's bureau, contractual services to business and industry, and free noontime lectures at city hall, the county courthouse, and the inner harbor central business district. It also helps businesses and industries organize their own EAPs ("Information," 1983; Mitchell, 1985).

Sheppard Pratt has set higher goals for the coming year, targeting three key populations: the general public (generalized interpersonal skills such as managing anger, managing stress, how to live with difficult people); business (employee motivation, productivity, creative leadership, for example); and health professionals and human services providers (Mitchell, 1985).

The "total EAP concept" is considered an extension of the hospital's philosophy, a conviction that the modern psychiatric center should, in the words of its president, Dr. Robert W. Gibson, "assume a leadership role in preventive education for all sectors of our society—for business communities, for organizations, for individuals—since a major answer for conquering mental illness *is* prevention" (quoted in Scherr and Tainter, 1982). The workplace is viewed as the most accessible place to intervene because "it is a potential source of anxiety and stress." It is also here that managers can "identify and influence the troubled employee at an early, constructive stage." When managers see the correlation between employee mental health and company well-being, they can be "more effective in improving the workplace" ("Information," 1983).

Vista Hill Foundation (San Diego) only recently began moving its two PPHs in the San Diego area—Mesa Vista, Vista Hill (and Vista Sandia in Albuquerque)—into day and evening chemical dependency programs. At last report, it had not yet moved into stress clinics, sleeping and eating disorder clinics, pain clinics, or other parts of what its vice-president of clinical programs termed "an endless range of special symptom programs." These would not, however, be hospital-based because hospitalized patients would not be involved (Moore, 1985).

Vista Hill has developed a five-tier plan for each of its PPHs that would include a residential treatment center for adults or children, a day hospital, a therapeutic group home (or board and care), and more organized outpatient care. The PPH would act as a hub for and administer the services.

The five-tier plan reflects a view of the "hospital of the future" that Vista Hill's Dr. Robert Moore has described (though he does not take original credit for it): an intensive care unit surrounded by clinics, general hospitals, or psychiatric hospitals. One of these clinics could serve as a stress clinic, or a clinic for patients with severe anxiety (Moore, 1984, 1985). Moore said he is not certain how to differentiate stress reaction from anxiety because they tend to run together. These units would be physically independent or freestanding because they would not have to be in the hospital.

PHILOSOPHICAL ISSUES

Twenty years ago, no one could anticipate the drastic changes in national health care policies, serious socioeconomic changes, inability of community mental health centers to fulfill their mission, the rise of private insurance coverage, the increase in the numbers of psychiatric units in general hospitals and of PPHs (including growth of the investor-owned chains), and new diagnostic techniques (Robbins, 1983). As new patterns of care have emerged, there has been a tendency for PPHs to rationalize them as better "on a scientific or clinical basis when in reality they have been responses to socio-economic and political pressures, prejudices,or idealistic wishes" (Robbins, 1983).

As PPHs respond to the needs of an increasing number of patients, and provide a wider range of services with less funding, improvement in psychiatric treatment, in or out of hospital, cannot be achieved by administrative arranging and rearranging. For Dr. Lewis Robbins, psychiatrist-in-chief emeritus of Long Island Jewish-Hillside Medical Center, improvement in patient care will come "basically from research into the causes and treatment of psychiatric illnesses, the innovative application of new knowledge and the evaluation of outcomes" (Robbins, 1983).

PPHs also will have to face the question of their identity. "Where does a PPH stop and something else begin?" asks Vista Hill's Moore. Why should treatment of stress reactions and other occupational mental health issues be taken as the wave of the future for PPHs? "It's not exactly a hospital role," he points out; "more perhaps for the governing body, the ownership, or the corporation" (Moore, 1985).

With only one PPH (South Oaks) now offering a program of occupational psychiatry as part of its regular services, and the remaining programs associated with a PPH only as separate corporate entities (Prairie View's Growth Associates, Charter Medical's EAS, Sheppard Pratt's Education Center, and Vista Hill's plans for its PPHs), occupational psychiatry would not appear to be the wave of the future for PPHs.

What, then, is the mission of the PPH? Traditionally, it has been to provide psychiatric hospital care. However, many such as those at Vista Hill now see that as obsolete. A PPHs mission now is to provide "good mental health care at whatever level of intensity it should be provided," and that, Moore admits, could include "all kinds of things" (Moore, 1985). "All kinds of things" would rather accurately describe the few PPH-related programs found in this survey who also have revised their views of their mission.

A PPH is not different from any other hospital that questions its mission as it becomes clear that the bulk of health care in the future is not going to be delivered either in or through hospitals (Goldbeck, 1984). Psychiatric hospitals began deinstitutionalizing some time ago, shifting their care from inpatient to ambulatory, and from institutional to community settings (Romano, 1978). As expected, benefits failed to materialize, however, deinstitutionalizing came under critical scrutiny. One critic has proposed psychiatric hospitals develop a "middle step" to fill the gap between the psychiatric ward and the community (Gould, 1981).

The role a PPH adopts in providing services for occupational stress could turn on how it views stress in the first place. Vista Hill's Moore thinks stress has a "faddism" about it that "bread and butter psychiatry" does not.

Eating disorders, anxiety disorders, phobias, and stress have all existed for years. However, as the biomedical view of mental disorders has received more emphasis, stress has received less emphasis (Moore, 1985).

Growth Associates "makes speeches" about stress, but is not convinced that speeches are helpful. It sees that its involvement with organizational problems may produce more results than just talking about stress. The difference, as it sees it, is the longer-term, closer work with the organization, rather than short-term presentations. It sees its strength in consulting on the issues that people hurt about within an organization, and helping them deal with the stress and the structures that add stress (Raber, 1985).

Contributing to the move to outpatient occupational psychiatric programs seen in the PPHs surveyed is the likelihood that the workplace is not a particularly significant source of problems that require psychiatric hospitalization. Moore, for one, does not think "an awful lot" of patients are in psychiatric hospitals because of a workplace problem. He does not deny that workplaces can be sources of considerable stress to many people, and that changing a workplace can make it less stressful. However, he is not prepared to say it is a significant reason for people to become ill enough to be hospitalized. Also, he does not feel admitting people to psychiatric hospitals will solve any problems in the workplace; any such idea, he advises, "might as well be abandoned" (Moore, 1985).

A view of stress like Moore's contrasts somewhat with the view expressed by Dr. Alan McLean that the external environment is a major factor in determining whether a specific stressor will produce symptoms, even though McLean considers the vulnerability of the individual is a more important factor (McLean, 1982).

The APA's Task Force on Psychiatry and Industry has suggested making the work organization the subject of psychiatric scrutiny, even identifying it as the patient. That includes the possibility that changes in an organization might be recommended by a psychiatrist for the desirable effects they would have on employee behavior ("Report," 1984).

Any individual or institution providing services relating to workplace stress and other mental health issues related to work organization has a responsibility never to use mental health programs to hide workplace dangers (Goldbeck, 1984). The workplace has been given even more of the causal burden for stress—more than a worker's home life—by the Institute for Labor and Mental Health in San Francisco. This group identifies the principal causes of workplace stress as the "many impediments to workers' full use of their skills and cooperative impulses that management erects to maintain its authority over the workforce" (Judis, 1980).

The potential for conflict between the psychiatrist, the PPH, employees, and management has also been noted. Psychiatrists who help in the workplace have been reminded that they must understand they are part of the system, and that they are there to *help* it achieve its purposes. The rules and the organizational hierarchy must be accepted, and psychiatrists must have a defined role. Psychiatrists must also be able to accept decisions that are not in harmony with their recommendations, but continue to monitor them and make recommendations accordingly (McLean, 1984).

Attention to workplace stress can be minimized, or even displaced, in favor of approaches deemed more fruitful, as already noted in the case of Growth Associates. Stress is characterized by the Associates' director as "a kind of theoretical notion" and he points out it is involved in "most any human problem." It is also "the buzz word these days." For him, the reason that more PPHs are not involved with the problem is because "big bucks are not involved in workplace stress" (Raber, 1985).

In sum, there are good philosophical reasons for questioning whether there is a future for PPHs in workplace stress management. The drastic changes in national health care, questions regarding the identity and the mission of the PPH, a growing recognition that stress does not usually require hospitalization or that admitting people to a PPH will change anything in the workplace, and the likelihood that a PPH can have little or no effect on how work is organized—all help explain why stress management programs are not viewed as a significant part of the PPHs market now or for the future. No geographical or other systemic differences were found among the institutions studied that would alter this conclusion.

MARKETING ISSUES

PPHs are going to have to become "very much involved" in motivating industrial workers to seek their help, Pasquale Carone has said. The workplace provides the best place to do that because an illness can be so subtle that the family fails to see it, while people not emotionally affected in the workplace can recognize a worker with a problem (Carone, 1985).

PPHs have to have "a gimmick," Carone has advised, or a specialty program as a drawing card. South Oaks began with alcoholism and now is dealing with cocaine abuse because, Carone explained, "we can appeal to a different economic-social stratum—the white collar worker." Other specialty programs might deal with gambling and posttraumatic neuroses.

People who have been transferred from inpatient to outpatient status after only three or four weeks can be another public relations and marketing potential, Carone has pointed out. When they realize a short stay is possible they will tell other workers. That, combined with regular speaking engagements and meeting with industry leaders on a personal basis has enhanced South Oak's recognition in industry. Carone considered it as much a marketing role as the activities of the hospital's own marketing staff (Carone, 1985).

South Oaks is situated on the border between two Long Island (New York) counties with a total population of 4 million. Industry is thriving and unemployment is lower than the national average. For South Oaks, it is an unusually large market for occupational psychiatry, with a definite percentage of people involved with workplace stress who are going to need inpatient care (Carone, 1985).

A principal reason Growth Associates was made a separate part of the corporate structure was that outside consultants showed them it was a significant marketing tool for their hospital. The work that Growth Associates does away from the hospital has benefited its referral base. As a result, Growth Associates has taken on an increased marketing role as part of its mission, "to make its link with the hospital more explicit" (Raber, 1985).

Although Sheppard Pratt's visibility in the Baltimore area has "increased tremendously" as a result of its education center programs, it has not been used as a marketing tool for the hospital. Occasionally, someone who comes to one of their programs will become a hospital patient, or recommend Sheppard Pratt to others. But there is no firm data on the effects of its extensive program on their hospital admissions (Mitchell, 1985).

St. Joseph Medical Center, on the other hand, uses its stress management center as a public relations tool, "the kind of thing we can go public with and use as the focus of advertising the entire institution" (Porter, 1985). The hospital uses the center as a loss leader in providing less-expensive services to the community. This has given it a competitive edge over other agencies in the community that provide stress management and other mental health services, and those agencies charge that St. Joseph is "undercutting" them.

Competition of another sort resulted when physicians at two other general hospitals in town asked St. Joseph to do stress assessments of their patients. The administrations of the two hospitals reportedly could not find a way to "credential" the St. Joseph people. Garry Porter understands: "They don't want us stealing their patients" (Porter, 1985).

PPHs are going to have to move in this direction because they must spread out their resource base and cannot depend on patient census to provide all their revenues. Since occupational psychiatry is primarily outpatient, PPHs are bound to compete and conflict with other mental health care agencies. For example, Vista Hill was competing with some of its own medical staff who were independently providing such services to the community. Vista Hill is also not interested in competing with clinics that are referral sources (Moore, 1985).

A PPH could move too aggressively into nonhospital programs and ruin its original market. That will depend, however, on the type of community it is in. A PPH could set up an array of special-symptom clinics in one community with little negative reaction while the same program could damage the hospital in another area. As we have noted, although the stress management clinic at St. Joseph operates on an outpatient basis, it is viewed by other mental health agencies in the community as undercutting them. Vista Hill's Moore has cautioned PPHs to think through what they are doing and not move impulsively (Moore, 1985).

PPHs contracting outreach services can expect to encounter the concern among employers about health care costs generally, but particularly costs for psychiatric disorders. The APA's Task Force described psychiatric disorders benefits as "the least concrete and least manageable benefit," representing for many employers "the most rapidly growing cost" ("Report," p. 1140, 1984).

Outpatient psychotherapy could offset other medical care costs, however. Mumford et al. (1984) feel their findings argue "specifically for the likelihood that mental health treatment may improve patients' ability to stay healthy enough to avoid hospital admission for physical illness." The effects they found were largely in the reduction of inpatient rather than outpatient costs, and in older rather than younger patients.

Occupational psychiatric programs, including EAPs, can be a source of PPH admissions, though conclusive data is lacking. A business or industry could become suspicious about a PPH taking hospital admissions from patients utilizing its contract program. In addition to putting caps on the amount they will spend for benefits, business and industry could require that a PPH not take such admissions (Moore, 1985).

A PPH could also end up working against itself if its outreach programs help people avoid hospitalization. The more successful their programs, the less their primary function of providing hospital care will be needed. Facing that kind of dilemma, a PPH might well be expected to change its orientation. It has even been suggested that some hospitals would have to close down so that a corporate ownership could stay in the mental health business. "PPHs have to be ready to do that, and that is very threatening" (Moore, 1985).

What brought psychiatry into schools, industry, and other social systems—and into these kind of conflicts—has been a model of psychiatry that is at the opposite pole from the biomedical view that tends to make psychiatry a small subset of internal medicine (Sabshin, 1981). The "socio-therapeutic" model, as it has been dubbed, with its social etiology and treatments, has broadened the boundaries of psychiatry, and has increased conflicts with other mental health agencies and disciplines (Sabshin, 1981).

An increased adversarial relationship between psychiatrists and medical doctors has been predicted if dollars must be taken from the medical providers to pay for new mental health benefits (Goldbeck, 1984). The same could be said about PPHs and general hospitals. If increased mental health care also leads to reduced need for medical services, then medical professionals might not be expected to support psychiatric benefits.

Affiliation with a corporate organization could conceivably mean higher costs for outreach programs of PPHs. When Vista Hill met with county officials about its plans to purchase a small company that operated transitional living centers with many county-supported patients, the first question raised by the officials was whether Vista Hill would pass on its administrative overhead to that operation and thus increase the cost to the county (Moore, 1985).

Even if a hospital were to decide not to require such an operation to pay administrative costs because it is not a break-even operation, Medicare auditors would disallow all costs not associated with the hospital. This could mean being left with unbillable administrative costs. "Maybe," mused Dr. Moore, "a mom and pop operation would do the job less expensively" (Moore, 1985).

Reimbursement can be expected to continue to be a question for any program like a PPH outreach program, and it will be there whether the reimbursement is private or public. A wait-and-see attitude has developed, with the knowledge that some belt-tightening is going to have to happen, the degree of which is uncertain (Carone and Krinsky, 1982; Carone, 1985).

When a study of insurance coverage for the inpatient stress management unit at St. Joseph was conducted after eight months of operation, Medicare or Medicaid coverage constituted close to 50 percent of total coverage, with private coverage amounting to 40 percent, and unintentional charity accounting for the remainder. However, in its outpatient stress management clinic, private insurance made up nearly 80 percent of the coverage while Medicare and Medicaid coverage was rare. The reason was *not* because St. Joseph excluded Medicaid patients; it has no particular target population. "Maybe," its director surmised, "Medicaid patients do not want to look at themselves that way" (Porter, 1985).

One caveat for any PPH thinking of establishing an industry outreach program: The staff will be working with a different type of patient than to which they are accustomed. These patients are not accustomed to the intensity of care that other psychiatric hospital patients are. South Oaks had to build staff commitment gradually to working with these new patients who came in frightened and displayed hostility as a protective mechanism. Some of these patients originally thought they could not afford PPH because it was private, and didn't realize that their insurance would reimburse the majority of the costs.

Two other problems relating to insurance have been indicated. Insurance companies are increasingly using professional or peer review organizations to determine whether a patient should be admitted and what the length of stay should be. For South Oaks, this has raised a problem of confidentiality (Carone and Krinsky, 1982), as it has for other PPHs who have occupational psychiatric programs. From the beginning, such programs, involving as they do nonhospital, nonmedical people, have had this problem (Carone and Krinsky, 1982), and it can be expected to continue.

Also, industrial workers are still unlikely to understand their employer insurance coverage completely. Attorneys are now encouraging employees to bring lawsuits against their insurance companies to secure appropriate benefits (Carone, 1985).

THE FUTURE

The present role of PPHs in stress programs is less than we thought existed, and it portends to be even less in the future. It appears that work stress, in and of itself, is treated in less-intensive settings than a PPH. A number of interventions seem to obviate the need for hospitalization into a PPH where intensive psychosocial treatment is provided. For example, EAPs that refer troubled employees to a variety of treatment settings seem to utilize the outpatient setting appropriately for the majority of their referrals. We also believe that a "commonsense" factor is involved; namely, those who are experiencing psychological problems from work stress are not psychiatrically ill to the same degree as are people for whom hospitalization is required. In short, those suffering from work stress are for the most part functional. They are hurting but are not debilitated.

From the industry side, stress management programs have been viewed as a marketing opportunity for PPHs. Dealing with stress was one of the most popular programs for Caterpillar Tractor's employees nationwide. Their former manager of health care planning, Ronald Hurst, has called it "the cutting edge of the new wave," and reinforced what we said above by pointing out that the day of the hospital " is behind us." The new concept, however, is alternatives to hospitalization, and if PPHs continue to think about filling beds, as Hurst declared, they may not see a place for themselves in this new era. "There are many ways of providing revenue other than putting people in a bed" (Hurst, 1985).

Seeking help from a PPH for a problem that is induced by workplace stress is probably not appropriate; rather, alternatives should be sought because the probability is quite high that the individual is not ill enough to warrant hospitalization. As the survey completed for this study strongly suggests, the PPHs themselves are not convinced that they are the ones to provide the help.

REFERENCES

Brody, L. S. ed. 1982. Perspectives on industrial and occupational psychiatry. *The Psychiatric Hospital,* 13(3): 73–76.

Carone, P. A. 1985. Personal communication, May 8, 1985.

Carone, P. A. and Krinsky, L. W. 1982. A program geared specifically to industry by the private psychiatric hospital. *The Psychiatric Hospital,* 13: 84–87.

Dawkins, J., Depp, F. C. and Selzer, N. 1984. Occupational stress in a public mental hospital: The psychiatrist's view. *Hospital and Community Psychiatry,* 35(1): 56–60.

Goldbeck, W.B. 1982. Psychiatry and industry: A business view. *The Psychiatric Hospital,* 13: 95–98.

———. 1984. Conference on psychiatry and business. Torrance, Calif. Videotape.

Gould, M. A. 1981. The effects of societal and legislative pressures on inpatient treatment. *Journal of National Association of Private Psychiatric Hospitals,* 12(1). 0–10.

Hurst, R. 1985. Personal communication, May 9, 1985.

"Information for Patient Referral." 1983. The Sheppard & Enock Pratt Hospital. Baltimore.

Judis, J. 1980. How therapy treats workplace stress. *In These Times,* 4(27): 2.

McDonald, M. C. 1982. Psychiatry and industry: Why is collaboration important? *The Psychiatric Hospital,* 13: 70–71.

McLean, A. A. 1982. Improving mental health at work. *The Psychiatric Hospital,* 13: 77–83.

———. 1984. Conference on Psychiatry and Business. Torrance, Calif. Videotape.

Mitchell, P. 1985. Personal communication, June 11, 1985.

Moore, R. 1984. Conference on Psychiatry and Business. Torrance, Calif. Videotape.

———. 1985. Personal communication, March 29, 1985.

Mumford, E., Schlesinger, H. J., Glass, G. V., Patrick C., and Cuerdon, T. 1984. New look at evidence about reduced cost of medical utilization following mental health treatment. *The American Journal of Psychiatry,* 141: 1145-1158.

Porter, G. 1985. Personal communication, May 22, 1985.

Raber, M. 1985. Personal communication, May 15, 1985.

"Report of the Task Force on Psychiatry and Industry." 1984. *The American Journal of Psychiatry,* 141: 1139-1144.

Robbins, L. L. 1983. The private psychiatric hospital: The impact of current trends. *The Psychiatric Hospital,* 14: 13-16.

Romano, J. 1978. Temples, asylums–hospitals? *Journals of National Association of Private Psychiatric Hospitals,* 9(4): 4-12.

Ross, E. A. 1982. Working with industry, a challenge to psychiatry. *The Psychiatric Hospital,* 13: 99-101.

Sabshin, M. 1981. Toward strategic planning for psychiatry in the 1980s. *Journal of National Association of Private Psychiatric Hospitals,* 12: 113-118.

Scherr, M. L. and Tainter, P. M. 1982. Health promotion in the workplace: The Sheppard experience. *The Psychiatric Hospital,* 13: 92-94.

Thornton, S. 1985. Personal communication, May 10 and June 20, 1985.

V   Summary

23 *Work organizations and health care: future directions*

Rabi S. Bhagat, James C. Quick, Jonathan D. Quick, and James E. Dalton, Jr.

Imagine the dawn of human history, and Homo sapiens are stepping out from their caves to watch the rising sun. Suddenly, one of them hears a rustling in the forest. A young Homo sapiens who had earlier drifted out of the cave is about to be attacked by a saber-toothed tiger. The older Homo sapiens's muscles tense, his heart pounds, his breath comes rapidly as he sharply eyes the tiger's movement in order to determine his immediate response. How to save the child? He reaches down, picks up a sharp rock, and hurls it at the animal. The tiger snarls but disappears into the forest and the child is rescued without any apparent harm. The man feels his body go limp, his breathing beginning to ease. He returns to his cave with the child.

Imagine now a modern-day scenario. It is the start of another working day and modern Homo sapiens step out of their homes to catch the rush-hour traffic on crowded expressways going downtown to work. One of them runs into a minor car accident and is three hours late in reporting for his work. There is an important sales meeting today that could determine the fate of his department's financial survival. He is the principal architect and the organizer of the sales meeting. Three hours late for work, he opens the conference room door to find everyone gone and the sales meeting postponed indefinitely into the future. The man feels his body go limp and his stomach churning. He sits down and experiences a sudden yearning for a scotch on the rocks.

The saber-toothed tiger is long gone in the evolution of human history but our modern jungle is no less perilous and stressful. The sense of panic over a missed sales meeting, a tight plane connection, reorganizational pressures during budget cuts and economic downturns—these are the new "tigers" of the modern world with which the modern Homo sapiens must somehow cope. These episodes can set the heart pounding, make muscles tense, and cause sweat to stream. These responses may have served our ancestors well, and they serve us as well in getting our attention focused and nerves ready for a sudden "fight or flight response" (often called the experience of distress). Stress has become an important part of our modern vocabulary and over the past 30 years, physicians and health officials have come to realize the dysfunctional effects of stress on the nation's state of health.

According to the American Academy of Family Physicians, two-thirds of office visits to family doctors are promoted by stress-related symptoms. The substantial increase in medical care expenditures in the United States from $26.9 billion in 1970 (5.3 percent of the GNP) to $234.4 billion in 1980 (9.4 percent of the GNP) and over $462.4 billion in 1985 (9.9 percent of the GNP) has generated considerable alarm in the various professions related to health care delivery systems. Our purpose in organizing the conference from which this book evolved, as has already been stated in Chapter 1, is to identify some systematic programs for long-range issues in research on work stress and its prevention by various available strategies. In Chapter 1, we presented a conceptual framework behind our organization of the three-day conference. In this penultimate chapter, our intent is to specify some of the future directions in research and prevention of work stress in today's organizations.

FUTURE DIRECTION 1: FOSTERING GREATER INTERDISCIPLINARY FRAMEWORKS

The need for developing interdisciplinary frameworks is rather urgent. In the past we have seen relatively little in the way of developing interdisciplinary frameworks to grapple with the complexity of stress-related phenomena in today's work organizations. Dominant traditions of social psychological research on work stress and cognition in organizations seem to rely exclusively on psychological measures and ignore the significance of contributions from biomedical sciences. In a similar vein, research on medical and clinical sciences has largely ignored important advances made in the domain of social psychological approaches to work stress and its prevention. We find such a state of affairs to be problematic in developing important findings in the field. Consider the stressful effects of budget cuts in organizations. The consequences of the cuts are best understood by a team of investigators that includes economists, health psychologists, organizational researchers, and medical specialists, as well as labor relations experts. A multidisciplinary research team would considerably aid in the identification of important sources of variance that are presently being given unidisciplinary and incomplete interpretations. There have been some important developments that encourage our belief that it would be possible to rely on more interdisciplinary frameworks in the future. A new interdisciplinary journal called *Quality of Life and Cardiovascular Care* has been launched; it grew out of a workshop organized by the National Heart, Lung and Blood Institute. The division of health psychology of the American Psychological Association and the division of medical sociology of the American Sociological Association foster development of interdisciplinary frameworks in further understanding the effects of work stress on psychological, adaptational, and health-related outcomes. As editors of this volume, we would like to see this trend become even stronger in the future.

FUTURE DIRECTION 2: TOWARD A BETTER UNDERSTANDING OF ORGANIZATIONAL CULTURE AND CHANGE-RELATED PROCESSES

As Robert Kahn notes in Chapter 24, perhaps the most effective strategy in terms of sustaining a long-term perspective in the prevention of stress is to encourage work organizations to change aspects of their environments that are inherently stressful. Literature reviewed by Murphy (1984) indicates that while worksite-based stress management programs are feasible in reducing physiological arousal levels and psychological manifestations of stress, the long-term effectiveness of such training programs is of questionable value. He noted that, despite some benefits to the employees, it is perhaps not wise to recommend these programs for all types of organizations. A major disadvantage of worksite stress management programs is that they are not often designed to eliminate the sources of stress at work, but only teach workers more effective coping strategies. Ganster et al., (1982) have described this as an "inoculation approach" and discuss the limited usefulness of such an approach. The point is simple: stress management programs that increase the individual's coping skills in the short term without necessarily being able to effect changes in the objective stressors in the employee's work and organizational environment are not particularly useful. There are some definite benefits in implementing therapeutic approaches in the management of stressful reactions in one's work environment. But we stand to gain a lot more leverage in eliminating harmful effects of work stress on employee health by focusing on those aspects of the work environment that are potentially located in the culture of how an organization is managed in the context of its own task and technological environment. We believe that the knowledge base on work and organizational stress is reasonably sufficient at this point of our theory development to initiate some long-term intervention programs designed to focus on changing permanently the noxious aspects of organizational stressors. Poor ergonomic conditions, heavy work load, shift work, and continuous changes in the organization's technology do affect health outcomes both directly and indirectly (Cooper and Payne, 1978, 1980; Quick and Quick, 1984). In addition, it is also known that these stressful factors become even more detrimental in the presence of stressful life events in the personal lives of the employees (Bhagat et al., 1985). Therefore, organizational techniques to bring about some permanent desired solutions in the management of stress and stressful reactions should include both preventive (those that focus on organization-wide changes) and therapeutic (those that focus on improvement of counseling and clinical systems) approaches. Chapters in this volume have clearly articulated this message and we need to reemphasize the need for this kind of combined approach in the management of stress and related health care services. In this connection, we would also like to underscore the importance of "policy vacuums" existing in organizations, which may account for a key reason why well designed programs, based on sound research findings, do not often have discernible influence on administrative practice. Policy vacuums are said to exist when a condition characterized by the absence of the following exists (Corwin and Louis, 1982):

1. An *organized* constituency of policy makers to whom research is directed.
2. Agreement among significant constituents and dominant coalitions on clear policy issues and identifiable research questions that need to be addressed.
3. Consistent policies pertaining to utilization of research findings in several areas of applications.
4. Coordination among independent agencies responsible for developing policies in various areas.
5. Concrete ongoing operational programs targeted to use research findings in the development of various programs.

Corwin and Louis (1982) note that these conditions are often overlapping in varying degrees. The notion of a policy vacuum is a particularly important one when we consider the state of utilization of research findings in the area of work stress and its prevention. As we have already mentioned, there exist important findings (as the chapters in this book would underscore) that could indeed be of considerable significance in improving the adverse impact of stress on health. We believe that important policy issues that need to be formulated are either not attended to or are attended to by the wrong person (that is, someone who might have the least inclination to formulate such policies). Issues that need to be translated into programs often fail to make it on to important agendas. We find that absence of clear-cut guidelines and procedures pertaining to evaluation of research findings makes it exceedingly difficult for the findings to be readily implemented into policies that do indeed matter. One gets the clear impression that managers who are most in need of useful information on work stress and its possible effects on employee health *do not readily want the information* that they almost ritualistically commission (Downs, 1965; Knorr, 1977).

Based on our careful assessment of the gap in the status of knowledge in the field of stress and health and its applied significance, we believe that the following conditions currently affect their use.

1. Researchers on organizational stress often do not have adequate understanding of the different mixes of organizational culture and policy vacuums that currently exist in contemporary work organizations. While they sincerely believe that their research findings would be actively sought after and implemented, such a desired state of affairs often does not exist.

2. The politics of organizational interventions (Pettigrew, 1982) are often not appropriately understood by either the researchers who create important research-based findings or the managers of work units who are supposed to be rather eager in their propensities to seek and implement such findings.

3. There is often a gap between knowledge that results from the application of rigorous theoretical frameworks to important research issues and the knowledge that might truly be needed (even though either the researcher or the practitioner might not be fully aware of what is needed) in the specific situational context of a client organization.

Unless genuine involvement on the part of ultimate users of such knowledge of work stress and health is either present or created through various persuasive meetings, chances are that the above conditions would prevent effective utilization of the findings of a book such as this one. Hakel et al., (1982) note that research with implementation in mind requires a very different orientation on the part of the organizational researcher compared to research where such objectives are not of crucial importance. One has to examine the motivation of the client system, the research subjects, and the senior administrators to provide valid data and to act on the conclusions of a programmatic research process. Perceived relevance of the research questions and instruments is sometimes as important and may even be more important than "scientific rigor." The observation that researchers and users belong to separate communities with different values and ideologies and that these differences impede utilization has been noted by several authors (Bhagat and Dutta, 1985; Dunnette and Brown, 1960, Duncan, 1974; Dunn, 1980; Serpa, 1983). Some writers on the utilization process (Archibald, 1970; Van de Vall, Bolas, and Kang, 1976) even suggest that such cultural gaps become most crucial and difficult to manage when the research is launched primarily by the academics.

At any rate, we urge researchers to attempt to understand and deal effectively with such issues pertaining to different mixes of organizational culture and policy vacuums existing in contemporary organizations. In this connection, it might be useful to employ some of the strategies as recommended by Kotter and Schlesinger (1979) in dealing with issues concerning "policy vacuums" and resistance to change and innovation.

1. First, there is the strategy of education and effective communication. Information on how various competing companies in the industry and in the community have either improved or are attempting to improve productivity by imple-

menting effective programs relating to management of stress and promotion of health in the workplace would be effective in bringing about the necessary changes. A recent book entitled *Health Promotion in the Workplace*, edited by O'Donnell and Ainsworth (1984), would be helpful in this regard. Edited by a director of health promotion services (O'Donnell) and a physician (Ainsworth), it relates various case histories of contemporary organizations that have succeeded in improving productivity and reducing dysfunctional effects of work stress. They describe assessment techniques for various types of health and fitness programs such as improvement of nutrition and diet, cessation of smoking and substance and alcohol abuse, and so on. There are examples of multimodal (psychological and medical) services and how company physicians and nursing staff might work and effectively communicate with researchers and consultants in the health promotion area. They also present strategies for integrating such programs into the overall structure of the organization. We believe that well-designed educational seminars also aid important key decision makers in removing inaccurate perceptions and in understanding the nature of ultimate benefits of such programs in terms of costs and benefits to the organization.

2. Participation and involvement of the employees who will benefit from such programs is the second strategy that we would recommend in the design and implementation of various health care systems in the workplace. It is important that individuals who would be eventual users of the programs participate in their design from the initial stages. In the implementation of management information systems, for example, managers are more likely to use the new system if they have some significant inputs (King and Rodriguez, 1981). It is needless to emphasize that this is a very important method for dealing with resistance to change as well as for uncovering some of the untested assumptions and symbolic significance of such programs in the context of today's organizations.

3. Finally there is the strategy of negotiation, consensus-building, and cooperation among key decision makers. Admittedly, this is a somewhat difficult process and university-based researchers may not be fully aware of the cultural forces at play in order to be able to employ this strategy effectively. Generally, these strategies are covert in nature and require that program planners attempt to win over the key individuals to smooth the implementation process without a great deal of confusion and resistance. We believe that as more collaborative projects are jointly undertaken by industry, university, and governmental officials, some elements of this strategy would naturally come to be implemented.

FUTURE DIRECTION 3: TOWARD A MORE DYNAMIC VIEW OF STRESS AND ADAPTATION

In the process of reviewing the programmatic themes of the chapters in this book, it became clear that researchers and practitioners alike adopt a relatively dynamic view of stress and adaptation in the workplace. Lazarus and DeLongis (1983) and Lazarus and Folkman (1984) encourage us to take precisely this stance. Different work environments clearly impose different adaptational demands; for example, the employees of a growth-oriented, successful, and well-managed work organization will obviously expend much less effort in coping with stress than those of an organization in the oil and gas industry facing severe economic downturns owing to sharp falls in oil and gas prices, as is the case in today's energy industry in Texas. Lazarus and his associates have long emphasized that processes of adaptation are best understood in a longitudinal framework—one that explicitly takes into account the transactional nature of encounters between the person and his or her immediate and distal environment—whether it is real or symbolic. Lazarus and Folkman (1984: 220) state that

few would argue that individual variations in personality, psychodynamics and behavior are fully encompassed within a view of society as an adaptation to natural environment. The overarching problem is how best to understand the relationships between the individual and society and the disturbances of that relationship that fall under the heading of stress.

They recommend the use of a paradigm that explicitly recognizes society as a shaper of the person and the groups in which the person is immersed. As societal values and structures change and force individuals into adaptational modes, society too undergoes some important changes in response to the collective version of such adaptational efforts originating with the individual. Therefore, whether the environment of an individual is merely the specific context of a stressful encounter such as pressure to learn a new type of video terminal on the job or organize layoff meetings during times of economic downturn, the transactions that characterize such processes are necessarily dynamic in scope. Although biological evolution is a slow process, social evolution or change has become rather rapid in modern times and the sources of stress are continuously shifting. Thus, if we incorporate Lazarus and his colleagues' suggestion in our research design, we necessarily need to view stress as a struggle between opposing forces—that is, demands that are always to some degree countered by effectiveness of coping and adaption-related mechanisms. The work stress created by excessive role overloads and conflicts, underutilization of one's skills and abilities, economic difficulties and budget cuts, adoption of new technological systems, and so on are ultimately embedded in the context of a society that is always undergoing important changes. Social and organizational changes often produce loss of anchors and identities on which individuals might have depended in the past, thereby creating a sense of powerlessness and inertia in being able to manage or control events that induce learned helplessness (Abramson, Seligman and Teasdale, 1978).

What is needed, then, is a perspective that attempts to analyze the dynamics of stress and coping with the changing circumstances of living in the employees' work and nonwork "domains." Theoretical frameworks that obscure these ubiquitous effects are therefore necessarily limiting in scope by design and cannot yield useful information. The main gap in knowledge, in our view, stems from the absence of systematic research on the process of stress and coping as they relate to the dynamic events that occur in organizational settings. When one chooses to observe the phenomena of stress and coping at an arbitrary point in time in the life course of an organization, the data that are gathered reveal a snapshot or a relatively static view of affairs in that organization's adaptational efforts. If one fails to examine relevant processes at several other points in time, one loses the sense of continuity and readjustments that are necessary for a dynamic view of the effects of work stress and psychological, behavioral and health-related outcomes. For example, consider changes in institutionalized patterns of work, observed among physicians (Sarason, 1977; Thomas, 1983), which can result in profound and long-term dissatisfaction with one's professional role. For a complete understanding of the factors that induce such dissatisfaction, one has to adopt a long-term perspective that incorporates the influences of both objective environmental events (real changes in the profession of medicine, in health claim payments) and subjective appraisal related processes (how one feels about them in terms of one's role). Almost all kinds of research on effectiveness of worksite programs that include hypertension screening and treatment, smoking cessation, weight loss, training for coping with technological changes, and so forth, are best conducted with a dynamic view of the organization and the individual. It is only then that we stand to gain fresher insights to further enhance their effectiveness.

FUTURE DIRECTION 4: FOSTERING A COLLABORATIVE STRATEGY AMONG MAJOR CONSTITUENTS

A collaborative strategy is different in scope from that of an interdisciplinary orientation (future direction 1). Here we emphasize the need for creating a synergy among academic researchers, practitioners, labor union leaders, industrial relations experts, and policy makers at various government agencies. The role of organizational research on work stress and health care is rapidly increasing and work in this area promises to expand further as we learn more about various mechanisms of behavioral and organizational influences on health-related outcomes. However, there exist some persistent dilemmas on how to effect changes at the individual level that motivate learning of healthy behaviors and at the organizational level that would sustain such gains in learning. Research on cessation of smoking, for example, depicts that by focusing on the effects and risks of smoking one often loses sight of the behavioral effects of cessation rates on individuals. A large percentage of ex-smokers eventually start smoking again as a result of the experience of irritability, sleep disturbances, inability to concentrate, and lack of other behavioral alternatives to smoking at home or at one's place of work. A collaborative team that includes researchers who focus on causes and consequences of smoking on health, concerned managers of work organizations, and perhaps the Surgeon General's office might be more effective in devising ways to better understand and, it is hoped, prevent the occurrence of this addictive behavior. Recent advances in biobehavioral research on common mechanisms and treatment of substance abuse (Shiffman and Willis, 1985) also lead us to emphasize that a closer collaborative relationship among various interested constitutents would be an important step in prevention of such abuse.

Research on work stress and its prevention provide an important interface for the concerns and interests of researchers, practitioners, and government agencies. We hope that with increased collaborative endeavors, we would be able to control much of the adverse impacts of work stress on employees and promote health care concerns in the workplace. To the extent the themes articulated in this volume along with this chapter and Kahn's concluding chapter help accomplish this goal, we would consider our efforts worthwhile. It is also our hope that the future Homo sapiens would be relatively freer from the threatening "tigers" of the modern world as a result of such synergistic collaboration among interested constituents.

REFERENCES

Abramson, L. Y., Seligman, M. E. P., and Teasdale, J. D. 1978. Learned helplessness in humans: critique and reformulation. *Journal of Abnormal Psychology*, 87: 49–74.

Archibald, K. A. 1970. Alternative orientations to social science utilization. *Social Science Information*, 9: 7–34.

Bhagat, R. S. and Beehr, T. A. 1985. Utilization and diffusion of knowledge on human stress and cognition in organizations: Constraints and perspectives. In Beehr, T. A. and Bhagat, R. S. (Eds.). *Human Stress and Cognition in Organizations: An Integrated Perspective*. New York: Wiley Interscience.

Bhagat, R. S., McQuaid, S. J., Lindholm, H., and Segovis, J. 1985. Total life stress: A multimethod validation of the construct and its effects on organizational outcomes and employee withdrawal behaviors. *Journal of Applied Psychology*, 70(1): 202–214.

Cooper, C. L. and Payne, R. (Eds.) 1978. *Stress at Work*. New York: John Wiley.

————. (Eds.) 1980. *Current Concerns in Occupational Stress*. New York: John Wiley.

Corwin, R. G. and Louis, K. S. 1982. Organizational barriers to utilization of research. *Administrative Science Quarterly*, 27(4): 623–640.

Downs, A. 1965. Some thoughts on giving people economic advice. *American Behavioral Scientist*, 9: 30–32.

Duncan, W. J. 1974. The researcher and the manager: A comparative view of the need for mutual understanding. *Management Science*, 20: 1157–1163.

Dunn, W. N. 1980. The two-communities metaphor and models of knowledge use. *Knowledge: Creation, Diffusion Utilization*, 1: 515–536.

Dunnette, M.D. and Brown, Z. M. 1968. Behavioral science research and the conduct of business. *Academy of Management Journal*, 11: 177–187.

Ganster, D. C., Mayes, B. T., Sime, W. E., and Tharp, G. D. 1982. Managing organizational stress: A field experiment. *Journal of Applied Psychology*, 67: 533–542.

Hakel, M. D., Sorcher, M., Beer, M., and Moses, J. L. 1982. *Making It Happen: Designing Research with Implementation in Mind*. Beverley Hills, Calif.: Sage Publications.

King, W. R. and Rodriguez, J. I. 1981. Participative design of strategic decision support systems: An empirical assessment. *Management Science*, 27: 717–726.

Knorr, K.D. 1977. Policy makers' use of social science knowledge: Symbolic or instrumental. In Weiss, C. (Ed.). *Using Social Research in Federal Policy Making*: 165–182. Lexington, Mass.: Lexington Books.

Kotter, J. P. and Schlesinger, L. A. 1979. Choosing strategies for change. *Harvard Business Review*, 57: 106–114.

Lazarus, R. S. and DeLongis, A. 1983. Psychological stress and coping in aging. *American Psychologist*, 38: 245–254.

Lazarus, R. S. and Folkman, S. 1984. *Stress, Appraisal and Coping*, New York: Springer.

Murphy, L. R. 1984. Occupational stress management: A review and appraisal. *Journal of Occupational Psychology*, 57: 1–15.

O'Donnell, M. P. and Ainsworth,T. H. (Eds.) 1984. *Health Promotion in the Workplace*. New York: John Wiley.

Pettigrew, A. M. 1982. Towards a political theory of organizational intervention. In Hakel, M. D., Sorcher, M., Beer, M., and Moses, J. L. (Eds.). *Making It Happen: Designing Research with Implementation in Mind*. Beverly Hills, Calif.: Sage Publications.

Quick, J. C. and Quick, J. D. 1984. *Organizational Stress and Preventive Management*. New York: McGraw-Hill.

Sarason, S. B. 1977. *Work, Aging and Social Change*. New York: The Free Press.

Serpa, R. 1983. Culture: The often ignored factor in knowledge utilization. In Kilmann, R. H. et al. (Eds.). *Producing Useful Knowledge for Organizations*: 121–132. New York: Praeger.

Shiffman, S. and Willis, T. A. (Eds.) 1985. *Coping and Substance Abuse*. New York: Academic Press.

Thomas, L. 1983. *The Youngest Science: Notes of a Medicine-Watcher*. New York: Viking Press.

Van de Vall, M., Bolas, C., and Kang, T. S. 1976. Applied social science research in industrial organizations: An evaluation of functions, theory and methods. *Journal of Applied Behavioral Science*, 12: 158–177.

24 *Work stress in the 1980s: research and practice*

Robert L. Kahn

The organization of the conference in work stress was clear and logical—the first day on causes of work stress, the second on preventive interventions, and the third on interventions that are curative or restorative in character. The papers and contributions (this book's chapters) to this conference, however, are not so neatly compartmentalized. This, I believe, was predictable and acceptable. All of us have our own theoretical orientations, have done our own research, and have accumulated our own experience in organizational life. We therefore have our own stories to tell, and we tell them in spite of topical boundaries. Indeed, if autonomy at work is an antidote against the effects of work stress, I hereby pronounce all of the authors safe from stress.

The rest of us, I suspect, are experiencing a phenomenon that systems theorists call information-input overload. The usual methods of dealing with this kind of overload are less than satisfactory. They include error, approximation, queuing, filtering, and "leaving the field." I propose a different method of dealing with our information overload: integration of a great deal of material around a few central questions and concepts. With respect to work stressors I propose to consider two main questions: (1) How much agreement have we reached on the conceptualization and identification of work stressors? (2) How much agreement have we attained on a theory of stress? This question, of course, has a number of components: How much agreement is there on the etiology and the pathways or mechanisms that lead from specific stressors to health or illness? How much agreement is there on the organizational and environmental causes of such stressors? On the subjective processes of perception and cognition that mediate their effects? And on other factors that may moderate the effect of stressors on individual well-being?

With respect to interventions to deal with stress, three main questions must be addressed: (1) How much agreement have we reached regarding the modes of preventive interventions? (2) How much agreement have we reached with respect to modes of therapeutic interventions? (3) To what extent are we agreed regarding the appropriate intervening agencies in American society for creating and sustaining these interventions?

CONCEPTUALIZATION OF STRESS AND IDENTIFICATION OF STRESSORS

The first of these issues is quickly disposed of; we do not agree on the use of *stress* as a concept nor on its definition. In this book the term "stress" has been used to refer to damaging stimuli in the environment, to the internal processes that result when individuals are exposed to such stimuli and attempt to deal with them, and to the immediate or longer range results of such stimuli and coping attempts. This scatter of implied definitions is by no means unique to the subject of this book; it is characteristic of the current diversity in use of the stress concept itself. These difficulties, I believe, are more terminological than profound, and they are easily avoidable. The solution of choice in my opinion is to drop the word "stress" from our scientific vocabulary. It is a useful word, but probably not a useful scientific concept now, if indeed it ever was. There is too much confusion about its meaning and too great a variety in its usage.

Like other terms—health, for instance—it is a great name for an institute or a conference, and it is more than satisfactory for describing broad societal goals (stress reduction, for example). It is also a useful term to describe broad clinical aspirations or outcomes (clients being enabled to deal more satisfactorily with stressful situations, for example). Research, however, requires more explicit criterion variables.

The main ambiguity in the stress term as employed by behavioral scientists is, as I have already suggested, its use to designate both an external force applied to some object and the effect of that force on the body. In physics and in engineering the first of these meanings is explicit and exclusive; stress is the external force and the term "strain" is used to describe its effects. Physical effects typically include deformation of structure or decrement in function. Whatever the dimension, strain is then defined as the ratio of the resulting change in the object to its original condition.

The dual meaning of stress, to refer ambiguously to both the stimulus and the response, appears first in physiology. Cannon (1932), in his discussion of subjects exposed to extreme variations in temperature, leaves us uncertain as to whether the term "stress" refers only to the external experimental variables of heat and cold, or whether it refers instead to the resulting conditions within the organism—lowered blood sugar or heightened anxiety, for example.

Selye (1976), perhaps the most influential of stress researchers, initially avoided this ambiguity in his own work by defining stress as the nonspecific response of the body to any demand made upon it and by proposing (much later) that the term "stressor" be used to refer to the external stimulus (event, force, or whatever) that evoked the "stress" response. Selye's stressor was thus identical with the physicist's or engineer's stress, and Selye's stress identical with the engineer's strain.

This was the confused conceptual state of the field when the behavioral scientists entered it, and we cannot claim yet to have resolved its ambiguities (Appley and Trumbull, 1967). My own conceptual preference is unambiguous. I propose to use the term "stress" as a descriptor of our field of interest. I propose to use the term "stressor" to refer to an external force or condition hypothesized or demonstrated to have negative (painful, damaging, incapacitating) effects on the organisms of interest. Such stressors can be either physical or psychosocial, momentary or prolonged, and temporary or permanent in their effects.

Defining stressors in these external terms clearly aligns us with those theorists who call themselves stimulus-based. It does not imply, however, a definition independent of all responses, nor should it. The demonstration that a given event or condition can properly be called a stressor assumes the previous study of its effects on organisms similar to those about to be the subjects of research. In that sense, and only in that sense, our definition of stress is "response-based." But the definition of a stimulus as a stressor is independent of the response of the specific organism under study. For example, if in the course of a stress experiment I subject a rat to an electrical shock of a certain magnitude, I do so knowing that other laboratory animals in other experiments have reacted to a shock of this voltage "as if it were stressful." If the particular animal I am now studying does not react to that shock, I am led to inquire about the special characteristics of this rat that made it "stress proof" or nonreactive; I am not led to define stress differently for each rat under study.

Defining stressors in external terms does not imply lack of interest in the internal states and processes of organisms as they respond to such stressors. On the contrary, attempts to understand the entire stress sequence should include explicit definition of the external force or condition, the conscious perception or unconscious "reception" of those external stimuli by the person, the cognitive processes by which the significance of the stimuli are understood and appraised, and the responses—physiological, psychological, and behavioral—that then occur. Some of these responses may be long deferred; as stress researchers we are interested in both short-term and long-term effects, in the coping cycles that are activated by stressors, and in the characteristics of individuals or situations that may moderate the relationship between stressors and their consequent effects.

The elements of a stress model that I have just described, leading from an external force or stimulus to short-term responses and enduring change, are much less in dispute among stress researchers than are the definitional issues. Similarly, there is more agreement on the nature of work-related stressors than on the conceptual labels by which they should be identified.

ON THE IDENTIFICATION OF STRESSORS

In the previous chapters, many specific stressors or negative stimuli were cited as occurring frequently in work settings. I think that those stressors can be understood in terms of eight main categories:

1. *Work deprivation* (job loss, job insecurity). The fact that the deprivation of work, actual or threatened,constitutes a demonstrated stressor serves to remind us that work has positive as well as negative consequences, and that the loss of work is almost invariably more stressful than the possession of even a relatively bad job.

Although these chapters emphasize the stresses of work, there was a common assumption about its desirability. People who lose their jobs speak of other concomitant losses: of no longer being in touch with friends, no longer engaged in worthwhile activity, no longer certain of what to do with their time. Brenner's suggestive work on the parallel epidemiology of unemployment and mental illness was taken seriously at the conference, as was the natural field experiment of Cobb and Kasl (1977) on the physical and psychological effects of plant closings.

In Part III, the stresses of job loss were emphasized by chapters concerned with preventive interventions—DeFrank and Pliner (Chapter 14) at the level of corporate policy and Winpisinger (Chapter 15) at the level of national policy. Their approaches to intervention are very different, but they begin with the same underlying assumption: Job loss, threatened and actual, causes physical and psychological symptoms of illness.

2. *Occupation.* Occupation is essentially a surrogate variable. When we show, for example, that farmers are more likely to have muscoloskeletal illnesses and white-collar workers more likely to have cardiovascular disease, we are using occupation as a marker for such job characteristics as lifting heavy weights, spending a great deal of time in sedentary positions, and the like.

The authors of previous chapters are interested in occupation primarily as a marker for more explicit stressors, an emphasis that is appropriate both for research and intervention. Stressors are not randomly distributed among jobs, and therefore occupational data can identify populations at risk. To understand *why* particular occupations are stressful and to intervene successfully, however, requires knowledge of the stressors themselves. Burke (Chapter 5); Rose (Chapter 10); and Baun, Bernacki and Herd (Chapter 16) utilize occupational data in this locational fashion, but then move to more specific stressors such as conflict, ambiguity, and lack of autonomy.

3. *Properties of the work itself* (intrinsic). Intrinsic characteristics of jobs include, for example, their hazardousness and ergonomic characteristics (such as postural constraint or exposure to VDT glare). Intrinsic properties of work also include such characteristics as complexity, repetitiveness, and lack of autonomy. All these were identified as stressors.

To call a job characteristic intrinsic does not imply that it is beyond modification. It does, however, remind us that the characteristic is inherent in the job function, the basic technology, or the nature of the materials. Being a lighthouse keeper is solitary work; being a police officer involves the risk of criminal attack; working with molten steel or uranium ore imposes hazards of other kinds; assembly-line tasks are by definition simplistic and repetitive; airport traffic controllers have an inescapable responsibility for the safety of others.

All these are job-intrinsic stressors, which must be dealt with either by a significant change in technology, reduced hours of exposure, or increased stress-resistance among job holders. The chapters by Burke (responsibility for things), Rose (responsibility for people), and Harrison et al. (job complexity; Chapter 7) exemplify concern with intrinsic job stressors.

4. *Role characteristics*. The distinction between intrinsic properties of the work and characteristics of the work role is not always easily made. However, conflict, ambiguity, overload, shift work, and chronic exposure to emotionally charged situations were cited as stressful characteristics of work roles.

The implicit assumption is that these characteristics of work roles reflect managerial decisions and choices, and that choices leading to less stressful role characteristics are feasible. Indeed, it is the argument of stress avoidability and managerial choice that makes these stressors subject to legal action and compensation payments, as Adams's Chapter (17) demonstrates.

5. *Interpersonal relations*. The quality of interpersonal relations, especially with supervisors and managers, was cited both as a source of strain (when the relationships were poor) and as a stress buffer or moderator (when the relationships were supportive).

This is not surprising; or at least it should not surprise us. Organizations are human enterprises, created, shaped, and maintained by the acts of their members. Most of the stressors we call organizational are imposed by individuals. The role stress of overload, for example, is typically experienced in the context of standards and deadlines imposed by a supervisor. Even ergonomic stressors like the postural constraint and visual glare of which many VDT operators complain are aggravated or relieved by the rigidity or flexibility of supervisors regarding rest periods and the willingness of co-workers to spell each other off. Most organizational stressors, in short, have interpersonal aspects.

6. *Lack of resources and equipment*. One of the most common forms of work stress—quantitative overload—can be viewed as a problem in resources and equipment. A secretary who is severely overloaded doing multiple revisions of long memoranda may be relieved by the purchase of a word processor and printer, which makes it possible to revise without retyping.

If we define resources to include human resources, as we should, the significance of this stressor is greatly increased. The "neuroendocrine effects of work stress" among air traffic controllers, described in Rose's chapter, are in part inherent in the task. But the "traffic effect," which shows greater physical symptoms in busier airports, is in part a problem in human resources. It might well be ameliorated by the allocation of more air traffic controllers to peak times and places.

7. *Work schedules*. The timing of work, and especially the requirement to perform shift work, was mentioned as a stressor. The requirement to work at night rather than during the day is demonstrably stressful, with effects ranging from gastrointestinal difficulties and disruption of sleep patterns to marital and familial strains. Nevertheless, some functions (police protection, communication, trans-

portation, hospital care) must be provided continuously, and others, because of the capital equipment involved, become economically feasible only on the assumption of shift work.

People differ in their sensitivity to shift work and proper selections can therefore reduce its damaging effects. Limiting the number of years in which a worker is required to do shift work could also limit its effects, as could the proper scheduling of rotating shifts. Research on the number of days required for adjusting to a new circadian pattern argues against the common practice of frequent shift changes, which spread the burden superficially and maximize strain by preventing full adjustment.

8. *Organizational climate.* Studies of climate have become frequent in recent years, despite the fact that the metaphorical term is usually undefined. Among the aspects of organizational climate that were cited as stressful in the course of the chapters were lack of career opportunity, competition between jobs, and the tendency to create what might be called "Type A" organizations and jobs.

We can properly ask whether these eight categories of stressors constitute a set; are they logically complete, or theory-derived? The answer must be no. They constitute a list, and the list is open ended. Moreover, it is a list generated partly by empirical research and partly by intuition and hunch. It is a beginning rather than a completed task, but it is enough of a beginning to generate great improvement in organizational life, if it is put to use.

TOWARD A THEORY OF STRESS

We have already referred to the elements of a stress model, a causal sequence that leads from some external force or stimulus to the perception and appraisal of that stimulus by the individual, and then to responses—physiological, psychological, and behavioral. We see this causal sequence as moderated at each of its links by enduring properties of the person and of the situation. We showed a good deal of agreement on the importance of this sequence and of its separate components. These matters are apparently much less in dispute than are the definitional issues, and I consider this to be a reason for considerable optimism. It implies that, despite differences in language, research workers and practitioners share an approach to the total process or causal sequence appropriate to stress research and intervention.

To be more specific, we agreed on three aspects that seem to me important for a full-fledged theory of stress. The first is agreement on the basic causal sequence that, in the case of work-related stress, involves six main categories of variables:

1. Organizational properties.
2. Job properties (objective stressors)

3. Perceived job properties (subjective stressors)

4. Appraisal (the demand of the stressor in relation to the ability or resources of the individual.

5. Response (psychological, physiological, behavioral)

6. Health and illness criteria.

The second area of agreement has to do with the importance of individual differences in any theory of stress. We saw individual characteristics as interacting with the stressors to which individuals are exposed. We spoke of host-resistance, of emotional sensitivity, of neuroticism, and of Type A personality characteristics as variables that moderated the effects of stressors on individuals. We spoke also of resilience, robustness, and of a general trait of stress resistance. We were not able to agree on how precisely to express or conceptualize these last three characteristics, nor on how to measure them. Chapters by Harrison et al. and Burke, and remarks by House (Chapter 4) emphasize the concept of person-environment fit. The chapter by Matteson (12) also emphasizes individual-organizational relationships.

A third area of agreement with respect to the requirements of a stress theory has to do with stress-moderating (or intensifying) situational characteristics. Two such characteristics were mentioned frequently in the chapters: social support and supervisory relations.

Finally, we were agreed on organizations themselves as a source of job stressors, although we were vague on the question of what attributes at the organizational level lead to the establishment of stressful jobs.

PREVENTIVE INTERVENTIONS AGAINST STRESS

Preventive interventions mentioned in the course of this book have been many. The list is long, miscellaneous, and reflects the varied experience of the authors. In principle, a preventive intervention could have as its primary target any of the elements in the causal sequence leading from organizational characteristics and objective stressors to immediate responses and outcomes of health or illness, and different practitioners have different preferences. These reflect their own areas of expertise, their assessment of costs and benefits of intervening at different points, and of the feasibility of any given interactions in the specific situation at hand. I think we will not do too much violence to the preventive interventions proposed at this conference—from physical fitness programs and team building to severance pay and assertiveness training—if we think of them in terms of four broad categories:

1. *Interventions intended to increase individual resistance.* These include physical fitness programs, biofeedback, assertiveness training, socialization programs, and

risk counselling. The chapters by Baun, Bernacki, and Herd (16), Burke (5), Matteson (12), and Seamonds (20), respectively, illustrate each of these approaches. In some respects, they are conservative strategies, in the literal sense of that term. They accept the organization as it is, so far as the imposition of stressors is concerned, and they assume that the job holders will remain in their jobs. What these approaches propose to change is the ability of the job holders to deal with the stressors of their jobs without damage.

2. *Improving the match between individuals and jobs.* Here we discussed methods of selection both in terms of initial assignment and subsequent transfer or relocation. Matteson (Chapter 12) discusses selection in this context, and DeFrank and Pliner (Chapter 14), although they are mainly concerned with job loss for other reasons, describe outplacement counseling in terms that apply to individual terminations for reasons of poor person-job fit. The main arguments are that choosing stress-resistant people for stressful jobs is humane and cost-effective, that such selection should be stressor-specific, and that unsuccessful selection often calls for transfer or outplacement.

3. *Job redesign.* Here we spoke of increased participation, autonomy and control, ergonomic changes in equipment and furniture, and the like. The chapters by Burke (5), Chesney (9), and Suskind (21) discuss various dimensions of job design; Matteson (12) is concerned explicitly with designs that increase participation. The common assumption is that, within any given organizational structure and technology, there are sufficient degrees of freedom to make jobs less stressful without decreasing overall efficiency.

4. *National and corporate policy.* Any of the preceding points could of course be made matters of national policy and legislation, and many of them could (and have) become the policies of specific corporations without the impetus of national urging. In this volume we discussed policies involving such issues as management education with respect to the effects of stress, the providing of severance pay and outplacement counseling to deal with technologically imposed unemployment, and the possibilities of full employment with the federal government as the employer of last resort.

Chapter 15 by Winpisinger is unique in its emphasis on national policy as an instrument for the prevention of work stress, but the importance of corporate policy for this purpose is implicit in many of the other chapters. Programs of job redesign, participation, and risk assessment, for example, do not diffuse and persist in corporate life without the sanction of corporate policy.

THERAPEUTIC INTERVENTIONS

Intrinsic to any therapeutic program is the assumption that a disease is already present. Damage has been done and therapy is undertaken to repair it. In the case of research on work stress, therapeutic interventions thus assume that one or more stressors are present and that they have at least created strains, if not outright illness. Our discussion of therapeutic interventions was as varied and individualized as the discussion of preventive interventions that preceded it. Among the broad issues emphasized were the following:

1. *Identification of stressors and evidence of strain through risk counseling.* The identificaton of stressors is not in itself therapeutic, but it can be considered an important first step. When management knows where damage is being done and what the damaging stressors are, the targets of therapy are indicated. Similarly, individuals who are helped to identify correctly the sources of stress are thereby put in a better position to make therapeutic choices.

2. *The providing of counsel or support* for individuals in trouble or with a strong potentiality for stress-related difficulty. Examples included the use of screening techniques for hypertension and subsequent regimens for the control of that disease.

A step beyond the identification of stressors and strains at work is the therapeutic interventions themselves. When aimed at the individual, such interventions typically attempt to moderate or eliminate entirely the effect of the stressors. Thus, the hypertensive employee in a job with severe time demands and personal responsibilities, who brings her blood pressure under control by means of antihypertensive drugs, continues to work under stress but without the same damaging effects.

Health advisory programs as described by Francek (Chapter 19), risk counseling as described by Seamonds (Chapter 20), and psychotherapeutic interventions as described by Harrison et al. (Chapter 7) exemplify this strategy of intervention. So do the brief and intensive therapies undertaken to deal with alcoholism and drug addiction, as Wolfe and Robischon point out in Chapter 22, and the programs designed to teach stress resistance and coping.

3. *Organizational Change.* The emphasis here was on team building and participation as ways of compensating for or buffering the effects of stressful job characteristics. The primary target in such interventions is the organization rather than the individual, which perhaps suggests stress prevention rather than therapy. Certainly organizational changes can eliminate stressful conditions, but they can also reduce the effects of such conditions. The chapters by Francek (19) and Numerof (13) are explicit in proposing that increased employee participation has stress-buffering effects.

CONCLUSION

I am forced to the conclusion that we have only scattered agreement with respect to interventions, both preventive and therapeutic. Our discussion suggests a melange of potential interventive actions, some at the macro level and some at the micro or individual level. Some are offered as general remedies for stressors of almost all kinds. (Risk counseling and team building were presented in these terms.) Other interventions were proposed in connection with very specific strains—biofeedback for hypertension, for example.

I would like to propose my own framework for thinking about modes of intervention with respect to stress at work. It seems to me the possibilities are basically four. We can propose that people simply "live with" the stressors imposed by work. This proposal typically involves not so much the advocacy of suffering as the hope that people will find ways of compensating in their off-the-job activities for the stressors to which they are exposed on the job.

A second strategy for stress intervention might be called "people matching." Selection, transfer, and, in a sense, termination are all examples of attempts to improve the match or goodness of fit between the person and the job.

A third intervention strategy we can label "people changing." These interventions emphasize ways in which individual characteristics can be altered in an enduring fashion. When we speak of giving information, of training, of counseling, or of establishing encounter or sensitivity groups, we are engaging in the strategy of reducing stress (stressors/strains) by changing individuals.

The fourth intervention strategy emphasizes organizational rather than individual change. Changing organizations can be thought of as involving the entire organizational structure or intervening more specifically with respect to certain jobs. Three basic kinds of organizatonal change seem relevant here: changes in the distribution of power or authority, changes in the allocation of rewards, and changes in the division of labor itself. The first two are perhaps clear enough to require no elaboration. The third (changes in the division of labor) includes efforts of the kind usually called job enlargement and job enrichment.

Of these several broad approaches to problems of intervention, I believe that the changing of organizations and jobs is the most promising. To advocate that, however, immediately raises the question of whether we know enough to bring about such changes constructively. I believe that the experiments that have been conducted along these lines are encouraging in their effects, although discouraging with respect to their widespread dissemination and diffusion. I believe also that the kinds of discussions that have characterized these chapters give promise for the fuller utilization of stress research and for the enlargement of that research enterprise. Both, I am convinced, will contribute to the quality of working life.

REFERENCES

Appley, M. H. and Trumbull, R. 1967. On the concept of psychological stress. In Appley, M. H. and Trumbull, R. (Eds.). *Psychological Stress: Issues in Research*. New York: Appleton, Century, Crofts.

Cannon, W. B. 1932. *The Wisdom of the Body*. New York: W. W. Norton.

Cobb, S. and Kasl, S. V. 1977. *Termination: The Consequences of Job Loss*. Cincinnati: Department of Health, Education, and Welfare (NIOSH), Publication No. 77–224.

Selye, H. 1976. *Stress in Health and Disease*. Boston: Butterworths.

Index